SAUNDERS SOLUTIONS IN
VETERINARY PRACTICE

SMALL ANIMAL
DERMATOLOGY

Commissioning Editor: Joyce Rodenhuis, Rita Demetriou-Swanwick
Development Editor: Sarah Keer-Keer, Louisa Welch
Project Manager: Jess Thompson
Designer/Text Design: Charles Gray/Keith Kail
Illustrations Manager: Merlyn Harvey
Illustrator: Deborah Maizels

SAUNDERS SOLUTIONS IN
VETERINARY PRACTICE

SMALL ANIMAL
DERMATOLOGY

Series Editor: **Fred Nind** BVM&S, MRCVS

Anita Patel

BVM, DVD, MRCVS
RCVS Specialist in Veterinary Dermatology

Peter Forsythe

BVM&S, DVD, MRCVS
RCVS Specialist in Veterinary Dermatology

With contributions from:
Stephen Smith

BVetMed (Hons.), CertZooMed, MRCVS
Resident in Avian and Exotics Medicine

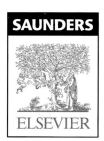

SAUNDERS

ELSEVIER

Edinburgh   London   New York   Oxford   Philadelphia   St Louis   Sydney   Toronto   2008

SAUNDERS
ELSEVIER

© 2008, Elsevier Limited. All rights reserved.

No part of this publication may be reproduced or transmitted in any form or by any means, electronic or mechanical, including photocopying, recording, or any information storage and retrieval system, without permission in writing from the publisher. Permissions may be sought directly from Elsevier's Rights Department: phone: (+1) 215 239 3804 (US) or (+44) 1865 843830 (UK); fax: (+44) 1865 853333; e-mail: healthpermissions@elsevier.com. You may also complete your request on-line via the Elsevier website at http://www.elsevier.com/permissions.

First published 2008

ISBN: 978-0-7020-2870-0

British Library Cataloguing in Publication Data
A catalogue record for this book is available from the British Library

Library of Congress Cataloging in Publication Data
A catalog record for this book is available from the Library of Congress

Notice

Knowledge and best practice in this field are constantly changing. As new research and experience broaden our knowledge, changes in practice, treatment and drug therapy may become necessary or appropriate. Readers are advised to check the most current information provided (i) on procedures featured or (ii) by the manufacturer of each product to be administered, to verify the recommended dose or formula, the method and duration of administration, and contraindications. It is the responsibility of the practitioner, relying on their own experience and knowledge of the patient, to make diagnoses, to determine dosages and the best treatment for each individual patient, and to take all appropriate safety precautions. To the fullest extent of the law, neither the Publisher nor the Authors assume any liability for any injury and/or damage to persons or property arising out or related to any use of the material contained in this book.

Neither the Publisher nor the Authors assume any responsibility for any loss or injury and/or damage to persons or property arising out of or related to any use of the material contained in this book. It is the responsibility of the treating practitioner, relying on independent expertise and knowledge of the patient, to determine the best treatment and method of application for the patient.

The Publisher

Printed in China.

your source for books,
journals and multimedia
in the health sciences
www.elsevierhealth.com

The
publisher's
policy is to use
**paper manufactured
from sustainable forests**

Working together to grow
libraries in developing countries
www.elsevier.com | www.bookaid.org | www.sabre.org

ELSEVIER   BOOK AID
International   Sabre Foundation

Contents

Acknowledgement

The authors would like to thank the veterinary surgeons in general practice for referring these cases, and colleagues in referral practice for their expert help with some of them.

Introduction

Saunders Solutions in Veterinary Practice series is a new range of veterinary textbooks which will grow into a mini library over the next few years, covering all the main disciplines of companion animal practice.

Readers should realize that it is not the authors' intention to cover all that is known about each topic. As such, the books in the *Solutions Series* are not standard reference works. Instead, they are intended to provide practical information on the more frequently encountered conditions in an easily accessible form based on real-life case studies. They cover that range of cases that fall between the boringly routine and the referral. The books will help practitioners with a particular interest in a topic or those preparing for a specialist qualification. The cases are arranged by presenting sign rather than by the underlying pathology, as this is how veterinary surgeons will see them in practice.

Each case also includes descriptions of underlying pathology and details of the nursing required, both in the veterinary clinic and at home. It is hoped that the books will also, therefore, be of interest to veterinary students in the later parts of their course and to veterinary nurses.

Continuing professional development (CPD) is mandatory for many veterinarians and a recommended practice for others. The *Saunders Series* will provide a CPD resource which can be accessed economically, shared with colleagues and used anywhere. They will also provide busy veterinary practitioners with quick access to authoritative information on the diagnosis and treatment of interesting and challenging cases. The robust cover has been made resistant to some of the more gruesome contaminants found in a veterinary clinic because this is where we hope these books will be used.

Joyce Rodenhuis and Mary Seager were the inspiration for the Series, and both the Series editor and the individual authors are grateful for their foresight in commissioning the Series and their unfailing support and guidance during their production.

DERMATOLOGY

Dermatological cases are common. A student once pointed out to me that every single case that she had seen during a full day of seeing practice in my first opinion clinic had had at least one dermatological manifestation.

These cases can also be challenging, confusing and frustrating. For most dermatological conditions, several treatment and/or management options are available, making the situation even more complicated.

It is hoped that this book will be a handy reference for some of these cases, and encourage the practitioner to pursue a definitive diagnosis and plan effective management even if the condition cannot be cured.

Because each case is, by and large, complete in itself, there is some repetition between chapters, especially when similar diseases are dealt with in different species. Conversely, because some conditions (e.g. cheyletiellosis) present differently in different species, they may be covered in more than one section. However, the authors hope that this form of presentation will make it quicker and easier for clinicians to find what they need to know about a particular presentation.

Fred Nind
Series Editor

1 The dermatology consultation

INTRODUCTION

The initial, most important step in achieving a satisfactory consultation and management of any dermatological condition is to obtain a thorough history. Taking short cuts in this step can lead to a misdiagnosis, affect the welfare of the animal, and add a lot of unnecessary expense and dissatisfaction for the owner.

The history should be obtained in a logical fashion, with the view of building up a picture of the condition and a list of differential diagnoses, while examining the patient. This book shows how to work up a case in this manner.

With computerized records in most practices, the age at onset, breed and sex of the individual animal should be readily available. This information provides some useful clues when formulating a list of differential diagnosis.

Age at onset:
- Parasitic problems such as pediculosis, otoacariasis, cheyletiellosis and demodectic mange are more commonly seen in puppies and adolescent animals.
- Genodermatoses can become progressive and, in some cases, are more apparent with age. They are usually established by 3 years of age.
- Of the allergies, atopic dermatitis has an age of onset of more than 6 months and below 3 years, and flea allergic dermatitis is more common in animals older than 5 years of age.
- Hormonal problems tend to manifest after the age of 6 years.
- Neoplastic conditions generally occur in older animals.

Breed predispositions:
- Demodicosis in Staffordshire bull terriers, Scottish terriers.
- Atopic dermatitis in Labradors, West Highland terrier and other terrier breeds, German shepherd dogs, whereas flea allergic dermatitis can occur in any breed.
- Dermatophytosis is more prevalent in Persian cats.
- Dilute coat colour in certain breeds, i.e. blue coat in Dobermanns may be responsible for colour dilution alopecia.

Sex: Note whether the individual is entire or neutered. This is of particular interest when dealing with skin conditions associated with sex-hormone imbalance. There are few other skin conditions where sexual predispositions are recognized.

HISTORY TAKING

History taking is divided into those enquiries that relate specifically to the skin's condition and those about the general history and management of the animal. In general practice, because time is limited, you could combine some of the questioning with the examination of the animal. If the condition is recurrent, much of the history will already be available on records and will just need confirmation from the owner.

Specific history – key questions:
- Date of onset?
- Is the condition seasonal or non-seasonal?
- If non-seasonal is it continuous and progressive or is it intermittent?
- Is the condition pruritic or non-pruritic? This should include licking, biting, scratching or rubbing. If pruritic, we need to know whether initially non-pruritic and subsequently changed or has always been pruritic.
- Distribution of the lesions now, and initially, and how they have progressed?
- Is there a smell associated with the condition?

- Are there any in-contact animals in the house or casual contacts and if so are they affected?
- Are any people in the house affected?
- Did the condition start following a visit to the grooming parlour, or to boarding kennels?
- Are there any fleas on any of the pets in the house?

Non-specific history: You should include questions relating to the animal's general health and management, and you may need to ask more specific questions as you build up a picture of the condition.

General health – key questions:
- Is the appetite affected and, if so, has it increased or decreased?
- Has there been any change in water intake?
- Has the exercise tolerance changed?
- Is there any cough, sneezing or breathing difficulty?
- Have there been signs associated with gastroenteric disorders?
- Are sexual behaviours or oestrus cycle affected?
- Is the animal on any medication for any other conditions, i.e. cardiac, arthritic?

Management – key questions:
- Diet, including titbits, should be noted.
- Is the animal kennelled or kept indoors, and if so where does it spend most of its time? For example, those sleeping in bedrooms would have higher exposure to house dust mites.
- Is the dog a pet or used to work?
- Is the cat kept indoors and/or outdoors and if outdoors is it a hunter?
- What sort of bedding is used?
- Is the house carpeted or not?
- Is the condition worsened after contact with certain things? For example, grass or after a walk.
- Topical and systemic treatments used and response.
- Travel history, ectoparasitic, endoparasitic and vaccination status.

CLINICAL EXAMINATION

For the clinical examination, it is good practice to establish a routine to include both a general physical and a specific dermatological examination.

General physical examination: All organ systems should be examined in a methodical manner. Certain abnormalities may be indicative of certain diseases:
- Bradycardia may be suggestive of hypothyroidism.
- Oral lesions may be consistent with autoimmune, immune-mediated or neoplastic conditions.
- Conjunctivitis or epiphora may suggest an allergic aetiology.
- Muscle atrophy is suggestive of either spontaneous or iatrogenic hyperadrenocorticism.
- Abdominal palpation may reveal a mass or other abnormality.

Dermatological examination: The examination involves a detailed inspection of the skin based on visual inspection and palpation followed by specific procedures such as coat brushings, skin scrapings, etc. (see Chapter 2). You are looking for different indicators from the different parts of the skin:
- Mucous membranes – petechiae, ulceration, vesicles, bulla, erosions, hypopigmentation.
- Coat condition – lustreless, greasy, matted, scaly, dry and brittle or alopecic.
- Elasticity of the skin – loss of elasticity is associated with hyperadrenocorticism.
- Skin surface – examine for lesions on the entire skin surface, not just the obviously visible area. Distinguish between primary and secondary lesions and note the distribution (focal or multifocal; symmetrical or asymmetrical). The lesions may be present singly or grouped, or in annular, linear, polycyclic, arciform or serpiginous configurations. In some animals, the coat may need to be clipped to appreciate the lesions.

Primary lesions:
- Macule – flat, circumscribed area of discoloration of 1 cm or less.
- Papule – solid, raised palpable mass of 1 cm diameter or less (Fig. 1.1).
- Plaque – solid, raised elevation of more than 1 cm diameter (Fig. 1.2).
- Pustule – pus-filled, raised circumscribed lesion of 1 cm or less (Fig. 1.3).
- Vesicle – serum-filled, raised circumscribed lesion of 1 cm or less (Fig. 1.4).
- Bulla – serum-filled, raised circumscribed lesion of more than 1 cm.
- Cyst – cavity which is lined with membranous lining and is filled with fluid or semi-solid material.
- Nodule – solid, raised palpable mass of more than 1 cm (Fig. 1.5).
- Tumour – large palpable mass.

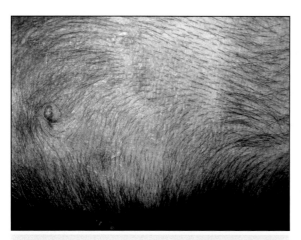

Figure 1.1 Papules in a dog with pyoderma.

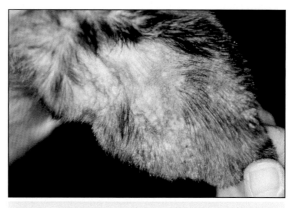

Figure 1.4 Vesicles on the concave aspect of the pinna.

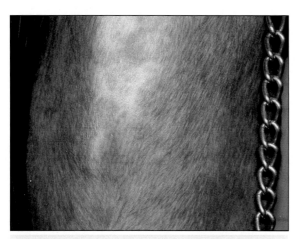

Figure 1.2 Plaques on ventral chest and abdomen of a dog.

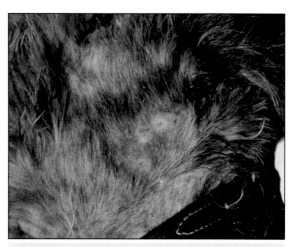

Figure 1.5 Nodules in a dog.

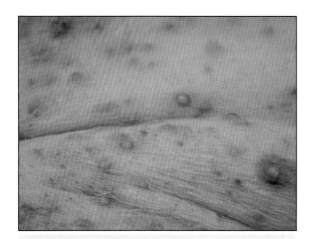

Figure 1.3 Pustules on glabrous skin.

- Wheal – oedematous, raised circumscribed lesion which blanches on diascopy (Fig. 1.6).
- Alopecia – loss of hair (this can be primary or secondary, i.e. self-induced).

Secondary lesions:
- Erythema – increased redness to the skin.
- Scale – superficial visible accumulation of loose corneocytes on the surface of the epidermis.
- Epidermal collarette – circular arrangement of scale with a central area of hyperpigmentation (Fig. 1.7).
- Crust – results from accumulation of dried cells and exudate (e.g. serum, blood, pus) on the skin surface (Fig. 1.8).
- Erosion – loss of the superficial epidermis without the loss of the basal layer (Fig. 1.9).

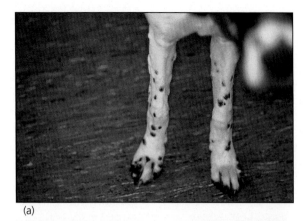
(a)

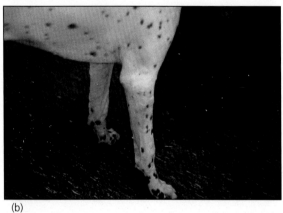
(b)

Figure 1.6 Wheals on the legs of a dog.

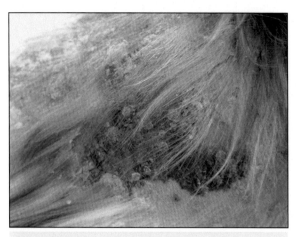

Figure 1.8 Crusts on the skin surface in a dog.

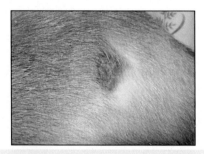

Figure 1.9 Erosion on the skin surface in a cat.

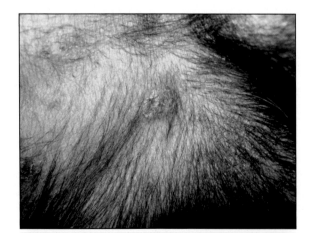

Figure 1.7 Epidermal collarettes.

- Ulceration – loss or the epidermis resulting in exposure of the dermis (Fig. 1.10).
- Fissure – a split or crack into the epidermis and dermis due to either trauma or disease.
- Scar – abnormal fibrous tissue which replaces damaged dermal and subcutaneous tissue.
- Lichenification – thickening of the skin resulting in exaggeration of the skin markings due to chronic inflammation (Fig. 1.11).
- Hyperpigmentation – darkening of the skin due to increased pigment in the epidermis and sometimes the dermis (Fig. 1.11).
- Hypopigmentation – reduction or loss of pigment in the epidermis.
- Comedone – dilated hair follicle blocked with sebum and other cellular debris (Fig. 1.12).
- Follicular cast – accumulation of keratin and sebum on the hair shaft and/or the hair bulb (Fig. 2.9).

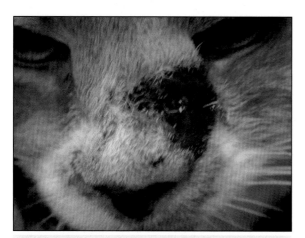

Figure 1.10 Ulceration of the skin exposing underlying soft tissue in a cat.

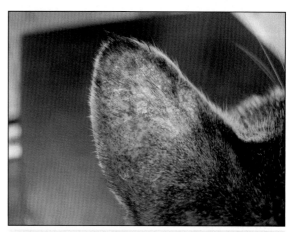

Figure 1.12 Comedones and scaling on the convex aspect of the pinna of a cat.

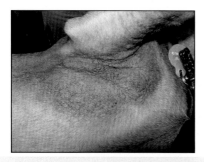

Figure 1.11 Lichenification and hyperpigmentation on the axilla of a dog.

Although all of the above are normally considered as secondary lesions, erythema, scale, crusts, comedones, follicular casts, hypopigmentation and hyperpigmentation may, in some skin conditions, be regarded as primary lesions.

It is good practice to examine the animal using a set procedure so that no part of the skin goes unchecked.

Unless the diagnosis is immediately obvious, which in the majority of cases it isn't, the next step is to list all the conditions consistent with the signalment, history and examinations – the 'differential diagnosis' – and then eliminate them by appropriate testing and therapeutic trials, to come to a definitive diagnosis. These tests and trials are discussed in Chapter 2.

2 Laboratory tests

INTRODUCTION

Unless the diagnosis is immediately obvious, many dermatology cases in veterinary medicine present something of a challenge to the clinician. In these more complex cases, consideration of the signalment, history and physical examination allows formulation of a differential diagnosis, and then various tests and therapeutic trials are employed to reach a definitive diagnosis. The tests available include those performed within the practice laboratory and those offered by external commercial labs.

The ideal diagnostic test is a procedure that gives a rapid, convenient and inexpensive indication of whether a patient has or has not a certain disease. Unfortunately, most diagnostic tests suffer from a problem of inherent unreliability and cannot always distinguish the normal from the abnormal, leading to false-positive and false-negative results. Biological variation, test methodology and the skill of the clinician all combine to account for test unreliability. It is important the clinician is aware of the limits of any diagnostic test, and test results should be interpreted in the light of the case history and clinical signs. This interpretation is of crucial clinical importance and is one of the most common sources of diagnostic error.

There are measures that the clinician can take to minimize the incidence of false-positive and false-negative test results. Firstly, take full histories and perform full physical and dermatological examinations and draw up a differential diagnosis (see Chapter 1). Whilst it is important to perform basic screening tests such as skin scrapes and cytology, diagnostic tests used should as far as possible be targeted to the diseases on the differential diagnosis list. The indiscriminate use of a wide variety of diagnostic tests will increase the likelihood of false-positive and false-negative test results. It is a common mistake to assume that because skin lesions look severe, autoimmune disease is involved. Statistically, the low prevalence of rare diseases will increase the chance of a false-positive test result, leading to an erroneous diagnosis. Much more frequently, severe skin lesions are just an unusual manifestation of a common disease.

DIAGNOSTIC TESTS FOR ECTOPARASITISM

Ectoparasitic diseases encountered in small animal practice are shown in Table 2.1. The tests available for the detection of external parasites are combings and coat brushings, the use of acetate strips, skin scrapes, hair plucks, a scabies IgG ELISA test and histopathological examination.

General principles for microscopy

Become familiar with the operation of your microscope. Apart from when using acetate strips, always apply a coverslip over any material to be examined microscopically. Having excessive material on the slide will make thorough examination difficult. Low power (×4 objective) is sufficient magnification for detection of ectoparasites, although a ×10 objective may be required for more detailed examination of specimens.

Combings

A flea comb may be used to collect material from the coat for gross examination. The test is useful for the detection of larger external parasites such as fleas and lice. If fleas are present in large numbers, they should be seen. However, fleas are only detected in around 60% of cases of canine flea allergy dermatitis and the figure is considerably lower in cats, who remove evidence of flea infestation by grooming. Thus, flea combing is an insensitive test for the diagnosis of flea infestation.

Table 2.1 Ectoparasites encountered in small animal practice

Insects	
Flea infestation	Common
Lice	Uncommon
Mites	
Sarcoptes scabiei	Common
Notoedres cati	Rare in cats
Cheyletiella spp.	Common
Otodectes cynotis	Common
Neotrombicula autumnalis	Common
Demodex spp.	Common
Endoparasites	
Pelodera, hookworms	Uncommon to rare

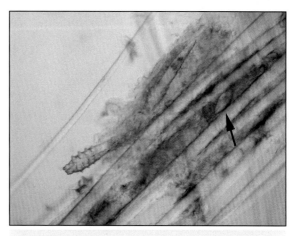

Figure 2.2 Hair pluck from a case of pododemodicosis with adult mites and egg (arrowed).

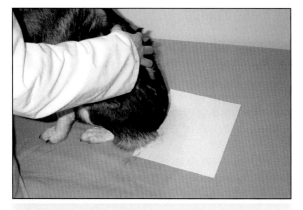

Figure 2.1 Collecting samples of scale for coat brush examination.

Coat brushing examination

This is a useful and moderately sensitive test for the diagnosis of surface and superficial parasites such as fleas, lice, harvest mites and *Cheyletiella* spp. mites. Scale is dislodged from the dorsal trunk (Fig. 2.1) onto a piece of A4 paper by combing or vigorous brushing with the fingertips. The paper is folded and tapped so that the material collected falls into the crease. Hair is removed and the material can be examined grossly for the presence of flea faeces, as well as larger parasites such as lice. The material should be collected onto clear adhesive tape, mounted onto a glass slide and examined under the low-power light microscope. The complete area under the adhesive tape should be carefully examined.

Hair plucks

Microscopic examination of hair plucks may be useful to detect *Demodex* spp. mites (Fig. 2.2) and *Cheyletiella* spp. or louse eggs. Hair plucks are very useful when taking samples from areas that are difficult to scrape, such as the feet in the case of pododemodicosis, when skin scraping would require sedation. Fifty to 100 hairs are plucked and mounted in liquid paraffin on a glass slide under a coverslip. The hair tips, shafts and bulbs should all be carefully examined. One study showed deep skin scraping to be more sensitive than hair plucks in cases of localized and squamous demodicosis, and therefore demodicosis should not be ruled out on the basis of not finding mites on hair plucks.

Skin scrapings

Skin scrapings are used to detect the presence of superficial and deep parasitic mites such as *Cheyletiella*, *Sarcoptes* and *Demodex* spp. Skin scrapings should be performed when there is evidence of erythema, scaling, crusting, alopecia, or a papular or pustular eruption. In cases of canine scabies, the hocks, elbows and pinnal margins are prime sites for finding mites. Avoid scraping areas that are excessively crusted or excoriated, as this may lead to false-negative results. Three to five different sites should be sampled (five in the case of suspected scabies or demodicosis).

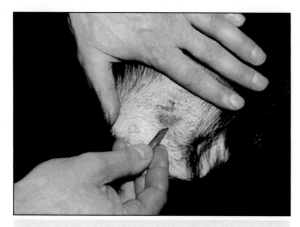

Figure 2.3 Deep skin scraping.

Hair should be clipped with a No. 40 clipper blade. When scraping for *Demodex* spp., it helps to gently squeeze the skin between thumb and forefinger, as this extrudes mites from the hair follicles. A small amount of liquid paraffin to suspend collected material (or water if using potassium hydroxide) is applied to the area to be scraped. A blunted No. 10 scalpel blade is used to scrape material from the skin surface. Deep skin scrapes resulting in capillary oozing should be made when looking for *Sarcoptes* or *Demodex* spp. mites (Fig. 2.3). Collected material is mounted onto a glass slide in liquid paraffin or potassium hydroxide. A coverslip should be applied. Examine samples for ectoparasites under the low-power objective and scan the entire area under the coverslip.

Canine *Sarcoptes* IgG ELISA

Commercial laboratories offer a *Sarcoptes* IgG ELISA test. This is a highly sensitive (~90%) test, although false-negative reactions may occur in early cases because sero-conversion may take up to 4 weeks following mite exposure. False-positive reactions may be seen in cases of canine atopic dermatitis due to house dust mite hypersensitivity because of cross-reaction between *Dermatophagoides* spp. house dust mites and *Sarcoptes scabiei*.

Histopathological examination

Histopathological examination is a very sensitive test for the diagnosis of demodicosis and if skin scrapes have been unrewarding, but demodicosis is still suspected, then histopathology would be the definitive rule out. Histopathologically, canine demodicosis results in interface mural folliculitis, perifolliculitis, folliculitis and furunculosis, and nodular dermatitis. Mites should be evident on histopathological sections. Histopathology is a highly insensitive test for other ectoparasitic diseases.

Interpretation of test results

With the exception of demodicosis, tests for ectoparasites are of low sensitivity but 100% specificity. *Sarcoptes* spp. mites are only found on skin scrape examination in around 50% of cases of canine scabies and *Cheyletiella* spp. mites may also be difficult to detect in some cases. Indeed, in multi-animal households, it can be helpful to check in contact (and frequently unaffected) animals for the presence of the parasite. Fleas are notoriously difficult to find, particularly in cats with any of the feline manifestations of pruritus.

Thus, other diagnostic tests (scabies IgG ELISA) or trial therapy should be performed where ectoparasitism is one of the differentials but external parasites cannot be detected.

Demodicosis

The situation is different in the case of demodicosis. Provided at least five carefully taken and thoroughly examined deep skin scrapes are negative, then the clinician can be confident in ruling out demodicosis as a cause of the skin disease, although there are rare exceptions. Possibly due to the thickness of their skin, it can be difficult to detect mites in the Shar Pei and occasionally mites can be difficult to find in cases of pododemodicosis. With such cases, histopathological examination is indicated to rule the disease in or out. Trial therapy is inappropriate for suspected demodicosis.

DIAGNOSTIC TESTS FOR DERMATOPHYTOSIS

Dermatophytosis is invasion of keratinized tissue usually by *Trichophyton*, *Epidermophyton* or *Microsporum* spp. of fungi.

Techniques available for diagnosis include:
- Wood's lamp examination
- Microscopic examination of hair shafts for the presence of spores
- Fungal culture
- Histopathology.

Wood's lamp: Wood's lamp is an ultraviolet light with a wavelength of 360 nm. Only lamps with two bulbs and a magnifier should be used. It is important to switch the lamp on and allow it to warm up for 5 minutes prior to examination. Examination of the animal should be

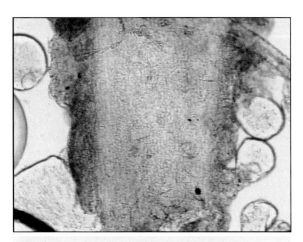

Figure 2.4 Hair shaft infected with dermatophytes. (Courtesy of Dr N. McEwan.)

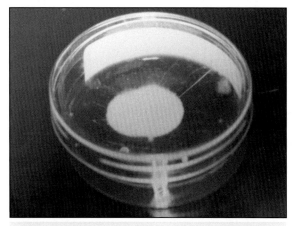

Figure 2.5 Dermatophyte test medium showing red colour change and white colony growth on the surface at 10 days. Note the darkly pigmented growth of saprophytic fungal organism on the edge of the plate.

conducted in a darkened room. Hair shafts infected with certain strains of *Microsporum canis* fluoresce an apple green colour under Wood's lamp examination due to tryptophan metabolites. Wood's lamp examination is a test with high specificity (100% in the right hands) but low sensitivity, as only 50% of strains of *Microsporum canis* fluoresce. Rare infections with *M. audounii*, *M. distortum* and *Trichophyton schoenlenii* may also result in fluorescence.

Direct microscopy: Most dermatophytosis cases in domestic animals involve ectothrix invasion of hair shafts by fungal spores which can be visualized under ×40 magnification using the light microscope. Fluorescing hairs or hairs from lesions may be plucked for direct microscopic examination. Samples should be mounted on the slide in liquid paraffin or potassium hydroxide. Hair shafts with distorted or damaged cuticles should be examined under higher power for the presence of fungal spores (Fig. 2.4). Although a test with high specificity in the right hands, this is not a sensitive technique for the diagnosis of dermatophytosis in the hands of the inexperienced clinician.

Fungal culture: Fungal culture is arguably the most sensitive test for dermatophytosis and should be performed whenever this disease is suspected. The simplest method of collection of material for culture is the MacKenzie brush technique. This is most commonly used for routine screening of cats for dermatophytosis. A new toothbrush is used and hair and scale are col-

lected on the bristles by brushing the hair coat for 30–60 seconds, paying particular attention to lesional skin. The shaft of the brush can be cut off and the entire head of the brush submitted to the laboratory. In addition to using the brush method, it is advisable to culture scale scraped from lesions and also hair plucks from lesion margins.

Dermatophyte test medium (DTM) is used as an in-practice growth medium for the diagnosis of dermatophytosis. DTM is Sabouraud's dextrose agar with various antimicrobials that suppress bacterial and some saprophytic fungal growth, along with phenol red as an indicator. Dermatophytes metabolize protein in the medium first, giving off alkaline metabolites which turn the pH indicator red (Fig. 2.5). This should happen within 10 days and should occur as the fungal colony grows. Saprophytic species of fungi metabolize carbohydrates first and the red colour change should only appear after 10 or more days and subsequent to colony growth. There are potential problems associated with the use of DTM. The agar should be inspected daily for evidence of fungal growth and colour change; some saprophytic species of fungi can induce a colour change within 10 days and *Microsporum persicolor* may produce a colour change after 10 days. Thus, the identity of any fungal mycelium should be confirmed by microscopic examination, which requires specialist knowledge. Furthermore, DTM may not be a suitable growth medium for the identification of some fungi that will only sporulate on Sabouraud's dextrose agar. Nevertheless, DTM culture remains a useful in-practice tool for screening for dermatophytosis, but the clinician should be aware of the limitations.

Histopathology: Fungal elements may be identified on histopathological sections and are more readily visualized with the use of special stains such as periodic acid schiff (PAS).

TRICHOGRAPHY

Trichography is the technique of microscopic examination of hair shafts. Apart from ectoparasite diagnosis, the microscopic examination of plucked hairs is also useful in the investigation of causes of alopecia in cats and dogs and in certain scaling disorders, particularly sebaceous adenitis.

Technique: Fifty to 100 hairs are plucked using a pair of haemostat forceps, the jaws of which are protected by drip tubing so as not to fracture the shafts. The hairs are mounted on a microscope slide in liquid paraffin under a coverslip. Hair tips, shafts and roots are examined under the low-power light microscope.

Interpretation: Normal hair tips taper to a fine point. Fractured hair shafts indicate self-trauma due to pruritus. This is a useful test in cases of feline symmetrical alopecia where it is not clear that the cause of the alopecia is due to self-trauma (Fig. 2.6).

Examination of hair bulbs: A club-shaped, well-pigmented bulb is characteristic of a hair in the anagen (growing) phase (Fig. 2.7). A thin, straight, non-pigmented, fully keratinized tapered root is characteristic of a telogen (resting) hair (Fig. 2.8). In general, both telogen and anagen hairs will be seen on trichography from healthy cats and dogs. Assessment of anagen-to-telogen ratios can be helpful in ascertaining the cause of alopecia, although care must be taken in interpreting these ratios. Breeds such as the chow-chow, samoyed, Pomeranian and husky retain large numbers of telogen hairs for a long period of time and are said to have 'telogen-dominated hair cycles'. Conversely, breeds including the

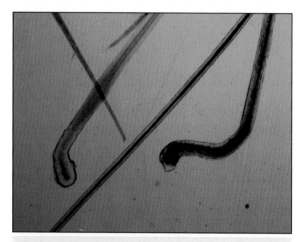

Figure 2.7 Anagen hair bulbs.

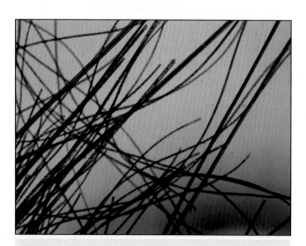

Figure 2.6 Fractured hair shafts from a cat with alopecia due to self-trauma.

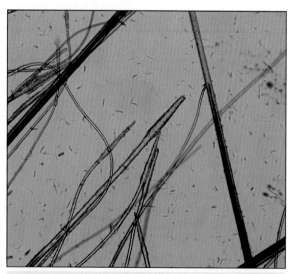

Figure 2.8 Telogen hair bulbs.

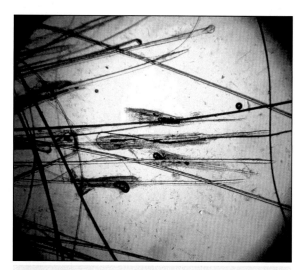

Figure 2.9 Follicular casts from a case of sebaceous adenitis.

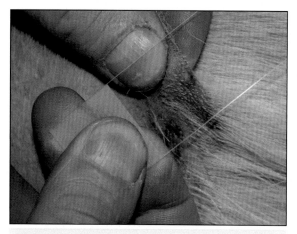

Figure 2.10 Taking an impression smear from a pustule.

poodle and Bichon Frise have 'anagen-dominated hair cycles', where the hair continues to grow. These are breeds that require hair cuts. Despite this breed variation, the absence of anagen hair roots in a trichogram would be suggestive of a hair growth cycle disorder such as an endocrinopathy. The presence of anagen bulbs indicates active hair growth and would make a hair growth cycle disorder less likely to be the cause of alopecia; self-trauma or a folliculitis would be more likely in such cases.

Follicular casts: The presence of follicular casts (accumulations of keratosebaceous material around the hair shaft) indicates a follicular cornification disorder of the hair follicle (Fig. 2.9). This is most commonly seen in the scaly form of sebaceous adenitis as seen in the Japanese akita and English springer spaniel.

CYTOLOGY

Cytology is a fundamentally important technique in veterinary dermatology that can be employed quickly, easily and inexpensively in a practice situation. Cytology frequently yields useful information on a case, and enables a more precise diagnosis to be made so that an accurate prognosis can be given. It will greatly enhance the chances of therapeutic success.

Cytology is useful in the diagnosis of:
- Bacterial skin diseases
- *Malassezia* dermatitis

- Otitis externa
- Eosinophilic granuloma complex in cats
- Pemphigus foliaceus
- Ulcers and non-healing wounds
- Nodules and swellings.

Indications for cytology:
- Pustules, macules, crusting and scaling lesions
- Vesicles and bullae
- Abscesses, cysts and draining sinus tracts
- Ulcers
- All suspected neoplasms, and other nodular, papular and plaque type lesions
- Atypical or unusual lesions.

Cytological techniques

In general, aim to take samples from fully developed lesions but before secondary changes have occurred. The best samples are from intact pustules, below crust, the leading edge of ulcers, and non-ulcerated tumours.

Glass slide impressions: Impressions may be taken from any exudative lesion. The lid of a pustule should be carefully opened with a fine needle before taking four or five impressions directly onto the glass slide (Fig. 2.10). Move the slide slightly before each impression to avoid too thick a build up of material. Be gentle when taking direct impressions, otherwise cellular damage will render the cytology uninterpretable. Where a direct impression is not possible, material may be transferred from the lesion to the slide by the use of a cotton bud.

Impressions of the underside of crust can be diagnostically valuable, particularly in cases of suspected pemphigus foliaceus.

Acetate strips: Dry, greasy or waxy lesions are sampled using tape strips. A piece of tape about 50% longer than a microscope slide is used. The middle of the tape is pressed onto the area to be sampled several times to collect surface cells and debris. Each end of the tape is attached to one end of a microscope slide, forming a loop, and stained. Wrapping the tape around both ends of the slide holds it firmly in position and facilitates microscopic examination under oil immersion.

Ear cytology: Cytological examination of an aural discharge should be a standard procedure when faced with otitis externa. The findings are invaluable when deciding on the treatment to use and monitoring response to therapy. Samples of cerumen or pus can be collected from the vertical ear canals using cotton buds. The swab should be gently rolled onto the slide. The same slide may be used for both ears.

Needle aspiration: Nodules or swellings can be sampled by fine-needle aspiration. Most animals will tolerate needle aspiration without any form of chemical restraint. The mass to be sampled should be sprayed with alcohol and held firmly to avoid movement. The needle, usually 21-gauge, is introduced into the lesion and moved backwards and forwards several times, redirecting the needle so that different areas of the lesion are sampled. If necessary, the needle can be attached to a 5-ml syringe and negative pressure applied while the needle is within the mass. The pressure should be released before withdrawing the needle.

The needle is withdrawn and quickly attached to a syringe containing a few millilitres of air. The contents of the needle are then expelled onto a clean slide, which is quickly and gently smeared using a second slide. Speed is of the essence to avoid the sample dehydrating. The sample should be air dried and stained with a rapid stain.

Staining

Diff Quik® or Rapi-Diff® are suitable stains for cutaneous cytology. Staining technique varies depending on the sample. For samples that air dry on the slide, such as pus, serum or blood, the slide is first air dried and then all three components of the rapid stain are used. Waxy or greasy samples such as ear cytology samples

should be heat fixed by passing through a Bunsen burner flame several times and stained without using the first component of the stain, which is an alcohol fixative. Similarly, tape-strip samples for *Malassezia* dermatitis are stained in just the red and blue dyes. Use of the alcohol fixative dissolves the waxy and greasy material in which the yeast organisms are found. Apart from when looking at tape-strip samples, contrast and definition are greatly improved by the use of a coverslip, which can be mounted on a drop of immersion oil or DPX.

Cytological interpretation
Normal cytological features

It is important to be aware of the normal features so that abnormalities may be recognized. Most skin surface preparations contain cells from the surface layer of the epithelium, known as corneocytes (Fig. 2.11). Corneocytes are large, polygonal, translucent cells. Corneocytes frequently contain round or slightly oval, black or brown melanin granules (Fig. 2.11), which should not be confused with bacteria that always stain a blue colour under Diff Quik®. Numerous dark blue cigar-shaped structures that are now thought to be root sheath remnants from hair follicles are seen on preparations from haired skin (Fig. 2.11). Hair shafts are usually seen in skin surface preparations. Occasional microorganisms may also be detected on skin surface preparations. These include yeasts (*Malassezia* spp.), bacteria (cocci and rods) and sometimes, particularly from the feet, saprophytic, non-pathogenic fungal spores, which are usually segmented

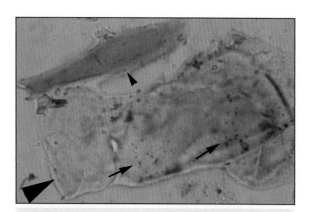

Figure 2.11 Stained tape-strip preparation showing corneocyte (large arrowhead), cell from hair follicle (small arrowhead) and melanin granules (arrow). ×1000 magnification. Diff Quik® stain.

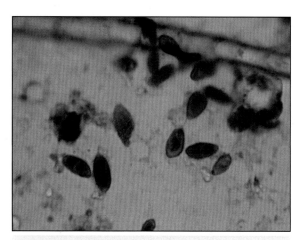

Figure 2.12 Tape-strip cytology from a dog's foot showing hair shaft and saprophytic fungal spores. ×1000 magnification. Diff Quik® stain.

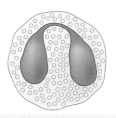

Figure 2.14 Eosinophil.

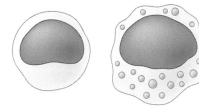

Figure 2.15 Macrophages. Activated cell on the right.

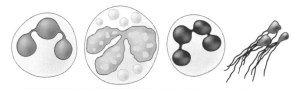

Figure 2.13 Neutrophils. Left to right: non-toxic cell, toxic neutrophil, pyknotic neutrophil and nuclear stranding.

and stain a green to blue colour (Fig. 2.12). Stain precipitate is frequently seen and appears as a blue or purple crystalline deposit.

Cytology from inflammatory lesions

Inflammatory cell types: Neutrophils, eosinophils, macrophages and lymphocytes may be seen in preparations from inflamed skin. It is important to be able to recognize these cells and be aware of their significance. Some inflammatory cells may take on different appearances depending on the disease process and ageing changes.

Neutrophils: Neutrophils (Fig. 2.13) are the most common inflammatory cell type seen in preparations from inflamed skin. They are seen in association with bacterial infections but may also be present in sterile disease processes. The presence of phagocytosed bacteria confirms an active bacterial infection. The distinction between a septic and non-septic aetiology may be

difficult in the absence of bacteria, but the presence of 'toxic' or 'degenerate' neutrophils with swollen pale nuclei is suggestive of infection. As neutrophils age the nuclei shrink, become hypersegmented and darker staining. These are known as pyknotic cells. Neutrophils may be damaged during slide preparation, resulting in purple-staining streaks of nuclear material across the slide.

Eosinophils: Eosinophils are easily recognized by their distinct red to orange granules (Fig. 2.14). There is considerable variation in granular morphology. Eosinophils are usually associated with allergic or parasitic diseases. They may be seen in large numbers from impression smears of feline eosinophilic plaques or indolent ulcers and from canine eosinophilic furunculosis. Eosinophils are also frequently seen in cases of canine deep pyoderma.

Macrophages: Macrophages are large mononuclear cells about one and a half times the size of a neutrophil. The cytoplasm of an activated macrophage takes on a foamy appearance due to the accumulation of proteolytic enzymes (Fig. 2.15). Macrophages are seen in some chronic inflammatory processes, often in association with neutrophils in pyogranulomatous inflammation, but may also be seen within a few hours of the initiation of inflammatory change. Therefore, their presence does not necessarily denote chronicity. The presence of pyogranulomatous inflammation even without evidence

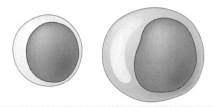

Figure 2.16 Left: lymphocyte. Right: plasma cell.

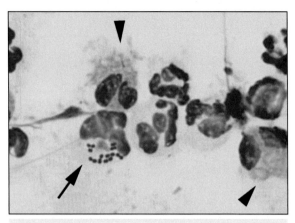

Figure 2.17 Neutrophil with phagocytosed cocci (arrow). Eosinophils (arrowheads).

of bacteria is often due to infection and is commonly seen in impressions from canine deep pyoderma lesions.

Lymphocytes and plasma cells: Lymphocytes (Fig. 2.16) are mononuclear cells and are slightly smaller than neutrophils. Plasma cells are B lymphocytes, which have started to manufacture immunoglobulins. Lymphocytes and plasma cells are seen in some longer-standing and immune-mediated lesions. Large numbers of atypical lymphocytes may be seen in impression smears of lymphoma.

Microorganisms

Bacteria: Bacteria are commonly found in cutaneous cytology preparations. An inflammatory infiltrate with the presence of phagocytosed bacteria denotes an active infection (Fig. 2.17). Thus, finding neutrophils with phagocytosed cocci from an intact pustule confirms a bacterial pyoderma. On occasion, large numbers of bacteria, frequently adherent to corneocytes, may be evident without a significant inflammatory infiltrate. This may be seen in cases of long-standing, poorly controlled atopic dermatitis and is known as bacterial overgrowth syndrome (Fig. 2.18).

Malassezia spp.: *Malassezia* spp., unipolar budding yeasts, usually stain a purple colour with Diff Quik® (Fig. 2.19). In some situations only the capsule of the yeast stains and these are known as ghost forms (Fig. 2.20). The significance of finding yeast organisms on a cytological preparation depends on several factors, including the anatomical site and the presence or absence of visible inflammation. Finding the occasional yeast organism from the feet (or ear canal) is consistent with normal skin. However, if the skin is inflamed or there is evidence of pruritus, and yeasts are seen in several fields, then antifungal treatment would be indicated.

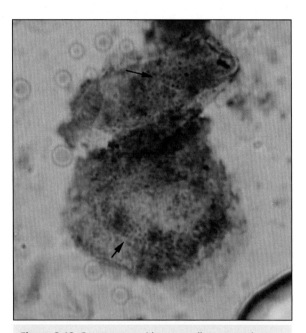

Figure 2.18 Corneocytes with many adherent cocci (arrows) from a case of bacterial overgrowth syndrome.

Acantholytic keratinocytes

Pemphigus foliaceus (see Chapter 17) results in the formation of pustules which contain large numbers of non-toxic neutrophils and acantholytic keratinocytes (Fig. 2.21). Less commonly, the pustule may also contain eosinophils. Acantholytic keratinocytes are nucleated keratinocytes from the stratum spinosum which have become detached from the epidermis and have a

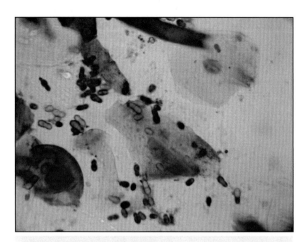

Figure 2.19 *Malassezia pachydermatis* organisms from a case of *Malassezia* dermatitis.

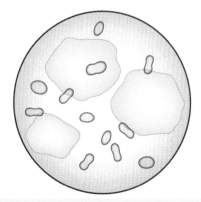

Figure 2.20 *Malassezia* ghosts.

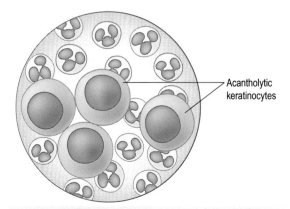

Acantholytic keratinocytes

Figure 2.21 Cytology from pemphigus foliaceus showing acantholytic keratinocytes and non-toxic neutrophils.

distinctive rounded appearance. Note that acantholytic keratinocytes may also be seen in other pustular and inflammatory dermatoses, including pyoderma and dermatophytosis.

Ear cytology

Cytological examination of any aural discharge should be a standard procedure when faced with otitis externa. The findings are invaluable when deciding on the treatment to use and monitoring response to therapy.

One of the most common primary inflammatory causes of recurrent otitis externa is atopic dermatitis. Frequently, in the early stages of atopic dermatitis, the dog may be presented with otitis externa and cytology reveals the presence of large numbers of corneocytes but no evidence of infection.

Occasional *Malassezia* organisms may be found in normal ear canals. Large numbers of yeasts will be seen in cases of *Malassezia* otitis externa. Cocci and/or rods will be seen in bacterial otitis and it is not uncommon to find a wide variety of microorganisms. If a rod infection is present, samples for bacterial culture and sensitivity testing should be taken prior to starting therapy. The presence of neutrophils and phagocytosed rods is very suggestive of infection with *Pseudomonas aeruginosa*.

BACTERIAL CULTURE AND SENSITIVITY TESTING

Canine and feline pyodermas are common presentations. In general, bacterial culture and sensitivity is not routinely performed in these cases because the antibacterial sensitivities of causal organisms are well known.

Culture and sensitivity testing are indicated where:
- Unusual organisms are seen on cytology.
- There has been a poor response to an antibacterial which is generally effective.
- In cases of canine deep pyoderma where long courses of therapy are required.

Technique: The best lesion to sample is an intact pustule, which is opened with a fine hypodermic needle and discharge is collected onto the tip of a bacterial swab. Prior to opening the pustule the area should be gently swabbed with surgical spirit to remove surface bacterial contaminants. If there are no intact lesions then a swab from the underside of a crust or any other exudative lesion may be used, although the results should be interpreted with caution and the organism isolated should correlate with the results of cytological examination.

In deep pyoderma, swabs may be inserted into draining sinus tracts or the lesion gently squeezed to exude pus, which is collected onto the swab. Deeper tissue samples may be harvested for culture using a biopsy punch or elliptical incision. Commonly, such material is submitted for both culture and histopathological examination. If mycobacterial infection is suspected, samples may be frozen and only submitted for culture if histopathological examination is suggested of mycobacteriosis.

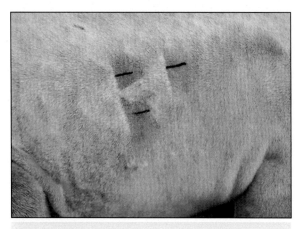

Figure 2.22 Lines drawn on skin at biopsy sites.

HISTOPATHOLOGY

Histopathological examination of skin biopsies is indicated in the following situations:
- Unusual skin diseases
- Erosive or ulcerative disorders
- Nodules and tumours
- In severe or life-threatening conditions
- Where a presentation is suggestive of a condition readily diagnosed on histopathology (zinc-responsive dermatosis, necrolytic migratory erythema, sebaceous adenitis, some immune-mediated diseases)
- Where there has been a poor response to treatment.

Histopathological examination is of little value in the investigation of most cases of pruritus.

Technique: Six- or 8-mm biopsy punches are suitable for most circumstances, although scalpel excision is necessary for larger or fragile lesions or when looking for evidence of panniculitis when there is a requirement to include the subcutis. Unless an area such as the pinna, footpad, lip or nasal planum is to be sampled, sedation and local anaesthesia are usually adequate. Local anaesthetic should not contain adrenaline, as this will cause vasoconstriction within the sample.

The biopsy punch should be considered a 'circular scalpel blade'. The punch should be placed perpendicular to the skin surface and a downward and rotational movement should be exerted to make the incision. The punch should not be rotated in both directions because this can induce artefactual changes in the sample.

It is important to biopsy lesions that are going to contain representative pathology. Suitable lesions include papules, pustules, vesicles, nodules, erosions or ulcers. Crusts are also of diagnostic value, but there is usually little to be gained from taking biopsies of chronic lichenified or excoriated areas. As a general rule, try and sample lesions at different stages of development. Take skin samples from the centre of the area of alopecia, as well as any advancing margin when sampling areas of alopecia.

Ideally, the excised tissue should be orientated for the pathologist so that the tissue can be sectioned in the plane of the hair follicles. This is most easily achieved by drawing a black line with an indelible marker in the direction of hair growth and taking the biopsy sample such that the line drawn bisects the sample (Fig. 2.22).

Sample submission: Dermatohistopathology is a specialized area and it is advisable to submit samples to laboratories with expertise in this field. To obtain the most useful information from the histopathologist, submission forms should be fully completed, giving signalment and a full history, including a description of disease progression, presence of any systemic signs, details of any previous diagnostic tests and results, and response to previous treatment. Only with this information will the pathologist be able to perform clinico-pathological correlation.

Interpretation of the histopathology report: Histopathology reports are usually divided into several sections. The first section details how many tissue sections were examined and gives the histopathological description of the lesions found. The next section gives the morphological diagnosis. This is a description of the histopathological reaction pattern. If the histopathological changes are pathognomonic then a specific diagnosis may be given, but it is more likely that the pathologist will discuss the changes and attempt to correlate them with the history given by the clinician.

PRURITUS WITH PAPULES AND/OR CRUSTING AND/ OR SCALING

3 Introduction to pruritus – pathogenesis and evolution of lesions

PRURITUS

Pruritus is a common presentation in small animal practice. A recently published survey (Hill P et al., 2006) showed that it accounts for 30–40% of all small animal dermatological consultations.

Broadly speaking, pruritus is defined as the sensation of itching, which may result in biting, licking, scratching and rubbing of the skin. It is triggered mainly by parasites, allergies and infections, but it can occur with almost any cutaneous disease. The pathophysiology of pruritus is not well understood. It is thought to result from the stimulation of cutaneous neuroreceptors by a range of mediators produced by inflammatory cells and by keratinocytes in the skin.

In many cases of pruritus, the cause is not immediately obvious and establishing the diagnosis is perceived to be a costly and time-consuming process. For this reason symptomatic treatment is often prescribed without first establishing the cause. This approach rarely leads to a cure and can often lead to complications, owner dissatisfaction and 'vet hopping'. Additionally, and apart from parasitic disease where a cure can usually be achieved, many cases of pruritus are likely to require long-term management, and this lack of a permanent 'cure' leads to further owner dissatisfaction. On the other hand, a specific diagnosis allows the clinician to give the owner an accurate prognosis. Furthermore, a detailed discussion of the therapeutic options and any potential adverse effects will help to maximize client compliance, thereby increasing the likelihood of successful long-term management.

The diagnostic process involves thorough history taking, full physical and dermatological examinations, and a series of diagnostic tests and therapeutic trials to rule out the differential diagnoses.

The information gleaned from a detailed and, hopefully, reliable history is of paramount importance when drawing up the list of differential diagnoses. It may help to ask an owner the same question in slightly different ways. Two different answers will make the clinician question the reliability of the history!

The owner should be questioned on the following:
1. Evidence of systemic involvement.
2. With reference to the skin disease:
   (a) Age of onset
   (b) Seasonality
   (c) Distribution of the pruritus
   (d) Initial appearance and distribution of any lesions, and how they have changed over time.
3. Management:
   (a) Environment
   (b) Diet
   (c) Evidence of contagion or zoonosis
   (d) Response to previous treatment.

Owners often only associate scratching with pruritus, and it is important to question them regarding rubbing, licking and biting, as well as scratching. All these actions can result in varying degrees of self-induced alopecia, excoriations and in some cases even ulceration. Other lesions commonly seen include papules, pustules, epidermal collarettes, scaling, crusting, hyperpigmentation and lichenification. Some of these lesions may be responsible for the pruritus, while in other cases they are a result of the pruritus. It is often difficult to establish whether the lesions preceded the onset pruritus or not, as unfortunately few owners will have noticed.

Different individuals show varying degrees of self-trauma associated with pruritus. The individual pruritic threshold and the effects of summation may explain this variation. Recognizing the cause or trigger factors in the chain of events is the key to the successful treatment and/or management of each patient.

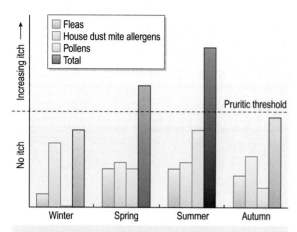

Figure 3.1 Variation of pruritic threshold.

PRURITIC THRESHOLD

It is thought that each individual animal only begins to show evidence of pruritus once the sum total of the allergen load passes its pruritic threshold. Each allergen produces a different level of pruritus, which when present at the same time in a pruritic animal will add up, causing the total pruritic stimulus to surpass the threshold. Conversely, if the sum total falls below the threshold, because for example the pollen season is over, the animal will cease to be pruritic (Fig. 3.1).

The aim of each chapter in this section on pruritus is to guide the reader through the approach to a variety of cases where pruritus was the main presenting sign. In each case the aim was to achieve a specific diagnosis with a view to prescribing specific treatments and management options to suit the patient and owner.

4 Sarcoptic mange

INITIAL PRESENTATION

Pruritus with erythema, alopecia, papules, crusting and scaling.

INTRODUCTION

Sarcoptic mange (also referred to as scabies) is a highly contagious, intensely pruritic and potentially zoonotic skin condition, due to an infestation of the skin by a sarcoptid mite *Sarcoptes scabiei* var. *canis*. The presenting signs of pruritus – papules, crusting, scaling, erythema and self-induced alopecia – are often confused with other dermatological conditions, such as staphylococcal pyoderma, allergic skin diseases or other ectoparasitic diseases.

CASE PRESENTING SIGNS

A 13-year-old uncastrated male samoyed was presented with severe pruritus, to the extent that the dog was continually scratching in the waiting room and during the consultation. It was also lethargic and exhibited erythema, alopecia, crusting and scaling.

CASE HISTORY

All dogs present with a history of intense pruritus, which in most cases fail to respond to increasing doses of glucocorticoids. The onset of pruritus tends to be sudden and severe, and the animal is usually presented shortly after onset, unless the individual has been intermittently treated with ectoparasiticidal products. A history of indirect contact with foxes is usually noted, especially in urban and suburban areas of the UK. Sarcoptic mange is contagious and of zoonotic importance, and evidence of contagion and zoonosis may come to light during the history taking.

The history in this case was as follows:
- The dog was acquired from a rescue centre 3 years prior to presentation.
- The dog had no previous history of skin disease, apart from having several sebaceous cysts removed surgically a few months before.
- The pruritus started about 2 months prior to presentation and had worsened over this period.
- The dog's environment and management had not altered over this period.
- There were no in-contact dogs, but there were foxes in the garden.
- The owner reported that the dog was lethargic and depressed.
- There was no zoonosis.
- The pruritus initially responded to oral prednisolone but, as the disease progressed, even increasing doses had no effect.
- Systemic antimicrobial therapy, for 7 days, was of no benefit.
- Flea control was sporadic.

CLINICAL EXAMINATION

The clinical signs can range from subtle lesions with marked pruritus to severe lesions. The primary lesions include erythematous and/or crusted papules, and secondary lesions include crusts, lichenification, scaling and hyperpigmentation. Initial lesion distribution tends to be on the ear margins, elbows, sternum and the hocks. If untreated the lesions can become widespread and often affect the demeanour of the dog, as in this case.

The physical and dermatological examination revealed:

- The temperature, heart rate and respiratory rates were within normal limits.
- Generalized skin lesions affecting the trunk, caudal aspects of the thighs, dorsal aspect of the tail and the feet (Figs 4.1 and 4.2).
- The lesions included scaling, crusting, erythema, papules and alopecia (Fig. 4.3).
- The skin was malodorous.
- There was a marked itch–scratch reflex.

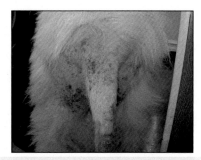

Figure 4.1 Crusting, scaling and erythema on the caudal aspect.

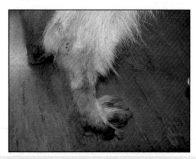

Figure 4.2 Erythema, crusting and secondary alopecia on the distal limb.

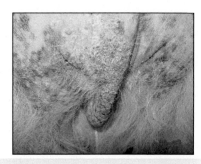

Figure 4.3 Close-up view showing the crusts.

DIFFERENTIAL DIAGNOSES

- Sarcoptic mange
- Staphylococcal pyoderma (either primary or secondary)
- *Malassezia* dermatitis
- Flea allergic dermatitis
- Adverse food reaction
- Hypothyroidism
- Pemphigus foliaceus
- Sebaceous adenitis
- Demodicosis
- Cheyletiellosis
- Cutaneous epitheliotropic lymphoma.

NB: Atopic dermatitis is usually a differential diagnosis for pruritus but was very unlikely given the age of this dog. Most dogs develop the condition by the age of 3 years.

CASE WORK-UP

The demonstration of a mite, eggs or faecal pellets on deep skin scrapes confirms the diagnosis but this test is only positive in around 50% of cases of canine scabies despite examination of scrapings from multiple sites. In those cases where mites are not seen, but the history and clinical signs are suggestive of infestation, a serological test to demonstrate the presence of anti-*Sarcoptes* IgG may further support the diagnosis. This test is reported to have sensitivity ranging between 83% and 92%, and specificity ranging between 89.5% and 92%.

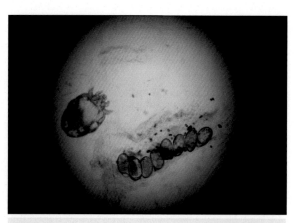

Figure 4.4 *Sarcoptes* mite, several eggs and faecal pellets.

The following tests were performed:

- In this case, mites, faecal pellets and eggs were demonstrated on skin scrapings (Fig. 4.4).
- Cytological examination of tape-strip preparations and smears from papules ruled out the involvement of *Malassezia*, but revealed staphylococcal infection.
- Gross and microscopic examination of coat brushings failed to reveal any evidence of fleas or other ectoparasites.

Flea allergic dermatitis remained a possible concurrent problem, given the distribution of the lesions. If the response to treatment for the sarcoptic mange and staphylococcal pyoderma were partial, one would need to either do further tests or monitor response to ongoing aggressive flea control.

Investigations into thyroid function were deferred, as the dog had been treated with prednisolone, which would affect the results. The test was performed after 8 weeks and was found to be within normal limits. The diagnoses of pemphigus foliaceus, sebaceous adenitis and cutaneous epitheliotropic lymphoma would be confirmed or ruled out by histopathological analysis of multiple skin biopsies but the first step was to treat the scabies. In this case, because of the complete response to the treatment, it was not necessary to subject the dog to further investigations.

DIAGNOSIS

A diagnosis of sarcoptic mange and secondary staphylococcal pyoderma was made based on the results of the skin scrapes and cytology.

PROGNOSIS

The prognosis is usually excellent for this condition provided there are no sources for re-infestations.

AETIOPATHOGENESIS OF SARCOPTIC MANGE

Sarcoptid mites belong to the family Sarcoptidae and are small (200–400 μm) and globose in shape. The mites mate in a moulting pocket on the surface of the skin and the fertilized female then burrows through the stratum corneum, laying eggs in a tunnel behind her. The eggs hatch into larvae and then nymphs, which burrow back to the surface of the skin to feed, or remain in a moulting pocket until they are mature. The life cycle

of the mite is 17–21 days. Mites tend initially to infest sparsely haired areas such as the elbow, hock, convex aspects of the pinnae and the ventrum.

The sarcoptid mite is a source of multiple antigens to which the host is exposed as it feeds, burrows and defecates. Exposure to the antigens induces humoral and cell-mediated immune responses. Even though spontaneous resolution is reported, most infected dogs go on to develop intense pruritus and lesions, caused by the burrowing of the mite in the epidermis and to a hypersensitivity reaction.

EPIDEMIOLOGY

The condition has a worldwide distribution, can occur at any time of the year, tends to be continuous and worsens over time. Even though the mite is an obligate parasite, it can survive, depending on the environmental temperature and humidity, off the host for up to 19 days. The incidence depends on contact with infected animals, fomites such as grooming implements, infected kennels (especially rescue kennels) and, in the UK, indirect contact with foxes would also appear to be a problem.

There is no age, breed or sex predisposition. Although infestation usually starts on lesser haired areas, it can become generalized and affect large areas of the body.

The infestation can spread to other dogs and in-contact humans. When exposed to an infested dog, people can develop a papular rash in areas of contact, such as the arms and the trunk, within 24 hours. These lesions tend to regress spontaneously once the affected animals are treated.

TREATMENT OPTIONS

Currently amitraz, moxidectin and selamectin are the only licensed preparations for sarcoptic mange in the UK. Moxidectin and selamectin are applied topically to the skin, through which they are absorbed. Most clinicians now favour these agents because of the ease of application and to avoid clipping the patient. The key to successful resolution is the concurrent treatment of both the in-contact animals and the environment.

Amitraz: Amitraz is licensed as a topical sponge-on preparation, applied every 7 days for 2–6 weeks. It exerts its effect by inhibiting monoamine oxidase. Clipping long-haired animals is advised prior to application of the product. It is contraindicated in chihuahuas at any age, in puppies less than 12 weeks of age and in nursing bitches. The product is toxic to fish and the manufacturer's guidelines should be followed. The side-effects of amitraz are transient sedation, lethargy, slow shallow breathing and bradycardia. These symptoms usually last for 24 hours, but if they persist, they can be reversed by the α2-adrenoreceptor antagonist atipamezole at the dose of 0.2 mg/kg, or the dog can be washed with a mild soap. Amitraz should not be handled by diabetic owners, as it could cause transient hyperglycaemia.

Moxidectin: Moxidectin is a second-generation systemic macrocylic lactone with broad-spectrum antiparasitic activity. It interacts with γ-aminobutyric acid (GABA) and the glutamate-gated chloride channels at the postsynaptic junctions, allowing an influx of chloride ions resulting in flaccid paralysis and death of the parasite. Moxidectin (2.5%) combined with imidacloprid is available as a spot-on preparation for the treatment of sarcoptic mange in puppies and dogs over 7 weeks of age. After topical application, moxidectin is absorbed percutaneously and reaches maximum plasma concentration after 4–9 days. The recommended dose is 2.5 mg/kg of moxidectin to be applied twice 4 weeks apart. Moxidectin is tolerated by collies and collie crosses; however, accidental ingestion in sensitive dogs can cause vomiting, salivation and transient neurological signs, such as ataxia, tremors, dilated pupils and nystagmus. Moxidectin is also reported to be toxic to aquatic organisms and therefore it should not be allowed to enter water.

Selamectin: Selamectin, a novel avermectin, is another safe broad-spectrum topical antiparasitic drug licensed for sarcoptic mange. It is easy to apply and is recommended for use at 6–12 mg/kg twice 30 days apart. Some dermatologists recommend applying the product three times at 14-day intervals. This advice is based on anecdotal reports of an improved response. However, even though the margin of safety is good, the owners should be warned of the extra-label use.

Milbemycin oxime: Three doses of milbemycin oxime given orally at 2 mg/kg every 7 days has been reported to have a variable efficacy ranging from 71% to 100%. It is available as a heartworm preparation in some countries and is not licensed for sarcoptic mange. It is expensive but can be used as a much safer alternative to ivermectin in ivermectin-sensitive dogs.

Ivermectin: Ivermectin given orally at 0.2–0.4 mg/kg three times 7 days apart, or injected subcutaneously twice 14 days apart, is effective against the mite. However, it is not licensed and is potentially toxic in ivermectin-sensitive breeds such as collies, collie crosses and other sheepdogs. The adverse effects include ataxia, tremors, dilated pupils, nystagmus, salivation, depression, coma and death.

Environmental treatment

The sarcoptic mite is able to survive in the environment, which can be a source of re-infestation. Because the dogs are intensely pruritic and scratch a lot, they often leave scale, crusts and hairs containing mites in the environment. Thorough vacuuming and the application of an acaricidal preparation are recommended as part of the treatment.

Treatment in this case

In this case the sarcoptic mange was treated with moxidectin combined with imidacloprid three times, 2 weeks apart (Figs 4.5 and 4.6) The staphylococcal

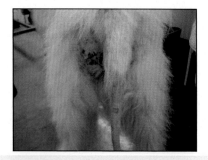

Figure 4.5 Caudal aspect 4 weeks post-treatment.

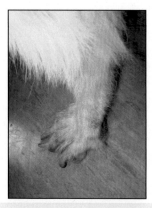

Figure 4.6 Distal limb 4 weeks post-treatment.

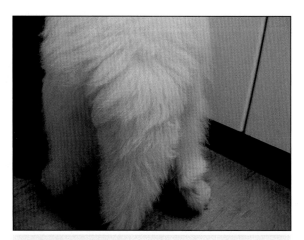

Figure 4.7 Caudal aspect 8 weeks post-treatment.

pyoderma resolved with 6 weeks of cefalexin (20 mg/kg). The environment was treated with a permethrin spray. There was complete response to the treatment and all the hair had regrown within 8 weeks (Fig. 4.7).

NURSING ASPECTS

Most dogs with chronic sarcoptic mange require an Elizabethan collar to prevent self-trauma. If the animal has been admitted into the surgery and kennelled whilst investigations are carried out, nurses must remember to clean the kennel thoroughly using an environmental ectoparasiticide spray before the kennel is used again. Clippers etc. and any potentially infected surfaces must also be thoroughly cleaned. Potentially infected dogs should be kept away from other animals in the waiting room.

CLINICAL TIPS

The prevalence of the disease varies with areas and therefore local knowledge of the area is useful. History of recent contact with foxes or rolling in fox faeces should alert the clinician. Often, individuals show a pinnal scratch reflex. In some cases the lesions may be subtle, especially if the individual has been regularly bathed or is being intermittently treated with flea preparations, which include miticidal drugs.

To increase the chance of demonstrating the mite on skin scraping, choose an untraumatized area with heavy scaling or crusted papules (usually the ear pinna or the elbow) to scrape. Scrape a wide area and collect all the material onto the slide. Allowing the slide to warm by the microscope light often activates the mite, making it easier to find. Placing a coverslip on the sample provides an even surface and makes it easier to see. Scan the entire slide under a ×4 or ×10 objective. Always treat all the in-contact dogs at the same time.

5 Flea allergic dermatitis

INITIAL PRESENTATION

Pruritus with papules, erythema, scaling and hyperpigmentation in a Jack Russell terrier.

INTRODUCTION

In some parts of the world, flea allergic dermatitis (FAD) is the most common allergic disease and a major cause of pruritus in dogs and cats. In other parts it is a significant problem only at certain times of the year. Although allergic dermatitis is the main condition associated with fleas, a distinction between pruritus resulting from severe flea infestation and a hypersensitivity response should be made. In very young puppies and kittens, severe flea infestations provoke varying degree of pruritus, but more often patients exhibit signs of weakness, lethargy and anaemia. Fleas are also vectors of infectious organisms such as *Bartonella*, *Rickettsia felis* and *Haemoplasma* spp.

CASE PRESENTING SIGNS

A 6-year-old female Jack Russell terrier was presented with severe erythema, pruritus, papules, alopecia and hyperpigmentation affecting the dorsum, feet, periocular skin, ears and muzzle.

CASE HISTORY

This varies between individuals but most pruritic dogs are presented with a history of pruritus and varying lesions affecting the lumbo-sacral region. As the flea life cycle is affected by environmental factors such as temperature and humidity, seasonal exacerbations may occur. Often flea control is only intermittently used and in-contact animals, especially cats, are inadequately treated. The history in this particular case was long and complex. The most relevant parts were:

- Long-standing history of non-seasonal pruritus involving face, feet and ventrum, and more recently the dorsal trunk had also become involved.
- The pruritus has been managed with intermittent methylprednisolone acetate injections, but these had become ineffective with severe deterioration in the dog's clinical condition.
- The dog was mainly fed on a commercial pet food and more recently an 8-week diet trial with a prescription hydrolysed hypoallergenic diet had failed to resolve the pruritus or the clinical lesions.
- The indoor environment was fully carpeted and the dog normally slept under the owner's bed.
- Outdoor access was to the garden only.
- Previous flea control had been intermittent, using fipronil and most recently selamectin.
- The three in-contact cats were unaffected and were intermittently treated for fleas with a pet shop product.
- The owner had seen fleas on one of the cats some weeks back and had treated it with proprietary flea product from the supermarket.

CLINICAL EXAMINATION

A whole range of clinical signs, from primary lesions such as papules and pustules, to severe secondary hyperpigmentation, lichenification and fibropruritic nodules are seen, depending on the chronicity of the disease. Self-induced alopecia due to over-grooming and secondary bacterial infection is often seen in affected dogs. Atopic dogs are predisposed to flea bite hypersensitivity, even those that have been well managed. Some dogs will present with pyotraumatic dermatitis on the rump, or at other sites.

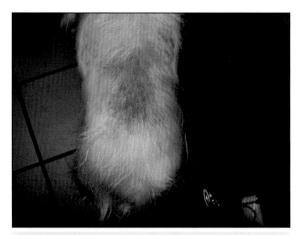

Figure 5.1 Erythema, papules and self-induced alopecia on the dorsum.

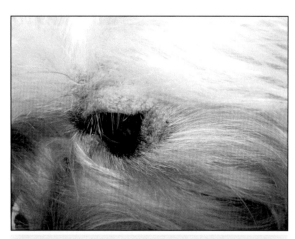

Figure 5.4 Periocular dermatitis.

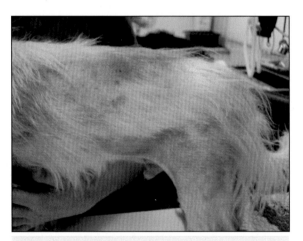

Figure 5.2 Lateral aspect on the trunk.

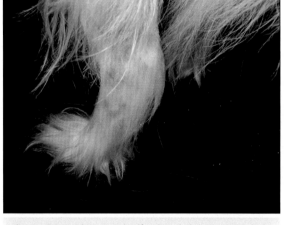

Figure 5.5 Erythema and self-induced alopecia extending to the distal aspect of the leg.

The clinical findings in this case were:
- Severe generalized erythema with papules, follicular papules and crusted patches on the trunk (Figs 5.1 and 5.2).
- Erythema, alopecia and papular rash on the ventrum and inguinal region (Fig. 5.3).
- The periocular skin was hyperpigmented, lichenified and erythematous, with evidence of excoriations (Fig. 5.4).
- Both the pinnae and vertical ear canals were erythematous.
- Erythema, self-induced alopecia, crusting and hyperpigmentation involving all four feet (Fig. 5.5).
- The skin was malodorous and greasy to the touch.

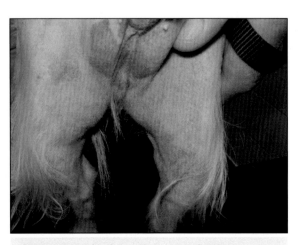

Figure 5.3 Papular dermatitis in inguinal regions.

- The peripheral lymph nodes were not enlarged and the other physical parameters were within normal limits.

DIFFERENTIAL DIAGNOSES

In this case, given the clinical signs and the distribution of the lesions, there was evidence for more than one type of hypersensitivity. The facial, pedal and ventral distribution suggested atopic dermatitis, and that affecting the dorsal aspect, flea allergy dermatitis. A concurrent adverse food reaction could also have been contributing to the pruritus. The other differentials included:
- Staphylococcal pyoderma
- Malasseziosis
- Sarcoptic mange
- Demodicosis
- *Otodectes* hypersensitivity
- Dermatophytosis
- Adverse drug reaction.

CASE WORK-UP

A number of the differential diagnoses were ruled out with simple in-house tests:
- Skin scrapes were performed to rule out demodicosis and to look for sarcoptic mange. Negative skin scrapes do not definitively rule out sarcoptic mange and therefore a *Sarcoptes* IgG ELISA test was performed, which was also negative.
- There was no fungal growth after 3 weeks of culturing of a sample obtained by the MacKenzie toothbrush technique.
- Tape-strip samples, obtained from crusted lesions, revealed clumps of coccoid bacteria, neutrophils and keratinocytes.
- *Staphylococcus intermedius* was isolated from a swab submitted for bacterial culture, which was sensitive to amoxicillin/clavulanate, cefalexin, enrofloxacin, marbofloxacin, clindamycin and trimethoprim/sulphonamide. It was resistant to amoxicillin, penicillin and tetracycline.
- Coat brushings failed to demonstrate any fleas or flea faeces.

In addition to atopic dermatitis, the history, clinical signs and distribution of lesions were suggestive of flea allergic dermatitis. The diagnosis of flea allergy dermatitis is supported with additional tests and with response to aggressive flea control. The simplest test is the demonstration of fleas or flea faeces using a flea comb; however, about a third of animals fail to show any evidence of fleas, for various reasons:
- Self-grooming removes the fleas and flea faeces
- Owners often groom or bath the animals before coming into the practice
- Intermittent flea control reduces the numbers, making it difficult to find them
- Exposure to the flea source may be intermittent.

In these cases further diagnostic tests may be of value; however, it is important to remember their limitations and ultimately a positive response to aggressive flea control is needed to confirm the diagnosis.

In vitro testing: In this case an *in vitro* Allercept IgE ELISA test using recombinant flea saliva revealed a markedly elevated flea allergen specific IgE concentration, which was consistent with flea allergy dermatitis and suggested current flea exposure. However, the specificity and the sensitivity of the testing are variable, and the test does not recognize those animals with cell-mediated hypersensitivity immune responses. It is useful as a diagnostic aid but a negative test should not necessarily rule out FAD. It is estimated that about 15–30% of individuals may show just cell-mediated immune responses. In addition, a serum IgE test for other allergens was performed (see Chapter 3) to assess the role of environmental allergens. This revealed high levels of IgE to house dust and storage mite allergens.

Intradermal testing: Intradermal testing with whole-body flea antigen or flea saliva may also support the diagnosis. This test produces immediate reactions (15–30 minutes), or late-phase reactions (4–6 hours) or delayed reactions (24–48 hours) to specific antigens injected intradermally. The test site should be examined at the appropriate times. Late-phase and delayed-type reactions are recognized either by an erythematous ring at the site of injection and/or a raised wheal. In this case this test was not deemed to be suitable for either flea antigen or other environmental allergens, because the last injection of methylprednisolone acetate had been given only 2 months prior to the initial examination by the dermatologist. The duration of action of this drug is anything between 4 and 6 weeks, and varies between individuals. Ideally, intradermal testing should be carried out not less than 12 weeks after the injection of a reposital glucocorticoid.

DIAGNOSIS

The diagnosis in this case was that of bacterial pyoderma, flea allergic dermatitis and atopic dermatitis.

PROGNOSIS

The long-term prognosis was good, provided the owner was able to maintain thorough long-term flea control on all the animals in the house and it was possible to effectively manage the concurrent atopic dermatitis. There may be flare-ups from time to time depending on the allergen load.

AETIOPATHOGENESIS OF FLEA ALLERGIC DERMATITIS

Although most cats and dogs have fleas at some point or other, not all develop clinical signs associated with hypersensitivity and it is probable that those that don't are not sensitized to the flea saliva. However, exposure, either intermittent or continuous, to flea bites is a predisposing factor in the development of the allergic response, as is atopic dermatitis. Sensitization can occur at any age and is usually lifelong.

Several allergenic proteins identified in flea saliva can result in an individual becoming sensitized. The proteins range from 12 to 50 kDa in molecular weight. Three types of allergic responses – immediate, late-phase and delayed-type responses – have been identified.

- Immediate-type hypersensitivity occurs within minutes of the flea bite and is associated with mast cell degranulation triggered by the chain of events following the binding of the allergen to the IgE.
- Late-phase reactions are associated with an influx of inflammatory cells in response to the release of pre-formed and newly synthesized inflammatory mediators including cytokines and chemokines. Infiltration of basophils, in particular, occurs in flea allergic dermatitis. Degranulation of basophils is associated with basophil hypersensitivity. This occurs at 4–6 hours after a flea bite.
- Delayed-type hypersensitivity is cell mediated; there is an influx of lymphocytes and macrophages associated with an interaction of several cytokines. This reaction shows clinical signs about 24–48 hours following a

flea bite and accounts for 15–30% of the flea allergic cases.

EPIDEMIOLOGY

There is no sex predisposition and sensitization can occur at any age, but appears to be seen mainly in older animals. Intermittent exposure is associated with increased sensitization, whereas continuous exposure may result in some tolerance.

The incidence of the disease is dependent on the presence of environmental conditions in which the fleas are likely to thrive and perpetuate. An ambient temperature of 18–30°C and high relative humidity of between 70% and 80% favours flea reproduction and survival; however, the flea's biology is such that it ensures its own and/or its intermediate stages' survival, even when the conditions are unfavourable. Although the flea itself is unable to survive cold temperatures, or high temperatures with low relative humidity, the pupal stage (Fig. 5.6) is able to endure them for up to 300 days. Then, when appropriate environmental conditions are encountered (see below), the adult flea emerges. The flea life cycle from egg to adulthood can therefore vary from 15 to 300 days depending on the environmental conditions.

The cat flea, *Ctenocephalides felis felis*, is the main species implicated in flea allergic dogs and cats. *Ctenocephalides canis* is also reported in some countries. Less commonly, flea species that normally infest other mammals and birds may be involved (Table 5.1). The female adult flea is an obligate parasite and needs a blood meal in order to produce eggs and, if the conditions on the host are ideal, it can lay up to 30–50 eggs a day. Feeding fleas can live up to 100 days and lay as many as 2000 eggs in their lifetime.

Fleas do not jump on and off animals, but tend to live on the host. The eggs fall into the animals' environ-

Table 5.1 Flea species and their main hosts

Flea species	Natural host
Ctenocephalides felis felis	Cats and dogs
Ctenocephalides canis	Dogs and cats
Pulex spp.	Humans
Echnidophaga galinacea	Birds
Spilopsysllus cuniculi	Rabbits
Archaeopsylla erinacei	Hedgehogs
Xenopsylla spp.	Small mammals

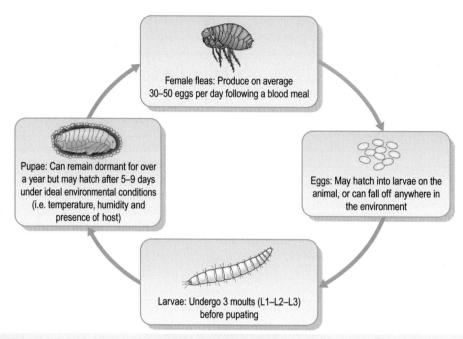

Figure 5.6 The flea life cycle.

ment during grooming or scratching, as they are non-adherent. The eggs hatch into the first larval stage, which burrow deep into crevices, carpet pile, etc., as they are photophobic and geotrophic. This stage feeds on flea faecal pellets and other organic debris in the environment. There are three larval stages and the third stage transforms into the pupa. This stage is a cocooned pre-emerged flea which is protected from environmental insults (including parasiticidal agents) and will only emerge if conditions ensure that its survival is more or less guaranteed by the presence of a host. These conditions include carbon dioxide, warmth and air movements, which indicate the presence of a host.

TREATMENT OPTIONS

Multiple therapies are usually required in the early stages of treatment of flea allergy dermatitis. They include those that limit pruritus, deal with any secondary infections and those that specifically kill the flea and its intermediate stages, both on the animal and in the environment.

Flea control: Both the treatment of all animals in the house and that of the environment should go hand in hand, at least during the initial stages. The treatment should be tailored to suit each case, depending on the number of animals within the household, the ability of the owner to use the products as indicated and the cost.

Fipronil: Fipronil belongs to the phenylpyrazole family and its mode of action is by blocking the pre- and post-synaptic transfer of chloride ions through the cell membrane, thus acting as an insect GABA antagonist. It has both insecticidal and acaricidal activity. It is available in spray and spot-on formulations and kills fleas within 24 hours, and tick and other insects within 48 hours. It is combined with s-methoprene, an insect growth regulator which inhibits the development of immature stages by mimicking the juvenile hormone.

Nitenpyram: Nitenpyram is used as a fast-acting, orally administered insecticide, which kills fleas on the animal as soon as 15 minutes after administration and has an efficacy of up to 100% kill within 24 hours. It acts by inhibiting specific nicotinic acetylcholine receptors. It is a useful product to achieve quick kill in cases such as this one, but is not designed to be used on its own. It can, however, be combined with lufenuron to provide integrated flea control.

Imidacloprid: Imidacloprid belongs to the group of chloronicotinyl compounds. Its mode of action is to bind to the nicotinergic acetylcholine receptors on the post-synaptic region of the insect nervous system, thereby stopping the acetylcholine from binding to the receptors. This results in the paralysis and death of the insect. Imidacloprid is effective against adult fleas as well as larval flea stages. It is available as a spot-on formulation and the label permits weekly use of this product.

Selamectin: Selamectin is a semi-synthetic avermectin with a broad spectrum of activity against endoparasites as well as ectoparasites. It is an adulticide with larvicidal and ovicidal properties. The product is absorbed percutaneously and then redistributed back to the cutaneous tissue via the circulation.

Metaflumizone: Metaflumizone belongs to the semicarbozone group of compounds and is available as a spot-on treatment against fleas. It is a sodium channel blocker which prevents the flow of sodium ions across the nerve cell membrane. This disrupts the transmission of nerve impulses and the eventual result is death by paralysis. For use in dogs, it is combined with amitraz to provide action against fleas and ticks. On its own, it is available for use in cats.

Pyriprole: Pyriprole belongs to the phenylpyrazole group of compounds. It is a spot-on formulation that has both insecticidal and acaricidal activity and its mode of action is similar to that of fipronil (see above). It is licensed for use against fleas and ticks in dogs only.

Pyrethrins: Pyrethrins are naturally occurring flea repellents and pyrethroids synthetic ones. A combination of permethrin, a pyrethroid and imidacloprid has a veterinary licence for use in dogs (contraindicated in cats).

Environmental control

Insect growth regulators: Insect growth regulators such as fenoxycarb, methoprene and pyriproxyfen are analogues of the juvenile hormone, which allows pupation when its concentration falls. Excessive concentrations prevent metamorphosis and thereby break the life cycle. These products are available as environmental aerosol sprays combined with an adulticide for effective control and in the case of methoprene as a spot-on treatment for the animal combined with fipronil.

Insect growth inhibitors such as lufenuron inhibit the synthesis of chitin, thus preventing successive larval moults.

Summary of environmental treatment: Aerosol sprays, pump sprays and foggers are available, which generally contain permethrin plus an insect growth inhibitor or regulator.
- Treat all the areas where the pet might visit (the whole house, cars, baskets, under beds, etc.).
- Clear out organic debris from the outside environment, as this can be a source for re-infestation even in the winter months.
- In cases where there is a severe infestation two treatments 2 weeks apart are necessary to eliminate newly hatched fleas.

Delivery methods for topical treatment of pets:
- Spot-on formulations
- Spray formulations
- Shampoos
- Dips
- Flea collars
- Systemic products.

Treatment in this case

In this case the long-term treatment also included allergen-specific immunotherapy for the management of the atopic dermatitis.

NURSING ASPECTS

Many clients will discuss their concerns with the nurse, or lay staff, rather than the vet. They should be able, tactfully, to reassure them and give them the correct advice. A good grasp of the flea life cycle, together with knowledge of the range of flea products on the veterinary market and their modes of action, is the key to giving correct advice to the client. Flea control within an individual household should be tailored to its needs. Many owners who are registered with the practice will call in to buy products during the summer months when the problem is most apparent. It is at this point, when they recognize the problem, that the client is most receptive to advice on supplementing topical therapy with environmental treatment.

The environment was treated twice 2 weeks apart with a spray containing permethrin and methoprene. The cats and the dog were treated with a spot-on solution containing fipronil and methoprene every 2 weeks for four occasions (extra-label use), then every 3–4 weeks. At the start of the treatment, all the animals (three in-contact cats and the dog) were given 3 days of nitenpyram orally to ensure quick kill and reduction in the flea population as soon as possible.

Antibiotic treatment: In this case cefalexin (15 mg/kg b.i.d.) was prescribed for 3 weeks, without any antipruritic treatment. At the end of the course, clinical examination and tape-strip preparations did not reveal any bacteria and antipruritic treatment was started (see below).

Antipruritic treatment: Given the severe pruritus and its effects on the animal's welfare, 1 mg/kg every 24 hours of prednisolone was prescribed for 7 days, after which it was reduced to alternate-day treatment. After 4 weeks it was reduced to 0.5 mg/kg on alternate days and stopped once the dog reached the maintenance phase of the allergen-specific immunotherapy.

FOLLOW-UP

Long-term flea control was maintained on all the animals in the household. The pedal pruritus persisted even after 1 year on allergen-specific immunotherapy and so 0.1 mg/kg of prednisolone was administered as a concurrent treatment. The dog has been successfully managed on this combination at the time of writing. It is possible that this dog has a concurrent adverse food reaction as well, but the owner was unwilling to repeat a diet trial.

6 Atopic dermatitis

INITIAL PRESENTATION

Pruritus with erythema, alopecia, papules and epidermal collarettes.

INTRODUCTION

Atopic dermatitis is a genetically determined pruritic dermatitis, associated with an immediate (type 1) hypersensitivity to specific environmental allergens. It is one of the most common causes of chronically recurring inflammatory skin disease and involves complex interactions of environmental, microbial, genetic, immunological and pharmacological factors.

The most common presenting signs are pruritus, erythema and secondary microbial infections. The distribution of the pruritus and the lesions typically involve the face, the ears, the ventral aspects of the abdomen, the perianal areas and the feet. The lesions vary from erythema and salivary staining, to self-induced alopecia, hyperpigmentation, lichenification, scaling, crusting and erosions. Otitis externa is seen in four out of five cases, usually involving the concave aspects of the pinna and the vertical ear canals. Recurring conjunctivitis, periocular dermatitis and sneezing may be evident in some cases.

Secondary microbial infections with *Staphylococcus* spp. or *Malassezia pachydermatis* are frequent findings in cases of atopic dermatitis and their importance should not be underestimated. Commonly, one of the first signs of the onset of atopic dermatitis is the development of a cutaneous yeast or bacterial infection, and infection is a major reason for the flare-up of pruritus in apparently well-controlled cases and one of the most common reasons for clients seeking veterinary attention. Clinical signs associated with staphylococcal infections include papules, pustules, epidermal collarettes, scaling and crusting. *Malassezia* dermatitis tends to cause erythema, greasy secretion and the matting of hair shafts over occluded areas such as the ventral neck, or between the digits.

It is common for the pruritus to be present initially only during the summer months, but with the passing of time it tends to become a year-round problem.

At least three of the following major and minor criteria should be satisfied to make a diagnosis of atopic dermatitis:

Major criteria
- First signs between 1 and 3 years of age (but may range from 6 months to 3 years)
- Pruritus that is generally glucocorticoid responsive
- Typical distribution of pruritus and lesions (facial, pedal, ventral and may involve perianal area)
- Otitis externa or bilateral erythema of the concave aspects of the pinna
- Chronic or chronically relapsing
- Genetically predisposed breed.

Minor criteria
- Bilateral conjunctivitis
- Facial erythema and cheilitis
- Recurrent staphylococcal pyoderma
- Seasonal or non-seasonal intermittent exacerbations
- Positive intradermal allergy test or elevated allergen specific serum IgE levels.

CASE PRESENTING SIGNS

A 23-month-old female Staffordshire bull terrier was presented for pruritus, erythema, papules, epidermal collarettes and alopecia.

CASE HISTORY

The main points of interest in the history were:

- It was acquired 9 months earlier, with mild dermatological signs already present.
- The pruritus had been intermittent; it was worse in the summer but was also present during the winter months.
- The pruritus mainly affected the face, ears, feet and ventrum.
- The owner was also concerned at the hair loss on the caudal thighs.
- There were no other animals in the house, but casual contact with dogs in the parks and with relatives' pets.
- Flea control had been used when the dog was first acquired, but not since.
- The dog was fed on a commercial proprietary diet, treats and table scraps.
- The pruritus, but not the rash, was glucocorticoid responsive.
- There was no history suggestive of systemic involvement.

In summary, this was a young dog, of a breed predisposed to atopic dermatitis, with a non-seasonal, glucocorticoid-responsive, facial, aural, pedal and ventral pruritus, and flea control was intermittent.

CLINICAL EXAMINATION

A full physical examination should be carried out prior to examining the skin. The dermatological examination should include all of the skin, extending from the tip of the nose to the tip of the tail and from the dorsum to the pads of the feet. One of the biggest pitfalls is to examine only the affected sites, thus missing other clues that could aid the diagnosis.

The early signs of atopic dermatitis can be subtle and there may be no other clinical signs other than pruritus, although, as in this case, many dogs will have erythema, self-induced alopecia, excoriations, papules, hyperpigmentation and other changes associated with secondary microbial overgrowth or infections. Some individuals will show erythema of the concave aspects of the pinna and the vertical ear canals without any history of ear disease.

The significant clinical findings in this case were:

- Papular rash on the ventral neck (Fig. 6.1).
- Small patch of acute moist dermatitis on the right side of the face.

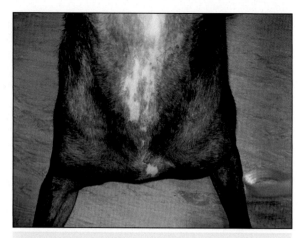

Figure 6.1 Papules, erythema, alopecia and excoriations on the ventral neck.

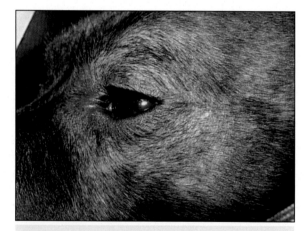

Figure 6.2 Periocular erythema and alopecia.

- Bilateral periocular dermatitis and alopecia (Fig. 6.2).
- Erythema of the concave aspects of both the pinnae.
- Hypotrichosis and erythema of the flexural aspects of the carpi and the extensor aspects of the elbows (Fig. 6.3).
- Alopecia, papules and epidermal collarettes on the ventral chest and abdomen.
- Non-inflammatory alopecia of the caudal thighs (Fig. 6.4).

DIFFERENTIAL DIAGNOSES

In all cases, unless there is an immediate diagnosis, it is best to formulate a list of differential diagnoses and methodically rule each one in or out. This list is drawn up from a consideration of the history and clinical signs, the latter comprising both the general pattern of disease as well as individual lesion recognition. This case is typical of many cases of pruritus in that the differential diagnosis list was quite extensive.

In this case the lesions consisted of inflammatory and non-inflammatory alopecia, hypotrichosis, papules, epidermal collarettes, acute moist dermatitis and erythema.

There were also two different types of hair loss. There were areas of self-induced alopecia and inflammation, and other areas of alopecia where the skin was not inflamed. In this case, the non-inflammatory alopecia over the caudal thighs was unlikely to have arisen because of self-trauma or a folliculitis (the common causes of inflammatory alopecia). This presentation of non-inflammatory alopecia is common in Staffordshire bull terriers with pattern alopecia, which is a poorly understood, non-inflammatory alopecia that results in so-called 'miniaturization' of hair follicles and in the well-recognized, breed-associated patterns of alopecia.

Differentials for the inflammatory alopecia/erythema/papules/epidermal collarettes

- Demodicosis
- Sarcoptic mange
- Secondary microbial infections
  - *Malassezia* dermatitis
  - Superficial staphylococcal pyoderma
- Atopic dermatitis
- Flea bite hypersensitivity
- Adverse food reaction
- Dermatophytosis.

Differentials for the non-inflammatory alopecia

- Pattern alopecia
- Demodicosis
- Dermatophytosis.

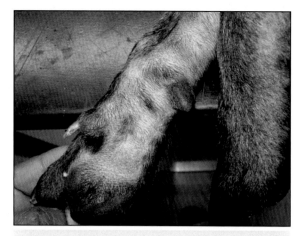

Figure 6.3 Alopecia and erythema on the flexural aspects of the carpus.

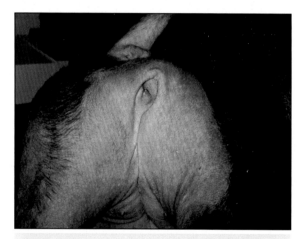

Figure 6.4 Symmetrical alopecia on the caudal thighs.

CASE WORK-UP

Staffordshire bull terriers are genetically predisposed to demodicosis; therefore, skin scrapings and hair plucks should always be performed on this breed, or in any case where there is evidence of papules, pustules, alopecia, crusting or scaling. Primary lesions such as papules are commonly associated with staphylococcal infections and/or sarcoptic mange. Cytology and response to therapy are used to confirm the involvement of secondary pyoderma and *Malassezia* dermatitis, both of which can contribute significantly to the degree of pruritus.

Diagnostic tests: The following diagnostic tests were performed:

- Skin scrapings, hair plucks and coat brushings, which were negative for *Demodex canis* and *Sarcoptes canis* mites.
- Hair plucks, which revealed both anagen and telogen hairs.
- Examination of coat brushings, which did not reveal any fleas, flea dirt or other ectoparasites.
- Examination of tape strip preparations from the ventral neck, which showed *Malassezia pachydermatis* and coccoid bacteria. Both organisms play a secondary role in the pathogenesis of the dermatitis and should therefore be treated.
- Fungal cultures from the hair plucks, which did not grow any dermatophytes.
- *Sarcoptes scabiei* mites are not always seen on skin scrapings in cases of scabies and likewise a failure to identify fleas or flea faeces on examination does not rule out the involvement of flea allergy dermatitis. Additionally, there was evidence of secondary yeast and bacterial infection that may have been contributing significantly to the level of pruritus. Therefore, despite the fact that this case satisfied sufficient major and minor criteria for the diagnosis of atopic dermatitis, it was important to rule out ectoparasitic disease and resolve the secondary yeast and bacterial infections before proceeding with the investigations into the underlying allergy. Prior treatment of concurrent and secondary diseases allows a baseline level of pruritus to be established before starting a diet trial.

Therapeutic trials: Initially, the following therapeutic trials were performed concurrently:
- The pyoderma was treated with cefalexin (20 mg/kg b.i.d.) for 3 weeks.
- The *Malassezia* dermatitis was treated by three times weekly baths with a shampoo containing 2% miconazole/2% chlorhexidine.
- To definitively rule out scabies or flea involvement, selamectin was applied three times at 2-weekly intervals, and the home was treated with a spray containing a combination of permethrin and pyriproxyfen.

Re-examination: On re-examination 4 weeks later, the pruritus had persisted but the papular lesions had resolved and no microbial organisms were seen on repeat cytology. The ongoing pruritus confirmed an underlying allergic aetiology.

Dietary trials: To rule out the involvement of an adverse food reaction, a hydrolysed diet was fed for 8 weeks. No other foods and only water to drink were allowed during this period. Weekly bathing with an antimicrobial shampoo was continued. Flea control was continued using imidacloprid every 4 weeks. The pruritus persisted during this period, with intermittent episodes of increased pruritus. In this case the diet trial ruled out an adverse food reaction as a cause of the disease.

DIAGNOSIS

This patient satisfied several of the major and minor clinical signs of atopic dermatitis, and there was no decrease in pruritus in response to the therapeutic and diet trials. Therefore, a clinical diagnosis of atopic dermatitis was made, which was supported by further testing.
- An intradermal test was performed and positive wheal and flare reactions to storage mites (*Tyrophagus putrescentiae* and *Acarus siro*), house dust mites (*Dermatophagoides farinae* and *D. pteronyssinus*), grass pollens (fescue and Timothy grass) and Lamb's quarter were elicited (Fig. 6.5).
- Skin biopsies were taken from the ventral abdomen and the caudal thigh. Histology of skin from the ventral abdomen revealed superficial perivascular dermatitis with mixed inflammatory cells, whilst that from the caudal thigh revealed miniaturized hair follicles containing short hair shafts of a reduced diameter with normal sebaceous and sweat glands.

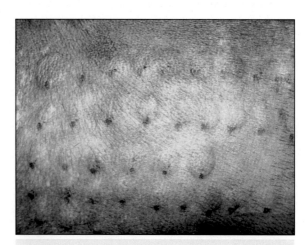

Figure 6.5 Intradermal test showing wheal and flare reactions.

The histopathology findings from the caudal thigh were consistent with pattern alopecia.

PROGNOSIS

Although the condition is not life threatening most atopic dogs require lifelong management. Severe microbial infections and long-term adverse effects of drugs used for the management could influence the patient's longevity. The owner was advised that there is no known treatment for the pattern alopecia.

AETIOPATHOGENESIS

A full review of the aetiopathogenesis of atopic dermatitis is beyond the scope of this section. However, the aetiopathogenesis is complex and multifactorial, and failure to recognize all the factors involved will probably result in unsuccessful management of the condition.

The primary event is the presentation of the allergen to the immune system that, through a chain of events, results in sensitization and subsequent hypersensitivity. A recent study showed that allergen exposure by either the percutaneous or inhalant route resulted in very similar lesion distribution and clinical signs. Other evidence supports the percutaneous penetration of allergens and the involvement of Langerhan's cells in the processing of the antigens, which are then presented to T-helper cells. In genetically predisposed individuals, this activates proliferation of TH2 cells that secrete cytokines such as IL-13, IL-5 and IL-4. IL-4 favouring the synthesis of IgE by B cells. This allergen-specific IgE binds, via the high-affinity Fc receptors, to dermal mast cells.

Subsequent re-exposure to allergens results in the cross-linking of adjacent IgE, leading to mast cell degranulation and the release of both preformed and newly synthesized inflammatory mediators. The release of preformed mediators, such as histamine, tryptase, chymase and heparin, results in the early signs of inflammation, such as erythema and pruritus. The newly formed mediators include the prostaglandins, leucotrienes, cytokines and chemokines. They are associated with the late-phase reaction that occurs about 4–6 hours after the initial event and are responsible for the recruitment of the inflammatory cells (TH2 cells and eosinophils) commonly seen on histological examination of the lesional skin.

One of the primary abnormalities in atopic dermatitis is a defective epidermal barrier function that aids penetration of allergens and irritants. Furthermore, atopic dogs have higher levels of bacterial colonization compared to healthy animals. Both these factors further exacerbate the pruritus which is also affected by the allergen load, which in turn depends on factors such as climate, season, indoor environment and geographical location. House dust mites, storage mites, grass pollens, weed pollens, tree pollens, mould spores, insect antigens and dander are all potential allergens in canine atopic dermatitis.

In animals in which the clinical disease is IgE mediated and is demonstrated by serum or intradermal allergy tests, the condition is referred to as atopic dermatitis. There is a subset of animals with clinical signs that satisfy the clinical diagnostic criteria of atopic dermatitis yet fail to demonstrate any allergen-specific IgE either by serum or intradermal testing; in these cases, the condition is referred to as atopic-like dermatitis.

EPIDEMIOLOGY

The exact incidence of atopic dermatitis is not known, although the disease is increasingly being recognized in general practice. The onset of clinical signs is usually between 1 and 3 years of age, and although there is an increase in the number of dogs being presented above 6 months, it is rarely seen in dogs under that age. Similarly, onset is not usually seen in dogs over 7 years old, unless there has been a change in environmental allergen load in a predisposed animal (e.g. a house move or exposure to novel allergens).

Genetic factors have been implicated in the development of the disease and breed predisposition is seen. Although atopic dermatitis can occur in any dog, certain breeds such as terriers, golden retrievers, Labradors, German shepherd dogs, English bull terriers and bulldogs are particularly predisposed.

CLINICAL TIPS

The definitive diagnosis of atopic dermatitis is based on major and minor historical and clinical features, and on ruling out all other possible causes of the pruritus. From a practical point of view, at least three or four major features should be present to satisfy the diagnosis and the minor criteria are used to further support the diagnosis.

The purpose of allergy (intradermal or serological) testing is to support the clinical diagnosis, to allow the selection of allergens for immunotherapy and, where possible, targeted avoidance of them. It also allows the introduction of measures to reduce the allergen load in the environment. A small subset of animals will have negative serum and intradermal tests (see 'Aetiopathogenesis' section).

Intradermal testing

Intradermal testing is preferred by dermatologists for determining which allergens the patient is sensitized to. The test is based on an immediate hypersensitivity response (10–25 minutes) to environmental allergens, resulting in an erythematous wheal at the site of a positive reaction. A positive histamine control and a negative control are always included. An objective scoring system may be used but experienced clinicians tend to use a subjective scoring system based on the diameter, erythema and the elevation of the wheal at each test site, comparing them to the reactions at the positive and negative control sites. Anti-inflammatory drug therapy interferes with the sensitivity of the test and therefore it is important to make sure that the timing of the test takes into account the withdrawal times of any medication the animal may have been taking. However, there are a number of other reasons for both false-negative and false-positive reactions, and up to 15% of individuals with typical clinical signs of atopic dermatitis are negative to intradermal (or serum) allergy testing.

False negatives

Common reasons for negative intradermal allergy tests, when a clinical diagnosis of atopic dermatitis has been made, are:
- Inadequate withdrawal times for drugs such as glucocorticoids and antihistamines
- Use of allergens that have lost their potency (improper storage/out of date)
- Incorrect dilution of allergen concentrate
- Insufficient allergen injected

- Subcutaneous injection instead of intradermal injection
- Stress.

False positives

Reasons for false-positive intradermal allergy tests:
- Test allergen may have irritant properties
- Too large an amount of allergen is injected
- Trauma due to poor technique
- Accidental injection of air with allergen
- Incorrect dilution of the allergen
- Dermatographism.

Serum allergy tests

Serum allergy tests measure the levels of allergen-specific IgE and several laboratories in the UK offer the test. They are performed using the high-affinity Fc receptor technology, or using monoclonal or polyclonal antibodies. The Fc receptor, found on the surface of mast cells, binds specifically to IgE with a high affinity. This test is considered the more reliable serological test, because it reduces the false-positive reactions that can be associated with the presence of IgG.
The main advantages of serological testing are convenience to the owner and clinician, because it does not require the patient to be anaesthetized or clipped. In the past it has been suggested that serum IgE levels are unaffected by drugs; however, more recent reports suggest that they do have an effect and therefore withdrawal times, similar to those in intradermal testing, should be followed.

False negatives

Common reasons for negative serological allergy tests, when a clinical diagnosis of atopic dermatitis has been made, are:
- Inadequate withdrawal times for drugs such as glucocorticoids and antihistamines.
- Degree of sensitivity is dependent on the reagents used.
- Timing of the allergy test – serum IgE concentrations decline rapidly if the patient is not being exposed to the allergen.
- Inappropriate allergen selection for that patient (most laboratories offer standard panels).
- Inherent genetic factors.

TREATMENT AND MANAGEMENT

The management of atopic dermatitis involves a combination of allergen avoidance, control of flare factors (such as secondary bacterial and yeast infections and ectoparasitism), allergen-specific immunotherapy and anti-inflammatory treatment. Frequently, a combination of treatments is a more effective way of managing this disease, rather than reliance on just one therapy. This approach also helps to minimize the use of those treatments which have severe side-effects.

Once atopic dermatitis is diagnosed, the client needs to understand that:
- There is no cure for the condition.
- The condition is most likely to require lifelong management.
- The clinical signs may wax and wane depending on environmental factors and on complications such as microbial infections.
- For a successful outcome, multiple management approaches and therapies may be required, which will vary according to environmental factors and individual needs.

The clinician needs to be prepared to tailor the treatment to the needs of the patient and the client at any given time.

Allergen-specific immunotherapy: The mechanism of allergen-specific immunotherapy is not known, but by presenting large volumes of allergen to the immune system by subcutaneous injections rather that very small amounts by percutaneous absorption, the aim is to alter the way the immune system responds to the allergen.

The treatment involves the administration of allergen extracts, identified either by intradermal testing or by serological testing, by subcutaneous injections in increasing amounts over several weeks (induction phase) until the maintenance dose is reached. Thereafter the main-tenance dose is usually injected monthly (maintenance phase), although this may vary between patients. There are a number of different induction protocols described depending on whether an aqueous or alum precipitated immunotherapy is used. These protocols are usually specified by the laboratory or company providing the therapy. The response may take 3–6 months to become noticeable; however, at least 10 months of treatment is recommended before making a final decision on efficacy. The reported success rates vary between 50% and 70%. In general, a third of patients may be expected to have their symptoms fully controlled, a third will require additional treatment to control symptoms and a third will derive no benefit at all from immunotherapy. It is evident in some patients that although they may require other treatment to control pruritus, the use of immunotherapy allows dosage reductions of these other treatments, which may have important cost and safety implications. Concomitant therapy may be required during the induction phase of treatment. Most cases require lifelong treatment and the majority of cases where immunotherapy is withdrawn because they are apparently cured tend to relapse months or years later. The frequency of injections can be tailored to individual needs. The therapy has few side-effects, is easy to administer and is cost-effective for long-term management.

Factors that influence the outcome of allergen-specific immunotherapy are:
- Owner compliance.
- Routine monitoring, which allows early identification and treatment of secondary microbial infections.
- Identifying other concurrent diseases such as sarcoptic mange, FAD, adverse food reaction and parasitic diseases in patients that have experienced a relapse during successful management.
- Tailoring the administration of injections to suit the animal's needs. For example, if the animal only gains relief from the injection for 2 weeks during the height of the allergen season, then during this season the injections can be administered every 2 weeks.
- Fluctuating environmental allergen loads, which vary with the ambient temperature, humidity and geographical area.

Anaphylaxis is rare; however, if it occurs emergency treatment is required. It is recommended that the patient should be kept at the veterinary surgery for at least 30 minutes following the injections during the induction phase.

Glucocorticoids: Glucocorticoids are highly effective in relieving pruritus and are often required in the early stages of the treatment to break the itch–scratch cycle. However, ideally they should not be used until all microbial infections have been treated. Anti-inflammatory doses of oral methylprednisolone or prednisolone are the drugs of choice and the treatment should be tapered to alternate days or every third day as soon as possible. Adverse effects include polyuria, polydipsia, polyphagia and recurrent pyoderma in some individuals. Most atopic dogs with non-seasonal pruritus require continuous therapy and, when glucocorticoids are used, it is best to inform the client of the potential long-term effects of these drugs and the dose should be adjusted to the lowest dosage that just controls the pruritus.

Ciclosporin: Ciclosporin has been recently licensed for the management of atopic dermatitis in dogs. It is an immunomodulating drug that inhibits the activation of T cells and consequently the cascade of immunological events that lead to clinical disease. It is reported to have a success rate of about 80% and experience has shown it to be a useful drug in the management of atopic dermatitis. It also appears to be a useful drug when used to control pruritus during the induction phase of immunotherapy. However, the drawbacks of this drug include its expense (especially for large dogs), the difficulty in administration to some dogs, vomiting, diarrhoea and abdominal pain. Other adverse effects include gingival hyperplasia, lameness, increased hair growth and papillomatosis. Unlike glucocorticoids, the long-term adverse effects of this drug are not yet known.

Antihistamines: The effect of this group of drugs is variable and is thought to benefit about 15–30% of dogs. They act on H1 receptors and therefore interfere with the action of histamine on blood vessels and histamine-induced pruritus. However, the complex pathogenesis of atopic dermatitis suggests that only a small proportion of the pruritus may be histamine induced. Therefore, antihistamines may be most successful when used in dogs during the early stages of the disease or before mast cell degranulation has occurred. Individual responses to antihistamines vary and therefore no universal drug is recommended (Table 6.1). Those individuals that fail to respond to the antihistamine the clinician is most comfortable using should undergo a trial treatment for 10–14 days with another. A recent review of published studies showed that a combination of chlorpheniramine and hydroxyzine may be the most effective way of using this group of drugs.

Table 6.1 Most commonly used antihistamines in dogs

Drug	Dose
Clemastine	1 mg/10 kg p.o. every 12 hours
Hydroxyzine	2 mg/kg p.o. every 8–12 hours
Chlorpheniramine	2–12 mg p.o. every 12 hours
Diphenhydramine	1–2 mg/kg p.o. every 8–12 hours
Promethazine	0.2–0.4 mg/kg p.o. every 8 hours
Alimemazine	0.5–2 mg/kg p.o. every 12 hours

Essential fatty acids (EFAs): Although, on their own, essential fatty acids have little effect in managing the pruritus, they have been shown to have synergistic action with corticosteroids and antihistamines. EFAs restore and maintain the epidermal lipid barrier, which may reduce the allergen penetration and episodes of microbial infections. In addition, they can alter the metabolism of arachidonic acid, resulting in production of anti-inflammatory prostaglandins and leucotrienes. The best response is thought to result from administration of EFA containing ratios of omega-6 fatty acids (evening primrose oil) to omega-3 fatty acids (marine fish oil) of between 5:1 and 10:1.

Plant extracts: Phytopica® contains an extract obtained from three plants, *Rehmannia glutinosa*, *Paeonia lactiflora* and *Glycyrrhiza uralensis*. It was shown to significantly reduce Canine Atopic Dermatitis Extent and Severity Index (CADESI) scores in approximately 25% of dogs in a study, although there was no significant reduction in owner assessment of pruritus between control and treated groups. The product is available as a powder which is sprinkled on food and is palatable.

TOPICAL TREATMENTS

Topical glucocorticoids: Topical glucocorticoids may be of value in some individuals early in the course of inflammation. There are a number of ointments, creams and gels available for veterinary use in the UK containing a combination of antimicrobial and a glucocorticoid with varying potency depending on the product. Although of benefit, particularly when treating focal lesions, they have their limitations because prolonged use of topical glucocorticoids can lead to atrophy of the skin, systemic

Table 6.2 Measures to reduce allergen load and exposure

Indoor allergens such as house dust mites and danders	Vacuum cleaners without bags recommended Keep patients out of bedrooms and off beds Dust mite-proof covers for pillows, quilts, etc. Keep patients on linoleum, tiled or wooden floors Keep bedding to a minimum and use plastic baskets which allow routine wet wiping Permethrin and/or insect growth regulators reduce the house dust mite burden in the environment
Outdoor allergens such as pollens	Keep off freshly cut grass Keep the patient in when grass cutting Keep the grass short and avoid walking in fields during the pollen seasons Avoid areas where offending weeds are found

absorption, and signs consistent with iatrogenic hyper-adrenocorticism. Furthermore, the presence of hair and the area affected also limit their use. However, recently a glucocorticoid spray containing 0.584% m/vol of hydrocortisone aceponate has been licensed for topical use in dogs. Its benefits include the ease of application even on haired skin, lack of systemic absorption and greatly reduced risk of cutaneous atrophy following topical application. At the time of writing the use of this product in clinical practice has been limited to clinical trials.

Tacrolimus: Tacrolimus is used topically in people with moderate to severe atopic eczema and its use has been reported in dogs to decrease erythema and pruritus in localized areas. It does not have the same atrophic effect on the skin as glucocorticoids. However, it is not licensed for veterinary use and necessary precautions should be taken if it is prescribed with written owners' consent.

Control of flare factors

In general, practical recommendations should be made to reduce allergen load in the pet's home environment and to reduce its exposure to them when out of doors (Table 6.2). Microbial infections must be treated

beyond clinical cure and measures to try to prevent further episodes of infection should be recommended. In addition, either specific therapy to alter the immune response to allergens or symptomatic treatment will be required.

Regular topical therapy in the form of shampoo therapy is recommended as an adjunct to allergen-specific immunotherapy and/or to systemic treatment. The type of shampoo used will need to be tailored to the patient's needs. For instance, antimicrobial shampoo may be recommended for a dog that is predisposed to developing secondary infections, while a shampoo containing colloidal oatmeal may be prescribed for a dog that suffers from dry scaling and pruritus.

Benefits of bathing allergic dogs are:
- It removes allergens from the skin and hair, thus reducing the allergen load on the animal.
- It rehydrates the epidermis and thus restores the epidermal barrier.
- It reduces the microbial burden or prevents microbial adherence and thereby reduces episodes of recurrent infections.
- It reduces pruritus and inflammation.

Treatment in this case

In this case the owner was advised that there is no known treatment for the pattern alopecia and that the allergic dermatitis would require long-term management, which in most cases is lifelong. The following treatments and control measures were recommended:

Allergen avoidance:
- It was advised that, as far as possible, the dog should be kept out of bedrooms and off stuffed furniture.
- Thorough and regular vacuuming of the home, using a HEPA-filtered vacuum cleaner.
- Treatment of the house environment three or four times yearly with a permethrin-containing acaricidal spray.
- A plastic bed should be used with hypoallergenic liner (Vetbed®), which should be washed at 60°C for 10 minutes, preferably every other day.
- As there were grass pollen allergies identified, pavement walking was advised during the summer months.

Allergen-specific immunotherapy: The dog was started on an allergen-specific immunotherapy, based on the results of the intradermal test. All the allergens identified from the test were included in the immunotherapy. It is not a licensed treatment in the UK and therefore requires a special treatment certificate for its use.

In this case concurrent treatment was also prescribed:

- During the induction phase of immunotherapy, clemastine was prescribed to reduce the pruritus
- Omega-6/omega-3 supplementation.

In addition, ongoing, thorough flea control using monthly applications of a spot-on adulticide was prescribed as well as the environmental treatment to control dust mites. Weekly baths with 2% miconazole/2% chlorhexidine shampoo were advised to help control recurrent microbial infections.

NURSING ASPECTS

Information on localized cleansing and/or total bathing should be given to owners. At this stage the frequency of the flea control should be adjusted, as the frequency of bathing will have an effect on the duration of the preparation's action. Routine ear cleaning following bathing and during management of atopic dermatitis is advised, as many dogs have concurrent otic disease. The nurses should be able to show the owners how to flush ears at home without damaging the ear epithelium. Some dogs may require Elizabethan collars to prevent self-induced dermatitis.

FOLLOW-UP

The dog has been managed with allergen-specific immunotherapy and weekly bathing for the last 3 years.

7 *Malassezia* dermatitis

INITIAL PRESENTATION

Pruritus with crusting, lichenification, erythema and alopecia.

INTRODUCTION

Malassezia pachydermatis is recognized as one of the major flare factors contributing to pruritus, especially in atopic dogs. Several different *Malassezia* species have been isolated but, of these, *Malassezia pachydermatis*, a non-lipid-dependent species, is the most studied in veterinary medicine. *Malassezia pachydermatis* is considered to be commensal on canine and feline skin, and can cause infections when the microclimate on the skin surface or in the ear is altered, or if the host immune responses are compromised. The lipid-dependent species *M. sympodialis* and *M. globosa* have been isolated from cats. The recognition of *Malassezia* dermatitis and its appropriate treatment was the key to successful management of atopic dermatitis in this case.

CASE PRESENTING SIGNS

An atopic 2-year-old castrated West Highland white terrier was re-presented with a history of recent pruritus, lichenification, hyperpigmentation and erythema affecting the axillae, extensor aspects of the elbows, and the groin.

CASE HISTORY

In most cases *Malassezia* dermatitis is associated with an underlying hypersensitivity disorder and the distribution of clinical signs may give an indication of the underlying condition. The relevant history to this case included:

- A diagnosis of atopic dermatitis had been made 1 year previously and was based on history, clinical signs, failure of response to an appropriate diet trial and intradermal reactivity to environmental allergens (house dust mites, storage mites and mould allergens).
- Response to allergen-specific immunotherapy was poor but remission of pruritus had been successfully achieved with ciclosporin (5 mg/kg on alternate days).
- There was no change in management or treatment before the flare-up.
- There had been a recent flare-up of pruritus that had coincided with very warm and humid weather.
- The flare-up had a duration of about 3 weeks, which did not coincide with the animal's regular visits to a grooming parlour.
- Good flea control was maintained with monthly applications of a spot-on fipronil and s-methoprene.

CLINICAL SIGNS

In dogs, the clinical signs of *Malassezia* dermatitis vary according to the intensity of the infection and the area affected. Infection can cause localized or generalized disease and pruritus is a common presenting sign. In most cases the skin lesions include erythema, scaling, hyperpigmentation, lichenification and crusting. Individual, or several concurrent sites such as ears, lips, muzzle, ventral neck, axillae, ventrum, perianal and feet may be involved. Dark brown waxy exudate in the ear canals or adherent to the nails is suggestive of *Malassezia* infection. Frequently, peripheral lymphadenopathy is also present.

Malassezia dermatitis is less common in cats. It has been associated with facial dermatitis and with otitis externa secondary to allergic skin disease. Generalized lesions in cats have been associated with immunedys-regulation in conditions such as the paraneoplastic syndromes.

In this case, the clinical signs included:

- Reactive lymphadenopathy of the pre-scapular and popliteal lymph nodes.
- Hyperpigmentation, lichenification, crusting and erythema on the axilla and the anterior aspects of the elbows (Fig. 7.1).
- Convex aspects of both ear pinnae and vertical ear canals were erythematous and oedematous (Fig. 7.2).
- Otic examination revealed erythematous-ceruminous otitis externa.
- The tympanic membranes were visible once the exudate had been flushed out using an ear cleaner.

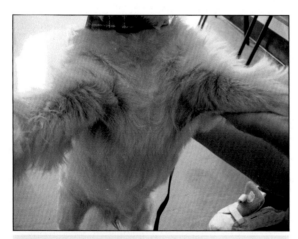

Figure 7.1 Erythema, hyperpigmentation and lichenification in the axilla.

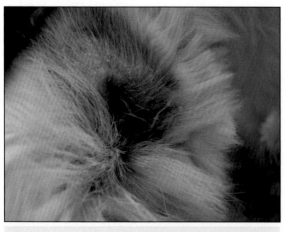

Figure 7.2 Erythema and yellowish waxy exudate in the ear.

DIFFERENTIAL DIAGNOSES

The differentials for the current cause of the pruritus and dermatitis were:

- *Malassezia* dermatitis
- Staphylococcal pyoderma
- Sarcoptic mange
- Flea allergic dermatitis
- Demodicosis.

CASE WORK-UP

This case shows a typical scenario, often encountered in practice, in which cases that have been well managed for an allergic disease suddenly flare-up. Microbial infections and ectoparasitic infestation are the most common flare factors contributing to a relapse in pruritus and the skin lesions. Hence, at this point a reassessment of the case history and clinical signs is required. Each of the resulting differential diagnoses should be ruled in or out by laboratory investigations.

Cytology: The cheapest, quickest and easiest way to demonstrate which organisms are involved is by cytological examination of tape-strip preparations, direct smears or scrapes stained with modified Wright's stain. *Malassezia* spp. are identified as oval- to peanut-shaped organisms under oil immersion. There is some debate about the significance of the number of yeast organisms seen on cytological examination. In the past, author's have stated that more than 10 organisms per high-power field are considered significant. However, in the author's experience and in more recent literature, just one organism per high-power field may be significant and justifies treatment if the clinical signs and history are suggestive of *Malassezia* infection.

Culture: *Malassezia pachydermatis* can also be cultured on modified Dixon's or Sabouraud's agar. In practice, however, this does not usually provide any more information than cytology.

Histology: *Malassezia* organisms may be seen on histological section with a variety of other diseases. Generally, in the absence of other diseases the histological findings include parakeratotic hyperkeratosis, acanthosis and superficial perivascular dermatitis.

In this case, *Malassezia pachydermatis* organisms were found on tape-strip preparations from the axilla and on otic cytology (Fig. 7.3).

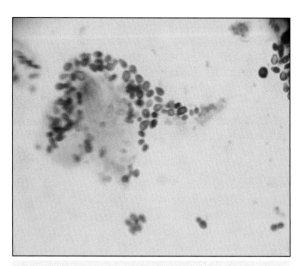

Figure 7.3 *Malassezia pachydermatis* demonstrated smear made from ear wax.

The routine use of flea control and the distribution of the lesions ruled out flea allergic dermatitis as a concurrent disease, and skin scrapings and coat brushings ruled out other ectoparasitic conditions. Although the skin scrapings failed to reveal *Sarcoptes* mites, a serological test was performed to rule it out completely. If this had not been done, a trial treatment with an appropriate product could have been an alternative method of ruling out scabies.

DIAGNOSIS

Malassezia dermatitis and otitis diagnosed as a flare factor in a dog managed for atopic dermatitis.

PROGNOSIS

The prognosis is favourable; treating the *Malassezia* dermatitis reduces the pruritus, making the management of the underlying allergic dermatitis more successful. The longer term prognosis is more variable. If an underlying cause for the yeast infection can be identified and corrected, then further episodes may be prevented. However, some dogs need ongoing intermittent or continuous therapy to prevent the infection recurring.

AETIOPATHOGENESIS AND IMMUNOPATHOGENESIS OF *MALASSEZIA* DERMATITIS

Malassezia pachydermatis are oval or round cells that reproduce by unicellular budding. Budding cells resem-

ble 'peanuts' or 'footprints' in shape. *In vitro*, *Malassezia pachydermatis* is grown on Sabouraud's agar incubated at 32°C, which does not require lipid enrichment. The organism is identified by its smooth white to cream convex colony growth after 3–5 days. With age, these colonies become darker and take on a brownish colour.

Malassezia pachydermatis has been found on dogs, cats, horses, foxes and ferrets. It has also been isolated from wild animals and birds. It is commonly isolated from the ear canals, lip margins, chin, periocular skin, interdigital skin, anus, anal sacs and vaginas of healthy animals. The mucocutaneous sites serve as reservoirs from which the organism is spread to other sites during licking and grooming. *Malassezia pachydermatis* is rarely isolated from the dorsum, groin or axilla of normal dogs.

For the organism to colonize any site it must attach itself to the host cells. Recent *in vitro* studies have shown that *M. pachydermatis* adheres to canine corneocytes in a dose- and time-dependent manner, by binding proteins, or glycoprotein, expressed on its surface to carbohydrate ligand on the corneocytes.

To understand how a normal commensal can become a pathogen in the case of *Malassezia* infections, the relationship between the host skin and the organism should be considered. For the organism to become pathogenic it must overcome the host defences and be able to colonize the skin. *Malassezia* organisms are known to produce enzymes (proteases, lipases, phospholipase, lipoxygenase and many others) which break down cells and trigger the release of inflammatory mediators. They also activate the complement cascade, all of which induces inflammation and recruits inflammatory cells.

A number of factors that provide a microenvironment conducive to the colonization of *Malassezia* of the host skin have been studied. These include anatomical features such as skin folds and areas with poor ventilation that provide a temperature and humidity suitable for the survival and proliferation of the organism. Underlying diseases that result in inflammation, exudation and/or pruritus contribute to changes in the skin's microclimate that favour colonization.

Studies have shown that *Malassezia* can invoke immune responses, despite the fact that it does not normally invade the stratum corneum. *Malassezia*-specific serum IgA and IgG concentrations in seborrhoeic basset hounds were higher when compared to healthy dogs, but these responses appear to provide little protection against infection. Further studies have demonstrated that serum *Malassezia*-specific IgE and IgG was higher in atopic dogs than in healthy individuals. Furthermore, immediate type hypersensitivity responses have been demonstrated by intradermal testing in atopic dogs.

Greater IgE responses to certain protein fractions of *Malassezia pachydermatis* have been demonstrated in atopic dogs with *Malassezia* dermatitis than in healthy dogs. It was suggested that proteins with molecular weights of 45 and 48 kDa might be major allergens, as they were recognized in most dogs with an atopic dermatitis and a concurrent *Malassezia* overgrowth, but much less frequently in healthy dogs.

EPIDEMIOLOGY OF *MALASSEZIA* DERMATITIS

Malassezia infections can occur in any breed; however, genetic predisposition appears to exist in breeds such as West Highland white terriers, basset hounds, German shepherds, cocker spaniels, miniature poodles and English setters. Although the reasons for these predispositions are not known, anatomical features and predisposition to underlying diseases may be important. There are no age or sex predispositions, but *Malassezia* dermatitis is usually associated with underlying conditions, such as atopic dermatitis in dogs and immunosuppression in cats. Some dermatologists consider that *Malassezia* dermatitis can occur in the absence of an underlying disease, particularly in basset hounds and cocker spaniels.

TREATMENT OPTIONS

Depending on the extent of the clinical signs, and client and patient compliance, topical and/or systemic therapy can be considered.

Topical treatment: 2% miconazole/2% chlorhexidine shampoo is the treatment of choice. Other topical antifungal preparations such as selenium sulphide, enilconazole and 1–4% chlorhexidine may also be useful. Shampoos, lotions and ointments containing antifungals such as ketaconazole, clotrimazole, miconazole and terbinafine, all of which are unlicensed preparations, may also be of some use.

Systemic therapy: Ketoconazole (2.5–10 mg/kg) or itraconazole (5–10 mg/kg, licensed for use in cats) once daily can be considered in some cases. These drugs are unlicensed and are expensive, particularly for large dogs.

Their side-effects include anorexia, vomiting, diarrhoea and hepatic dysfunction. In some cases reducing the dose may help with the gastroenteric signs. If they are to be used in the long term, then monitoring of hepatic function and haematology is advisable.

For successful long-term control of recurrent infections, it is necessary to identify and manage the underlying condition that predisposes the animal to *Malassezia* infections.

Treatment in this case

This case was treated with a combination of topical and systemic medications. Oral ketoconazole at 7.5 mg/kg was prescribed for 3 weeks, together with ciclosporin. Written owner consent was obtained for the use of ketoconazole. However, because the serum half-life of ciclosporin is doubled because of drug interaction with ketoconazole, the initial dose of ciclosporin (5 mg/kg e. o.d.) was reduced to 1.5 mg/kg every 24 hours while the *Malassezia* dermatitis was being treated.

NURSING ASPECTS

- Nursing care includes advising clients on regular bathing and demonstrating ear cleaning techniques.
- Nurses can also be usefully involved in routine monitoring for early signs of infection.

CLINICAL TIPS

- Always warn the client that this is in many cases a secondary infection, and successful management requires both controlling the underlying disease and the infection itself.
- Monitor routinely for microbial infections, as early recognition reduces the likelihood of severe consequences.
- Monitor response to the allergy therapy. Many therapies are immunosuppressive in nature.

FOLLOW-UP

The clinical signs resolved after the 3-week treatment. The dog was then switched back to 50 mg of ciclosporin three times a week and bathed in 2% miconazole/2% chlorhexidine shampoo weekly. Monitoring such cases every 8–12 weeks is crucial in managing the pruritus.

Cheyletiellosis

INITIAL PRESENTATION

Pruritus, papules and scaling.

INTRODUCTION

Cheyletiellosis is a common ectoparasitic disease affecting dogs, cats and rabbits. It is caused by *Cheyletiella* spp. of mites and results in a pruritic, papular and variably scaling skin disease predominantly affecting the dorsal trunk, although the pruritus can be generalized. As with all parasitic diseases, demonstration of the mite confirms the diagnosis, although in about half of all cases that won't be possible and trial ectoparasitic therapy will be necessary.

CASE PRESENTING SIGNS

A 3-year-old spayed female cross-bred was presented with dorsal scaling and pruritus.

CASE HISTORY

The dog had been in the owner's possession since it was a puppy. It was regularly wormed and vaccinated annually. Its diet consisted of a proprietary complete chicken- and rice-based dried food, with occasional scraps, biscuits and dog chews.

Over the previous year, there had been a progressive onset of, initially mild, dorsal pruritus, then increasingly severe scaling. There was no seasonality to the symptoms.

Other important history was as follows:
- The dog had been treated intermittently with a per-methrin spot-on preparation.
- There were no other pets in the household.

- The owner reported that, over the past year, she had developed pruritic papular eruptions over her forearms (Fig. 8.1). She had attributed this to the stress of a house move.
- The dog had free run of the house and slept in a basket in the owner's bedroom.
- The dog was exercised in nearby fields that contained a large population of rabbits.
- There had been a partial reduction in the level of pruritus, but no change in the degree of scaling, with the use of long-acting glucocorticoid injections.

CLINICAL EXAMINATION

There were no abnormalities detected on physical examination. Examination of the skin revealed:
- A mild papulocrustous eruption with diffuse scaling (Fig. 8.2) over the dorsal trunk.
- Gentle stimulation of the affected area resulted in a marked scratch reflex (Fig. 8.3).
- No other areas of skin were affected.

DIFFERENTIAL DIAGNOSES

This was a long-standing dorsal pruritic skin disease in a young dog, which made ectoparasitic disease very likely. It would be very unusual for atopic dermatitis, or an adverse food reaction, to result in pruritus confined to the dorsal trunk. The degree and distribution of pruritus was not consistent with scabies, but was entirely consistent with cheyletiellosis. There was no history of direct contact with other dogs, or cats, but ectoparasitic disease could not be ruled out on this basis alone, as indirect transmission does occur. There was history of exposure to rabbits, which can carry *Cheyletiella* spp. of mites.

There was also a history of possible zoonosis, and pruritic papules on the forearms in an owner are suggestive of scabies or cheyletiellosis. Heavy flea infestations can also result in bites to owners, but they are usually on the distal limbs.

The differential diagnoses included:

- Cheyletiellosis
- Flea allergy dermatitis
- Ectopic otodectic mange
- Pyoderma
- Cutaneous adverse food reaction
- Atopic dermatitis.

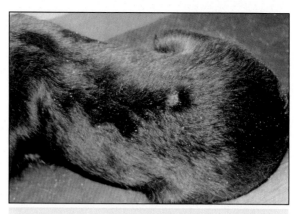

Figure 8.2 Diffuse scaling over the dorsal trunk resulting from cheyletiellosis.

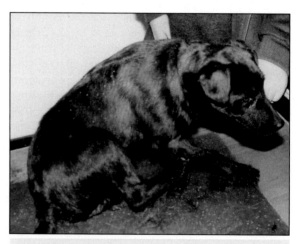

Figure 8.3 Scratch reflex elicited by gentle digital stimulation over the dorsum.

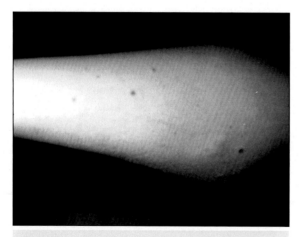

Figure 8.1 Papular lesions resulting from the bites of *Cheyletiella* spp. mites over the forearms of the owner.

CASE WORK-UP

The first step was to rule out any involvement of ecto-parasitism. Close visual inspection, flea combing and coat brushing examinations are useful for the detection of fleas and flea faeces. Tape strips, microscopic examination of coat brushings and skin scrapes are useful for finding evidence of *Cheyletiella* spp. mites. A recent study reported a vacuum cleaning technique as also a very effective method of identifying *Cheyletiella* mites. The following tests were performed:

- Microscopic examination of tape-strip preparations from the hair coat showed no evidence of ectoparasitism.
- Microscopic examination of coat brushings showed a few *Cheyletiella* spp. mites (Fig. 8.4) and their eggs attached to hair shafts (Fig. 8.5).

Cheyletiella spp. mites were also seen on examination of skin scrapes from the affected area (see Chapter 2). It was not possible to identify the exact species of mite involved.

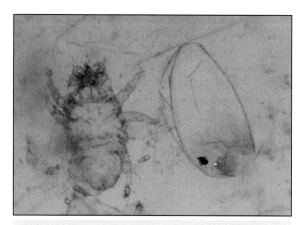

Figure 8.4 Adult *Cheyletiella* spp. mite and empty egg case found on microscopic examination of coat brushings and scale.

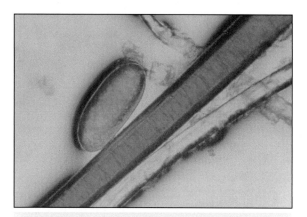

Figure 8.5 *Cheyletiella* spp. egg attached to hair shaft found on microscopic examination of coat brushings and scale.

DIAGNOSIS

A diagnosis of cheyletiellosis was confirmed. Humans in contact with pets carrying *Cheyletiella* spp. are at risk of becoming transiently infested themselves. The lesions are characterized by a pruritic papular dermatitis, mainly affecting the arms and chest. The limbs and buttocks are also, but less frequently, affected. *Cheyletiella* spp. are not capable of reproducing on humans and treatment of the pet host should result in resolution of symptoms on the in-contact owner, making treatment unnecessary. The owner was informed that this was likely to be the cause of her pruritic skin disease and that it would resolve with treatment of the dog.

PROGNOSIS

Although cheyletiellosis can be a challenging infestation to eliminate, especially in multi-animal households, the disease is completely curable and an excellent prognosis was given.

AETIOPATHOGENESIS OF CHEYLETIELLOSIS

Cheyletiella spp. mites are large (500 µm × 350 µm) obligate parasites that live on the skin surface. There are three commonly encountered species in veterinary dermatology: *Cheyletiella yasguri*, *C. blakiei* and *C. parasitovorax*. In the dog, cheyletiellosis is most commonly caused by *C. yasguri*, whereas *C. blakiei* and *C. parasitovorax* are most commonly encountered in the cat and rabbit respectively, although they are not host specific and may transfer readily between dogs, cats and rabbits. The mites have a 3- to 5-week life cycle spent entirely on the host. Eggs are bound to the proximal hair shafts by means of a cocoon-like structure of finely woven threads.

Cheyletiellosis most commonly results in a combination of scaling and pruritus. The degree of the pruritus is variable, although it is usually mild to moderate. Interestingly, it is recognized that the degree of pruritus often seems to be inversely proportional to the numbers of mites present. This may be due to the presence of a hypersensitivity response to the mite.

EPIDEMIOLOGY

Transmission is by direct contact with an infested animal or, given that the mites can survive for up to 10 days off the host, indirectly via fomites such as leads and grooming implements or via other environmental contact. Eggs bound to shed hair shafts can also act as an environmental reservoir of infection. Asymptomatic carrier states are also commonly encountered in multi-animal households amongst unaffected in-contacts.

The disease is a zoonosis and can result in a pruritic, papular eruption in owners, predominantly over the arms and trunk. There is great variation in the reported incidence of zoonosis in cases of cheyletiellosis (20–80%).

TREATMENT OPTIONS

Currently, there is no veterinary licensed treatment for cheyletiellosis in the UK, but various therapeutic protocols have been described. Given that the mite lacks host specificity and that there may be asymptomatic carriers in multi-animal households, it is imperative to treat all the in-contact animals. Additionally, as the mite can survive for up to 10 days off the host, it may also be necessary to decontaminate the environment, although adequate duration of treatment may obviate this requirement. Treatment duration should be at least 6 weeks and is to some extent influenced by the severity of the infestation, the number of animals involved, the acaricidal product chosen and whether or not there is concomitant environment treatment.

Lime sulphur: A lime sulphur dip is now available in the UK and this should be an effective and safe, if somewhat messy, treatment. Dips would need to be repeated on a weekly basis for a minimum of 6 weeks.

Fipronil: Fipronil spray, administered as a single application and combined with environmental decontamination using permethrin, was shown to be effective in one small study in one puppy and one dog. In a more recent report, a single application of a fipronil spot-on preparation was shown to be effective in the treatment of naturally occurring feline cheyletiellosis.

Macrocyclic lactones: Avermectins and milbemycins are macrocyclic fermentation products of various *Streptomyces* spp. Avermectins differ from each other chemically in side-chain substitutions on the lactone ring, whilst milbemycins differ from the avermectins through the absence of a sugar from the lactone skeleton.

Available avermectins in the UK include ivermectin, selamectin and moxidectin, a milbemycin. These drugs are active against a wide range of nematodes and arthropods.

Selamectin: Selamectin is an avermectin endectocide that combines both anthelmintic and ectoparasiticidal activity. In the UK it is licensed for the treatment of fleas, otodectic mange and sarcoptic acariasis, as well as gastrointestinal parasites, at a dosage of 6 mg/kg given at 4-weekly intervals. It has been reported to be effective for the treatment of cheyletiellosis in the dog and cat. One study investigated the efficacy of selamectin for the treatment of cheyletiellosis in dogs and found that it was safe and effective if used at fortnightly intervals. This is a convenient treatment for owners to administer and would be the author's first choice treatment for cheyletiellosis.

Moxidectin: Moxidectin is one of the milbemycins and is a fermentation product of *Streptomyces cyanogriseus*. It is a second-generation systemic macrocylic lactone with broad-spectrum antiparasitic activity. Moxidectin (2.5%) combined with 10% imidacloprid is available as a spot-on preparation for the treatment of sarcoptic mange in puppies and dogs over 7 weeks of age. At the time of writing, there is no published information as to its efficacy in treating cheyletiellosis, but it should also be an effective product although, like selamectin, it may need to be administered fortnightly.

Ivermectin: Ivermectin is a fermentation product of *S. avermitilis*. In the UK, it is an unlicensed product for the treatment of cheyletiellosis, but it is an economical and effective treatment when administered at a dose of 200–400 µg/kg (p.o., q7d or s.c. and pour-on, q14d) for a minimum period of 6–8 weeks. Apart from being an unlicensed product, the main drawback of ivermectin used in this way is that neurotoxic adverse reactions are common, particularly in herding breeds, although acute toxicity due to accidental overdosage may occur in any breed.

Amitraz: Amitraz is an acaricide/insecticide of the formamidine family. Amitraz is thought to act at octopamine receptor sites in ectoparasites, resulting in neuronal hyperexcitability and death. The undiluted product consists of a 5% w/v concentrated liquid. Used as a weekly dip, at a concentration of 250 ppm, it is a highly effective treatment for cheyletiellosis. Side-effects to amitraz include sedation, bradycardia and hyperglycaemia, which can be attributed to monoamine oxidase inhibition and α2-adrenergic agonistic activities, but are rare in dogs when used at this concentration.

Chosen treatment: In this case, after discussion with the owner, treatment was started with fortnightly applications of spot-on selamectin.

The house environment was thoroughly vacuumed and the entire floor area and car were treated with a permethrin spray.

The dog's bedding was washed weekly at a temperature of 60°C.

CLINICAL TIPS

In some cases of cheyletiellosis, the mite or its eggs can be extremely difficult to find. In a study comparing skin scraping, tape strips applied to clipped areas of skin and vacuum cleaning, these tests gave positive results in 41%, 73% and 100% of previously confirmed cases respectively.

The degree of pruritus often seems to be inversely proportional to the number of mites present. This is likely to be due to the presence of a hypersensitivity response to the presence of the mite, but can lead the clinician to suspect that some in-contact animals may not be carrying the mite and thus do not require treatment. This is not likely to be the case and all in-contacts should receive the same thorough treatment.

In multi-animal households, when it has not been possible to demonstrate the presence of mites on a symptomatic animal, it can be rewarding to take samples from an in-contact unaffected pet. In the authors' experience, it is often possible to demonstrate the presence of the mite from these animals.

Regardless of whether mites have been identified, trial ectoparasiticidal therapy is indicated if cheyletiellosis is one of the differential diagnoses. In the situation where it has not been possible to find mites or eggs, the clinician should aim to use the most effective treatment available, so that cheyletiellosis can be ruled out with confidence if there is no response.

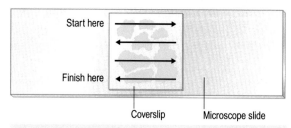

Figure 8.6 Examination of the area under the coverslip on a skin scrape preparation.

and the slide should be examined as shown in Fig. 8.6.

Once the diagnosis has been made and treatment started, owners frequently call back after only a week or two to report that their pet is still pruritic. In these situations, the treatment protocol should be reaffirmed with the owner and they should be advised that it may be several weeks before the pruritus can be expected to finally subside.

NURSING ASPECTS

Nurses may be given samples of scale or skin scrapes to examine from pruritic animals. Familiarity with the appearance of the mite is important. The mite is easily recognized by its large size, characteristic hooked mouthparts and four long pairs of legs that project well beyond the body margins of the mite (Fig. 8.4).

When given a skin scrape or tape strip to examine, it is important to examine the whole area under the tape or coverslip. The mites are easily identified under the low-power ×4 objective

FOLLOW-UP

Treatment was continued for a 6-week period. On follow-up examination after 6 weeks, the pruritus and scaling had resolved and the papular eruption over the owner's forearms had also cleared up. As it was possible that the infestation had been acquired from contact with rabbits, which was likely to continue, continued monthly applications of a selamectin spot-on were recommended. Follow-up 1 year later revealed no recurrence of the pruritus or scaling.

9

Dermatophytosis in a Jack Russell terrier

INITIAL PRESENTATION

Pruritus with crusting and scaling.

INTRODUCTION

Dermatophytosis is a fungal invasion of keratinized tissue of the stratum corneum, hair or claws by *Trichophyton*, *Epidermophyton* or *Microsporum* spp. In small animals, dermatophytosis is most frequently associated with infections caused by *Trichophyton* or *Microsporum* spp. Dermatophytosis results in variable alopecia, erythema, scaling, crusting and pruritus. This case report describes a case of pruritic dermatophytosis caused by infection with *Trichophyton erinacei*.

CASE PRESENTING SIGNS

A 10-year-old, entire female Jack Russell terrier was presented with progressive crusting and scaling and marked pruritus.

CASE HISTORY

There are aspects of the history that might alert the clinician to the possibility of dermatophytosis. These would include: breed predispositions to dermatophytosis (see 'Epidemiology' section); a history of exposure to a zoophilic or geophilic source of infection, such as a terrier breed hunting hedgehogs; evidence of contagion in contact animals or lesions on the owner suggestive of zoonosis; and the onset of skin disease in an animal with no previous history of skin problems. If there is pruritus, the appearance of alopecia or scaling prior to the onset of pruritus would suggest that this was not an allergic aetiology. A poor response to glucocorticoids, antibacterial or antiparasitic therapy could also be suggestive of dermatophytosis.

The relevant aspects of the history were:
- The initial sign was a patch of alopecia and scaling over one hindquarter.
- New lesions consisting of alopecia, erythema, crusting and scaling had subsequently appeared over the face, limbs and tail.
- Moderate to severe pruritus had been evident and had become apparent after the onset of alopecia.
- Slight weight loss had been noted over the past month, but the dog had remained bright and active.
- One other dog and a cat were part of the household. The dog had developed a similar lesion over the bridge of the nose, although this had resolved spontaneously.
- There was no evidence of zoonosis.
- Previous treatment with several weekly amitraz dips at a concentration of 500 ppm and various 7- to 10-day courses of systemic antibacterial therapy had not resulted in any clinical improvement.
- The dog had a history of hunting for hedgehogs.

CLINICAL EXAMINATION

There was mild peripheral lymphadenopathy, but there were no other abnormalities on general physical examination.

Examination of the skin revealed extensive patches of relatively well-demarcated alopecia, erythema, hyperpigmentation, and crusting and scaling over the muzzle, periorbital skin, the left dorsal trunk, the lateral thighs and the forelimbs (Figs 9.1, 9.2 and 9.3).

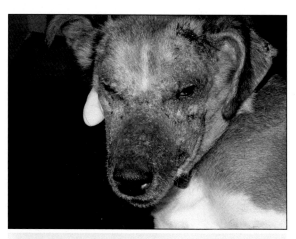

Figure 9.1 Well-demarcated alopecia, hyperpigmentation, scaling and crusting over the face. The nasal planum is unaffected.

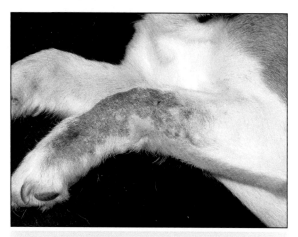

Figure 9.2 Well-demarcated patch of alopecia, erythema and hyperpigmentation over the left carpal area.

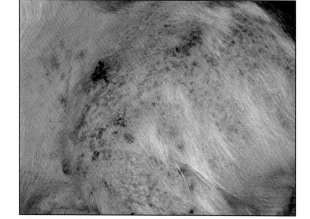

Figure 9.3 Patchy alopecia, multifocal post-inflammatory hyperpigmentation and erythema over the left hind limb.

DIFFERENTIAL DIAGNOSES

Multifocal patches of apparently spreading alopecia are suggestive of a folliculitis. The three common causes of folliculitis are demodicosis, pyoderma and dermatophytosis. In this case, the signalment, history and clinical presentation were highly suggestive of dermatophytosis resulting from infection with a *Trichophyton* spp.

The list of possible differential diagnoses included:

- Dermatophytosis
- Demodicosis
- Pyoderma
- Pemphigus foliaceus (although the lack of involvement of the nasal planum made this less likely).
- Epitheliotropic cutaneous lymphoma

In a case like this, hypothyroidism and hyperadrenocorticism, or another underlying immunosuppressive disease, might predispose it to the development of pyoderma, demodicosis or dermatophytosis.

CASE WORK-UP

Multiple deep skin scrapings should be performed in any case where demodicosis is suspected. In this case there were crusting lesions and cytology was also indicated to identify the presence or absence of bacterial infection.

The following diagnostic tests were performed:
- Microscopic examination of multiple deep skin scrapings, which failed to reveal the presence of *Demodex* spp. mites.
- Cytological examination of stained impression smears from the underside of the crusts (Fig. 9.4), which revealed degenerate neutrophils and small numbers of intra- and extracellular cocci. Small numbers

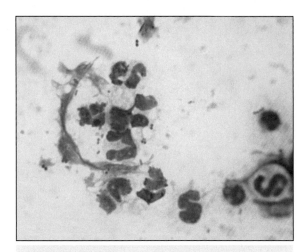

Figure 9.4 Cytology from a crusting lesion showing neutrophils, cocci and occasional rods.

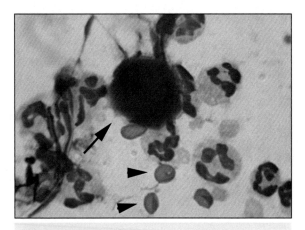

Figure 9.5 Cytology from a crusted lesion showing neutrophils, erythrocytes (arrowheads) and a single acantholytic keratinocyte (arrow).

of acantholytic keratinocytes were also evident (Fig. 9.5).

- Trichographic and Wood's lamp examination, which did not identify any fungal elements.
- Fungal culture on material collected using the MacKenzie brush technique, together with plucked hairs and scrapes, which grew *Trichophyton erinaciei*.
- Routine haematological and biochemical examinations, including basal thyroxine and endogenous TSH, and routine urinalysis, which did not reveal any abnormalities.

DIAGNOSIS

The history, clinical signs and fungal culture were consistent with a diagnosis of dermatophytosis, due to an infection with *Trichophyton erinaciei*.

PROGNOSIS

In general, the prognosis for treating dermatophytosis is good, but persistent infections do occur, particularly where there is immunosuppression. In cases of dermatophytosis resulting from *Trichophyton* spp., scarring resulting in permanent loss of hair over severely affected areas is a common sequela.

AETIOPATHOGENESIS OF TRICHOPHYTOSIS

Depending on their adaptation to soil, animal or man, dermatophytes may be classified as geophilic, zoophilic or anthrophilic respectively. The most commonly isolated dermatophyte pathogens in dogs and cats are *Microsporum canis*, *M. gypseum* and *T. mentagrophytes*. Infection requires direct transmission of spores to a susceptible host and transmission varies with the species of fungi. In the case of *M. canis*, it is usually by direct contact with an infected cat, or via contact with infected grooming utensils, fomites or an otherwise contaminated environment. Infection may also be acquired from direct or indirect contact with an infected or carrier person. *Trichophyton* spp. infection usually results from contact with an infected animal (in this case a hedgehog) and *M. gypseum* through contact with infected soil. Fungal spores are extremely resistant and the spores of *M. canis* may last up to 18 months within the environment.

Dermatophytes have been isolated from the skin and hair coat of healthy cats and dogs, reflecting asymptomatic carriage of the fungus. Thus, mere exposure to the fungus does not mean infection. Factors that favour the establishment of an infection include exposure to an increasing mass of fungal spores, increased skin humidity, mechanical disruption of the stratum corneum and compromised host immunosurveillance.

In an experimental model of *M. canis* dermatophytosis in cats, the time from inoculation to establishment of the lesion was in the region of 7–14 days. Dermatophytes require a source of newly synthesized keratin to survive and therefore invade the hair shaft or, in the case of *M. persicolor*, the keratinized cells of the stratum corneum. Fungal hyphae invade the hair follicle ostia, proliferate on the surface of the hair shaft and migrate downwards towards the hair bulb. Most infections involve ectothrix invasion of hair shafts, where fungal spores accumulate on the surface of hair shafts. The fungus produces keratinases that allow invasion of the hair shaft. Invasion of the hair shaft continues up to the keratogenous zone known as Adamson's fringe. The fungus then reaches a state of equilibrium with hair growth until the hair is eventually expelled. The initial growth and invasion of the fungus in the hair shaft must be 'faster' than loss of keratin tissues to prevent it being shed.

Spontaneous resolution of an infection is dependent on the host mounting an effective cell-mediated immune response. To check this response, some fungi produce substances (mannans) that inhibit cell-mediated immunity.

EPIDEMIOLOGY

In UK small animal practice, dermatophytosis is an uncommon skin disease. Various epidemiological factors have been recognized that tend to increase the incidence of dermatophytosis. They are:

- Hot humid climates
- Communally housed shelter cats (as opposed to individually housed, privately owned animals)
- Young animals, reflecting poorly developed innate and adaptive immunity and also different biochemical properties of skin secretions and differences in hair growth
- Immunosuppressed animals
- Long-haired animals
- Yorkshire terriers have an increased susceptibility to severe forms of *M. canis* infection
- Jack Russell terriers are more susceptible to *T. mentagrophytes* infections, reflecting their hunting behaviour.

It should be borne in mind that *M. canis* infections are more common in animals from urban areas, whereas *T. mentagrophytes* and *M. gypseum* infections are seen more frequently in animals from rural environments.

TREATMENT OPTIONS

Although dermatophytosis in healthy dogs and cats can undergo spontaneous remission within 3 months, a case of generalized dermatophytosis requires systemic anti-fungal therapy. There is little published information on the treatment of dermatophytosis caused by *Trichophyton* spp., but anecdote and clinical experience indicates that this disease may be more refractory to treatment, compared to infections with *Microsporum canis*. The current options for systemic antifungal therapy include the azoles ketoconazole, itraconazole and fluconazole, and the allylamine terbinafine. Griseofulvin is no longer available as a licensed treatment in the UK (Chapter 28).

Azoles: The azoles inhibit fungal lanosterol 14-demethylase, a cytochrome P-450 enzyme. They also inhibit intracellular triglyceride, phospholipid and cell wall chitin synthesis. Their potency and potential toxicity are related to their affinity to bind to fungal, versus mammalian, cytochrome P-450 enzymes. Ketoconazole, itraconazole and then fluconazole show increasing specificity for fungal as opposed to mammalian enzyme systems, and therefore itraconazole and fluconazole show increased antifungal potency and decreased side-effects compared to ketoconazole. Because of their effects on mammalian cytochrome P-450 enzymes, azoles have the potential to inhibit the metabolism of other medications and there is a significant potential for drug interactions. The azoles, particularly itraconazole, are lipophilic and keratinophilic and achieve persistent high concentrations within the stratum corneum and hair follicle, which makes them suitable for pulse therapy.

For the treatment of canine dermatophytosis, *ketoconazole* is administered at dosages of 10–20 mg/kg/day either as a single dose or divided twice daily. Absorption is enhanced by administration with food, to achieve an acid gastric pH. The most common adverse reaction is gastrointestinal disturbance with vomiting and/or diarrhoea, but higher doses may result in hepatotoxicity. *Itraconazole* is more expensive than ketoconazole but has less potential for toxicity. It may be administered at a dosage of 5–10 mg/kg q24 for the treatment of canine dermatophytosis.

Allylamines: Terbinafine, an allylamine, has been shown to be effective in the treatment of dermatophytosis; however, it is not licensed for this use in the UK. It inhibits the synthesis of ergosterol, an important component of fungal cell walls. It is also lipophilic and keratinophilic, and reaches high concentrations in the stratum corneum and in hard keratin structures such as nails. The dosage in dogs is 20–30 mg/kg every 24 hours. Elevation in ALT has been observed at this dosage, although there were no signs of clinical toxicity.

Topical therapy: Topical therapy is also indicated for the treatment of dermatophytosis as it may hasten the resolution of infection and prevent environmental contamination with fungal spores. The decontamination of the affected animal is also important to decrease the incidence of zoonotic infection.

Clipping, particularly of long-haired animals, should be considered as part of the treatment of dermatophytosis. Clipping reduces environmental contamination with fungal elements and is particularly helpful in the treatment of *M. canis* infection (see Section 3, Chapter 24).

Chosen treatment: Because there was evidence of pyoderma, and pending the results of the fungal culture, antibiotic treatment was started using cefalexin at a dosage of 25 mg/kg b.i.d., along with twice weekly chlorhexidine and miconazole shampoo therapy.

Following confirmation of the diagnosis, systemic antifungal therapy was introduced using itraconazole at a dosage of 10 mg/kg s.i.d. per os.

As this was a short-haired dog, clipping was not performed, but weekly chlorhexidine and miconazole shampoos were continued.

CLINICAL TIPS

Dermatophytosis has a very varied clinical appearance. Historically, dermatophytosis has been over-diagnosed because the classic, 'ringworm' lesion consisting of a circular patch of alopecia with an erythematous margin is much more likely to be due to a pyoderma than a fungal infection. However, dermatophytosis should be considered in the differential diagnosis of any annular, papular or pustular eruption.

Cytology in this case showed the presence of acantholytic keratinocytes in addition to neutrophils. This cytology is suggestive of pemphigus foliaceus (see Section 2, Chapter 13). However, acantholysis is recognized to occur in some cases of dermatophytosis, particularly that caused by *Trichophyton* spp. infection, because of the production of fungal enzymes that result in acantholysis. The same phenomenon is seen in some cases of pyoderma and so a diagnosis of pemphigus foliaceus should never be made on the basis of cytology alone. Another clue in this case

that it was a dermatophyte infection, rather than pemphigus foliaceus, was that the nasal planum was unaffected. Dermatophytosis usually results in a folliculitis and there are no hair follicles on the nasal planum.

NURSING ASPECTS

Dermatophytosis is a contagious, zoonotic disease. The fungal spores are very resistant and will last up to 18 months in the environment. It is therefore important to take every precaution to avoid accidental inoculation with spores from infected animals, and to avoid both environmental contamination and spreading the infection to susceptible animals.

If they have to be hospitalized, infected animals should be kept in suitable isolation facilities. Nurses handling these animals should wear disposable overalls, gloves and hats that are removed and carefully disposed of before handling animals in other areas of the practice. All bedding, grooming utensils, clippers, cages and so on should be vacuumed, scrubbed and washed with hot water, detergent and a suitable disinfectant after use. Current recommendations for environmental decontamination are to use either a concentrated chlorine bleach solution (1 : 10 to 1 : 100) or Clinafarm® (enilconazole) environmental spray (licensed for cattery use in most of Europe), or the detergent–peroxide-based product Virkon-S®.

Clipping of long-haired animals is recommended as an aid in the treatment of dermatophytosis, because it speeds resolution of infection and reduces environmental contamination. Clipping should be done carefully and great care should be taken to avoid excoriating the skin with the clipper blades, because inoculation and infection of excoriated areas is highly likely.

FOLLOW-UP

Antibacterial therapy was discontinued after 4 weeks of treatment. After 2 months of systemic antifungal therapy, there was a significant clinical improvement, with resolution of all the scaling and crusting, but the alopecia and

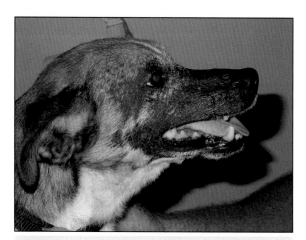

Figure 9.6 After 2 months of therapy with itraconazole. Active inflammation has resolved but hyperpigmentation and alopecia persist over the face.

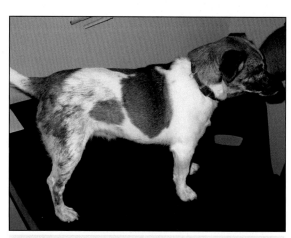

Figure 9.7 After 2 months of therapy with itraconazole. Active inflammation has resolved but hyperpigmentation and alopecia persist over the hindquarters.

hyperpigmentation remained on the previously affected areas (Figs 9.6 and 9.7).

No dermatophytes were grown on a repeat fungal culture and treatment was continued for a further 4 weeks. Another repeat fungal culture was again negative and so systemic treatment was withdrawn. It has been shown that clinical cure occurs prior to complete elimination of fungal elements from the skin, and two negative fungal cultures at an interval of 1 month should be obtained prior to withdrawal of therapy.

Follow-up a year later revealed that there had been some further hair regrowth over the previously affected areas, but partial alopecia remained. There had been no further episodes of skin disease.

10 Dermatophytosis in a guinea-pig

INITIAL PRESENTATION

Alopecia, crusting, scaling and pruritus.

INTRODUCTION

Ringworm is a relatively common disease of guinea-pigs seen in practice, but is often overlooked, or simply dismissed as 'mites'. In clinical cases, *Trichophyton mentagrophytes* is the most common isolate. *Microsporum canis* and other *Microsporum* species have occasionally been reported, and have been used to induce infections experimentally.

CASE PRESENTING SIGNS

A 4-year-old male, entire guinea-pig (*Cavia porcellus*), weighing 760 g, was presented with a long history of untreated skin disease. Initially, the owner reported hair loss on the face and around one eye. The guinea-pig otherwise seemed fine, so no treatment was sought. Gradually, over a period of several weeks, crusts and scaling developed and the lesions become more severe and mildly pruritic. At the time of presentation, the alopecia and scaling had also extended along the dorsum.

CASE HISTORY

As mentioned previously, thorough and comprehensive history taking is vital, since many diseases in small mammals are related to poor general husbandry. It is not wise to assume the owner knows the specific requirements of their pet, even if they have kept them for many years.

The guinea-pig was purchased at 9 weeks of age from a pet shop. He was kept with another male guinea-pig from the same litter that was also purchased at the pet shop. There were also dogs and cats in the house, but they had no direct contact with the guinea-pigs.

The guinea-pigs were housed in large hutches in the owner's garage at night, and allowed access to a large run in a private area of the garden during warm days. Their diet comprised a muesli-type guinea-pig mix, fed ad lib, along with constant access to hay. Each evening they were also given a selection of raw vegetable trimmings from the owner's meal preparations. No preventative healthcare was carried out and there was no previous medical history. There were no other general health problems; appetite, urination and defecation were all normal.

Several weeks previously, the owner noticed a thinning of the hair on the face, specifically around the left eye. No veterinary advice was sought, but the lesions gradually became worse. By the time of presentation, the lesions had progressed and extended along the back. The owner thought the guinea-pig seemed slightly itchy at this point. The other guinea-pig seemed fine.

CLINICAL EXAMINATION

A careful physical examination should always be carried out to evaluate for any other diseases or additional problems. This guinea-pig was bright, alert and vocal on presentation, and general physical examination was unremarkable, other than the dermatological abnormalities.

Dermatological examination showed marked crusting and scaling around the left eye (Fig. 10.1), with evidence

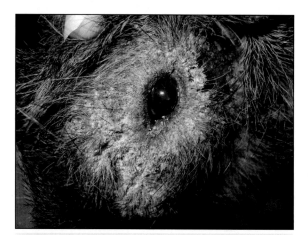

Figure 10.1 Extensive alopecia, crusting and scaling around the left eye. Notice also the inflammation of the skin below the pinna.

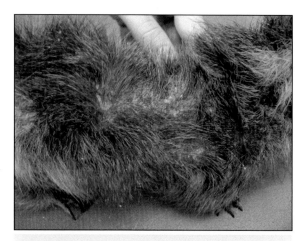

Figure 10.2 Patchy alopecia and scaling of the dorsal body.

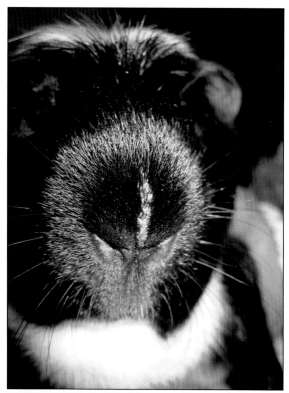

Figure 10.3 Small area of scaling and alopecia on the nose of another guinea-pig. Lesions like this may be the only initial signs of dermatophytosis, although no diagnosis was made in this particular patient.

of inflammation of the skin below the left ear. There was also extension of patchy alopecia and scaling onto the dorsum (Fig. 10.2).

The clinical signs associated with dermatophytosis in guinea-pigs vary. Lesions often begin with circumscribed or coalescing oval to patchy areas of non-pruritic scaling and alopecia, usually affecting the nose (Fig. 10.3), ears and face. However, in advanced cases lesions may spread to involve the neck, limbs and body. If untreated, then the lesions can become inflamed and infected with bacteria. This secondary infection will manifest as pustules, papules and crusts, usually with an increase in the pruritus, although the level of irritation does differ between individuals. Dermatophytosis can occur concurrently with *Trixacaris caviae* infestation; in these cases, the pruritus tends to be severe.

DIFFERENTIAL DIAGNOSES

- Dermatophytosis
- *Trixacaris caviae* infestation
- *Chirodiscoides caviae* infestation
- Pediculosis
- Rubbing against something in the cage
- Barbering by cage mates
- *Cryptococcus neoformans* infection
- Storage mite infestation (*Acarus farris*).

CASE WORK-UP

Because of the history and the nature of the lesions, dermatophytosis was suspected, although ectoparasitic infestations needed to be ruled out.

Skin/hair scrapes: Multiple skin scrapes were taken from around the left eye and the dorsum. These were mounted in liquid paraffin on a microscope slide with a coverslip and examined under ×40 magnification. No ectoparasites were seen. This absence does not entirely rule out ectoparasites and, in general, it may be useful to repeat the tape strips, or even consider prophylactic antiparasite treatment.

Further investigations aimed towards diagnosing dermatophytosis:

Wood's lamp examination: This was performed and was negative. Wood's lamp is an ultraviolet light that should be allowed to warm up for 5–10 minutes prior to use because the stability of the light's wavelength and intensity is temperature dependent. When exposed to ultraviolet light, hairs invaded by *M. canis* will show apple-green fluorescence in approximately 50% of isolates. The fluorescence is due to tryptophan metabolites produced by the fungus and hairs should be exposed for 3–5 minutes. Fluorescence is not present in scales or crusts, and illumination of debris should not be mistaken for fluorescent hairs. *Trichophyton* spp. will not fluoresce under ultraviolet light, therefore Wood's lamp examination is not often helpful in guinea-pigs and a negative result does not exclude dermatophytosis.

Hair plucks: Examination of hairs from the affected areas may demonstrate infected hair shafts. This is a difficult technique, requiring experience and a high-quality microscope. The hairs should be mounted in liquid paraffin or potassium hydroxide, covered with a coverslip and examined under ×400 magnification. Fungal hyphae may be seen, or arthrospores may be apparent within infected hair shafts. No fungal elements were seen in this case.

Skin/hair scrapes: Scrapes taken from the periphery of lesions can be examined as above for infected hair shafts. In rare cases of *Trichophyton* spp. infection, hyphae may only be present in the stratum corneum.

Fungal culture: This test enabled definitive diagnosis and identification of the dermatophyte species. Hair pluck and skin scrapes can be used from the lesions. The differences and limitations of in-house versus external testing are described below. In this case, samples were taken for external laboratory fungal culture, and 2 weeks later the results were reported as positive for *T. mentagrophytes*.

In-house testing: In-house dermatophyte test medium (DTM) kits are available and often used. These comprise a small culture plate containing Sabouraud's dextrose agar with cyclohexamide, gentamicin and chlortetracy-cline as antifungal and antibacterial agents. They also contain a phenol red colour indicator. Growing dermatophytes initially use proteins, producing alkaline metabolites that turn the indicator from yellow to red. Often, contaminant fungi use carbohydrates first, producing acidic metabolites which leave the indicator yellow. However, when the carbohydrates are used up, protein metabolism then causes the red colour change. Black or grey colonies are not clinically significant, whatever the colour change.

Hairs (and scale) from the lesion should be collected and inoculated onto the agar, with the lid replaced loosely to allow entry of air. Some dermatophytes take longer than others to produce the red colour change (10–14 days), so the test kit needs to be checked daily for 10 days. In addition, some non-pathogenic dermatophytes will cause the red colour change (e.g. *Aspergillus* spp.).

Since the presence of fungal growth and colour change is not entirely reliable, microscopic examination is essential to prevent an incorrect presumptive diagnosis.

Once grown, the plate should be sent to an external laboratory for identification. This allows the clinician to be sure what species is causing the problem, and may suggest the source of infection. For example, if *M. canis* was identified you might consider sampling the house cat.

External laboratory testing: Commercial laboratories use similar culture media but without the colour indicator. Some of the additives to the Sabouraud dextrose agar may inhibit the growth of certain pathogens; therefore, laboratories use plain agar, which sometimes makes the diagnosis of dermatophytosis easier. In addition, the greater experience of laboratory technicians at interpreting culture results and the possibility of extended culture under controlled conditions if required enables more accurate identification of the dermatophyte. Even with in-house DTM kits, the dermatophyte should still be sent to a lab for identification, so sending to the lab in the first place may well save time and be more accurate.

The relative costs of in-house DTM kits and external laboratory fungal culture tend to be fairly similar.

Sterile toothbrush: Samples may be obtained for microscopy or culture by grooming the hairs on and around the lesions with a sterile or new toothbrush.

Skin biopsy: Diagnosis can be made with skin biopsies submitted for histopathology. Fungal elements may be demonstrated with PAS (periodic acid–Schiff) or methenamine stains. Biopsies were not required for diagnosis in this case.

DIAGNOSIS

A definitive diagnosis was made from the positive fungal culture. In other cases, repeated cultures may be necessary to reach a diagnosis. Other factors to raise suspicion might include failure to respond to treatment for ectoparasites, lesions of multiple in-contact animals and lesions affecting the owner.

PROGNOSIS

Prognosis is good and treatment should be continued until two negative cultures 2–4 weeks apart have been achieved. If finances preclude this, then it is advisable to treat for 2–3 weeks past clinical cure.

Therapy in guinea-pigs is more challenging than in cats and dogs. Therapy usually lasts longer than with other patients, due to the difficulty in preventing self-licking or scratching. Also, owner compliance can be variable when challenged with having to bath and medicate a small mammal daily for an extended period. In very stressed individuals it may be an option to perform topical treatment twice weekly under sevoflurane (Sevoflo; Abbotts) or isoflurane (Isoflo; Abbotts) anaesthesia.

ANATOMY AND PHYSIOLOGY REFRESHER

Handling guinea-pigs: Guinea-pigs are friendly, sensitive creatures that may dash around the table to avoid capture, and often emit a piercing shriek at the slightest stimulus. They should be grasped rapidly and firmly around the shoulders with the hind feet supported by the other hand (Fig. 10.4). Grasping them firmly around the abdomen should be avoided as it can cause liver rupture.

Vitamin C and guinea-pigs: Guinea-pigs lack the enzyme to convert glucose to ascorbic acid (due to a mutated gene for L-gulono-γ-lactone oxidase) and are incapable of endogenous synthesis of vitamin C. For this reason, guinea-pigs require a daily intake of vitamin C

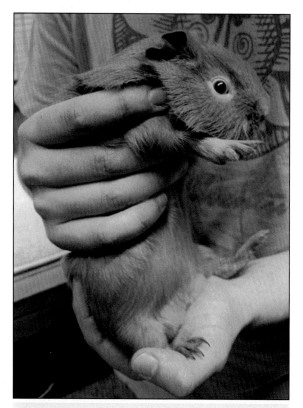

Figure 10.4 Correct restraint of a guinea-pig, with support being provided to the back legs.

of approximately 10 mg/kg, increasing to 30 mg/kg/day during pregnancy. A variety of commercial diets are available with varying vitamin C content and quality. Some forms of vitamin C supplement oxidize readily, so foods traditionally contained high quantities (800 mg/kg) to try to offset this, albeit unsuccessfully. Stabilized forms of the vitamin are now used in several of the leading brands of commercial diets in the UK, and these often have lower quantities of vitamin C (200–300 mg/kg) as less is lost during storage. The manufacturers' recommendations for shelf-life of the diet should be adhered to, and the diet supplemented with plenty of hay and fresh vegetables.

EPIDEMIOLOGY

Guinea-pigs are commonly affected by ringworm. Young animals are more susceptible, because of their incompletely developed immune systems and the lower concentration of fungistatic fatty acids in their sebum. Severe infections have been associated with mortality in neonates.

Non-clinical, asymptomatic carriage can occur, with risk of transmission to other animals, including humans. Therefore, the disease is an important and common zoonosis, especially because of the close contact between guinea-pigs and family members, especially children. *Trichophyton mentagrophytes* can be isolated from approximately 15% of healthy guinea-pigs. Disease normally occurs secondary to overcrowding, poor husbandry, systemic illness or other causes of stress. High temperature and humidity can also be predisposing factors.

Transmission of the organism occurs easily by direct contact with fungal spores on hair, bedding, soil and fomites. Concurrent infestation with mange mites (*Trixacaris caviae*) can also occur, and cases of dermatophytosis may be missed when mites are discovered first.

TREATMENT OPTIONS

Treatment of dermatophytosis should be attempted with topical therapy to remove spores from the hair shafts and systemic therapy to act at the hair follicles. Clipping of lesions may be beneficial in some cases, but was not carried out in this case.

In the past, griseofulvin was commonly used as systemic therapy for dermatophytosis. However, according to the veterinary cascade, itraconazole should now be the first choice drug since it is licensed for use in cats. The dose of itraconazole is 5–20 mg/kg once daily for 3–4 weeks.

Where griseofulvin is used, the dose is 15–25 mg/kg once daily orally for 14–28 days. Efficacy is reported to be improved if the drug is suspended in an oral liquid fatty acid supplement. Griseofulvin should be used with caution in young animals and is contraindicated in pregnant females due to its teratogenic effects. Other reported uses of griseofulvin include the paediatric suspension at 250 mg/kg orally every 10 days for three treatments and 1.5% griseofulvin in DMSO topically for 5–7 days.

Other oral antifungal drugs reported for the treatment of dermatophytosis include:
- Ketoconazole (10–40 mg/kg p.o. once daily for 2 weeks)
- Terbinafine (10–30 mg/kg once daily for 4–6 weeks, or 40 mg/kg once daily for 9 days)
- Fluconazole (16–20 mg/kg once daily for 14 days).

Focal dermatophyte lesions can also be treated until resolved with local topical therapy using either miconazole cream or clotrimazole cream once daily.

Other recommended treatments include washing with shampoo containing 2% miconazole and 2% chlorhexidine once or twice weekly. Also, topical 0.2% enilconazole can be applied daily or every other day with a toothbrush or used weekly as a dip. Enilconazole can be toxic if ingested. Some anecdotal reports of using lufenuron at 135–200 mg/kg orally every 30 days suggest it helps resolve difficult cases, but this is not supported by scientific data. Lime sulphur dips are also very useful for controlling ringworm.

Contaminated areas can be vacuumed and cleaned with a 1:10 solution of bleach and water. Carpets need to be fogged with enilconazole, since steam cleaning alone will not kill the spores. Animals in close contact should also be treated to prevent reinfection.

TREATMENT

The guinea-pig was treated with a combination of systemic and topical therapy. Treatment comprised topical treatment of the periocular lesion with 2% miconazole cream once daily for 6 weeks and twice weekly shampooing with miconazole/chlorhexidine shampoo for 8 weeks. Bathing guinea-pigs can be quite stressful for them, so this should be kept as brief as possible (remembering a 10-minute contact time is required) and the water kept warm enough to prevent chilling. Special care must be taken to ensure they are dried well after and do not become hypothermic.

Oral antifungal medication was given with itraconazole at 10 mg/kg once daily for 6 weeks. Due to increasing requirements during times of stress, vitamin C was given orally at 50 mg per day. To treat the secondary infection, trimethoprim/sulphamethoxazole was given at 15 mg/kg orally twice daily for 21 days. The in-contact guinea-pig was also treated with miconazole/chlorhexidine baths, oral itraconazole and vitamin C, but the cream was not used since there were no focal lesions. The owner was advised to wear gloves during treatment due to the zoonotic potential of dermatophytosis, and they were also advised that the children should wear gloves during handling.

During treatment the hutches were disinfected weekly with a 1:10 solution of bleach and water, and all bedding was discarded daily. Treatment was continued for 6 weeks (8 weeks for the shampoo), by which time the lesions had resolved and two consecutive fungal cultures were negative.

NURSING ASPECTS

As previously mentioned, whilst being easy to handle, guinea-pigs often emit a loud shrieking noise, even with the mildest restraint. It is worth warning the owners of this, although most will have already experienced it first hand during handling at home. Ensure they are handled confidently around the shoulders, using the other hand to support the back feet. Overzealous handling will cause pain and bruising, and can even result in liver rupture.

Since guinea-pigs are prey species, when in the veterinary practice consider their reaction to the environment. They should not be left to wait in a busy waiting room full of barking dogs, or sat in a carrier directly across from a hungry-looking cat. The same applies when hospitalized; where possible, they should be kept out of sight, sound and smell of predator species. During hospitalization, guinea-pigs will feel more secure with a deep bed of hay or shredded paper, with somewhere to hide. Retreats can easily be made by cutting a door in any small cardboard box; this can then be discarded after used, maintaining good hospital bio-security. If guinea-pigs are kept in pairs, then hospitalization of both may prove less stressful for each individual.

Remember that guinea-pigs need to receive vitamin C in their diet. Feeding rabbit food to guinea-pigs in the hospital is not appropriate. It is also worth remembering that some guinea-pigs eat pellets and some eat the muesli-type mixes; therefore, both need to be stocked for in-patients. Alternatively, you can have the owner bring in some of the guinea-pig's normal food.

CLINICAL TIPS

Vitamin C supplementation

In any sick guinea-pig or specifically where signs of vitamin C deficiency are present (rough coat, anorexia, diarrhoea, teeth grinding, lameness, delayed wound healing, infections), supplementation of vitamin C is recommended at a dose of 50 mg/animal/day. Initially, this can be given by injection, then by oral vitamin C at the same dosage (Fig. 10.5). Specially formulated guinea-pig treats, generic chewable vitamin C crumbled over the food or in the drinking water at 200–400 mg/l fresh daily can be used, although the latter method may be unreliable as vitamin C is degraded by light and metal. Other good sources of vitamin C include kale (125 mg/100 g), cabbage (60 mg/100 g), oranges, peppers and broccoli.

Antibiotic use

Antibiotics may be used in cases of ringworm if there is secondary bacterial infection present. Selection of an appropriate and safe antibiotic is very important if adverse effects are to be avoided. Broadly speaking, guinea-pigs possess a predominantly Gram-positive gastrointestinal flora. Disruption may allow proliferation of clostridial species, leading to a change in lumen pH and increased production of volatile fatty acids. The volatile fatty acids inhibit the normal bacteria further and cause production of iota toxin by the resident *Clostridia* sp. These toxins destroy the mucosal epithelium and will cause diarrhoea and enterotoxaemia, which often leads to more serious disease and even death. Narrow-spectrum antibiotics with action against Gram positives are more dangerous and oral use is considered high risk due to the drugs acting locally on the gastrointestinal tract flora. Amoxicillin, amoxicillin/clavulanate, ampicillin, bacitracin, cephalosporins, clindamycin, erythromycin, lincomycin, oxytetracycline and other penicillins are capable of causing antibody-associated diarrhoea when given orally to guinea-pigs. Gentamicin can also cause problems, so care should be taken to prevent grooming and ingestion after topical application. Procaine is toxic in guinea-pigs and streptomycin can cause an ascending paralysis and death.

Antibiotics that are reportedly safe in guinea-pigs include enrofloxacin, ciprofloxacin, marbofloxacin, trimethoprim–sulpha combinations and chloramphenicol.

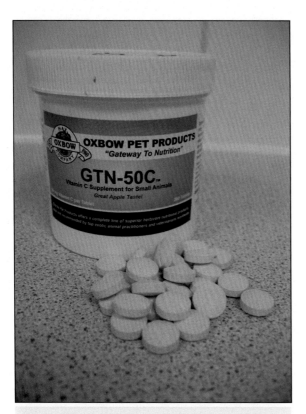

Figure 10.5 An example of apple-flavoured palatable vitamin C tablets specifically marketed for small mammals.

Stress

Being a prey species, guinea-pigs are prone to stress and subsequent immunosuppression. During treatment any stressors should be identified and removed, while the stress of treatment should be minimized as much as possible.

11 Adverse food reaction

INITIAL PRESENTATION

Pruritus with erythema, scaling, papules, crusting and otitis in a German shepherd.

INTRODUCTION

The term adverse food reaction describes an abnormal clinical response to an ingested food or food additive, and encompasses both immunological and non-immunological reactions. The clinical signs are variable and can involve both cutaneous and gastrointestinal systems. Whilst the concept of an adverse food reaction may be relatively easy to understand, the diagnosis in any individual animal can be challenging, because the clinician depends on the pet owner to comply with measures that need to be taken in order to achieve a definitive diagnosis, and because of the different pathomechanisms that may be involved.

Dogs and cats with adverse food reactions are usually presented with a history of non-seasonal pruritus that, anecdotally, may be poorly responsive to glucocorticoids and to ciclosporin. A history of intermittent pruritus could occur if the allergen is only fed now and again, i.e. if associated with a certain treat. There is no specific distribution, or lesion type, associated with adverse food reactions; however, there is a history of a recurrent otitis in many canine cases and, in cats, a head and neck distribution of pruritus has been reported. Some animals will have signs of gastrointestinal abnormalities of varying degrees, ranging from diarrhoea, vomiting, tenesmus and colitis, to just an increased frequency of defecation. In rare cases respiratory signs and epileptic seizures have also been reported.

CASE PRESENTING SIGNS

A 16-month-old German shepherd dog was presented with pruritus, follicular papules, bilateral otitis externa and malodour.

CASE HISTORY

As in all skin consultations a detailed history is essential, and in any case involving pruritus where a dietary trial may be required, full details on all dietary components are particularly important. A history of vomiting, diarrhoea or more than four bowel movements daily would increase the index of suspicion for an adverse food reaction. In this case the relevant findings were:

- The pruritus was non-seasonal, started at about 5 months of age, and was mainly confined to the ears and ventral abdomen. Pedal pruritus was not reported.
- There had been four episodes of otitis externa and an antibiotic-responsive ventral rash.
- The dog had a history of passing three to five bowel movements daily but had no systemic signs of illness.
- Thorough flea control had been maintained with monthly applications of fipronil since puppyhood.
- There had been no response to a trial treatment for sarcoptic mange with selamectin, three applications, 2 weeks apart.
- The dog was fed on a commercial complete dry food, containing various meat proteins and meat by-products. Table scraps and other titbits were also fed.
- The in-contact dogs and cats were unaffected.

CLINICAL EXAMINATION

The clinical signs of adverse food reactions are variable and range from non-lesional pruritus to severe self-induced excoriations and ulceration. The lesion distribution may be localized, such as an acral lick dermatitis in large breeds of dogs, or generalized. The most common primary signs are erythema and papular reactions. Secondary lesions include excoriations, crusts, lichenification, hyperpigmentation and scaling. Secondary recurrent bacterial pyoderma and *Malassezia* dermatitis is common. Recurrent otitis externa and/or media are reported in up to 80% of dogs with an adverse food reaction.

The clinical examination in this case revealed both ear disease and more generalized skin involvement.

Ear disease:

- Erythema, yellow crusts and patchy hyperpigmentation of the concave aspects of both pinnae (Fig. 11.1).
- Excoriations on the skin at the entrance of the ear canals.
- Yellowish exudate in the vertical and horizontal ear canals.
- Erythema of the epithelial lining.
- Tympanic membranes visible in both ears.

Skin lesions:

- Follicular papules and epidermal collarettes on the ventral abdomen (Fig. 11.2).
- Hyperpigmentation, lichenification, erythema and self-induced alopecia on the sternum and axilla (Fig. 11.3).
- Erythema of the anal area.
- Mild scaling on the dorsum.

DIFFERENTIAL DIAGNOSES

As with most cases of long-standing skin disease, it was necessary to differentiate between the primary, or underlying, disease and secondary infections and/or infestations.

The differentials considered for the underlying causes of pruritus (i.e. primary diseases) were:

- Adverse food reaction
- Atopic dermatitis
- Demodicosis
- Primary idiopathic recurrent pyoderma
- Sarcoptic mange, cheyletiellosis, flea allergy dermatitis and otodectic mange were differentials for this presentation but were unlikely in view of the ongoing and recent ectoparasitic therapy.

The differentials considered for the *secondary condition* were:

- Superficial staphylococcal pyoderma and/or *Malassezia* dermatitis
- Bacterial or yeast otitis externa.

CASE WORK-UP

As with any pruritic skin disease, it was necessary to rule out parasitic infestations and secondary microbial diseases before investigation of other causes.

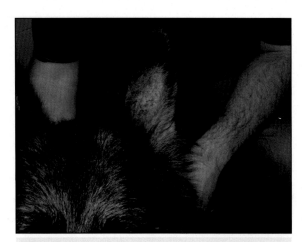

Figure 11.1 Hyperpigmentation and crusting on the concave aspects of the pinna.

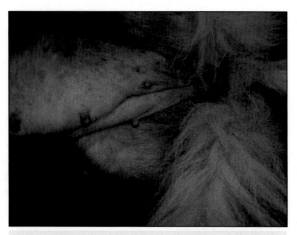

Figure 11.2 Papules and epidermal collarettes on the ventral abdomen.

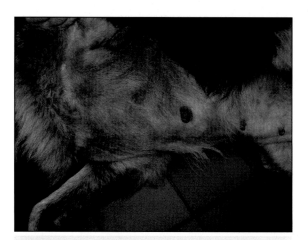

Figure 11.3 Hyperpigmentation, lichenification and alopecia on the ventrum.

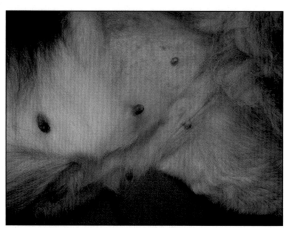

Figure 11.4 Ventral abdomen post-treatment.

In this case, the following tests were performed at the first visit:

- Microscopic examination of coat brushings, which did not reveal any flea dirt or *Cheyletiella* mites.
- Microscopic examination of skin scrapes, which ruled out demodicosis and failed to reveal *Sarcoptes* spp. mites.
- Liquid paraffin mounts of ear wax were examined to rule out *Otodectes cynotis* mites in the ears.
- Cytological examination of the otic discharge, which revealed an overgrowth of coccoid bacteria; of tape-strip preparations, which ruled out *Malassezia pachydermatis* organisms on the axillae and inguinal skin; and of papule smears, which revealed mainly neutrophils with intra- and extracellular coccoid bacteria.

Ectoparasitic disease was ruled out on the basis of the negative tests and ectoparasitic therapy. The clinical signs and the initial laboratory findings confirmed the involvement of a secondary superficial staphylococcal pyoderma and otitis externa. Empirical treatment for pyoderma and otitis was started immediately (clindamycin 10 mg/kg b.i.d.; daily acetic acid/boric acid ear cleaning and twice daily applications of a fucidic acid-containing product). The case was reassessed after 4 weeks, at which time the pyoderma and otitis had resolved (Figs 11.4 and 11.5), but pruritus persisted. In addition, the concave aspects of the pinnae and ventral inguinal skin were still mildly erythematous, supporting a probable allergic component. The next stage was to start a diet

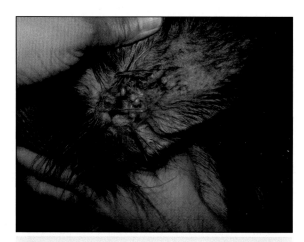

Figure 11.5 Concave aspect of the pinna post-treatment.

trial to investigate the involvement of an adverse food reaction.

Diet trials

The response to a restricted diet trial is currently the only effective diagnostic test for an adverse food reaction. The purpose of the trial is to establish whether the change of food results in a decrease in pruritus. Thus, a baseline level of pruritus needs to be established before starting the diet trial. This necessitates prior, thorough, treatment of all concurrent pruritic diseases such as ectoparasites and microbial infections.

Choice of diet: There are two choices of food, either novel protein and carbohydrate (i.e. ingredients to which the animal has not previously been exposed) or a hydrolysed protein. The selection of ingredients for a novel protein diet is based on the previous dietary history. Unfortunately, more often than not the exact ingredients within a commercial diet are unknown. In the UK, chicken, beef and wheat are common ingredients in dog foods, while fish, chicken and wheat are common ingredients in cat foods. Treats and table scraps given to the pet should also be taken into account. Hydrolysed diets usually contain chicken or soy protein that has been enzymatically degraded to break large protein molecules into smaller peptide molecules, rendering them, in theory, non-immunogenic. Although undoubtedly convenient, there is still a lack of data in veterinary dermatology as to whether dogs allergic to the parent protein will not react to the hydrolysed molecule. Novel protein and carbohydrate diets may be either home-cooked or proprietary preparations. All other foodstuffs including treats, chews, flavoured toys and toothpastes should be avoided. The choice of which diet to feed is based on an assessment of the previous dietary history and a discussion of the implications of the various options with the owner. In general, it is good practice to feed a type of diet which maximizes owner compliance. Although home-cooked diets are considered to be the 'gold standard', ultimately clients often find home cooking too much of a chore. Owner compliance is the major limitation in dietary trials.

Advantages of home cooking:
- Known protein and carbohydrate content without contamination
- Palatable to most pets
- Rules out potential reactions due to additives or preservatives.

Disadvantages of home cooking:
- Compliance issues because of the amount of work involved and the prolonged trial period
- Weight loss during the trial
- Gastrointestinal disturbances
- Expensive.

Advantages of commercial diets:
- Much more convenient than home-cooked diets, which improves owner compliance
- Apart from hydrolysed diets, they are usually less expensive than home cooking

- Meets nutritional requirements.
- Lower incidence of gastrointestinal disturbance.

Disadvantages of commercial diets:
- Some dogs find them unpalatable
- Limited ingredients may not be appropriate (although a hydrolysed diet gets around this problem)
- Contamination of the diet during processing can occur
- N.B. Some animals that have responded to a home-cooked diet are known to have relapsed when fed a commercial food containing the same ingredients.

Duration of food trials

Although empirical, most dermatologists advise a 6-week diet trial but there is some evidence that dogs may require up to 12 weeks of dieting to fully respond. The decision on whether to prolong the diet period or not depends on the clinical signs and additional diagnostic tests – e.g. you may decide to prolong the trial if an animal does not meet the major and minor criteria required to make a clinical diagnosis of atopic dermatitis, or if it has had a negative intradermal or serum allergy test for environmental allergens.

Dietary challenge

If the animal responds to the diet by showing a reduction in pruritus (>50% improvement), or complete resolution, the diagnosis has to be confirmed by challenge with the original dietary ingredients by re-introduction of the foods fed prior to the diet trial. This will result in increased pruritus within a week to 10 days if an adverse food reaction is involved. On occasion, there may be an obvious increase in pruritus within 24–48 hours of the dietary challenge. If the diet challenge does result in increased pruritus, the restricted diet is then re-introduced and the level of pruritus should subside again. Only then can a diagnosis of an adverse food reaction be made. A diagnosis of an adverse food reaction cannot be made if there is no increase in pruritus following challenge with the original food.

Provocation tests

Once a definitive diagnosis of an adverse food reaction has been made, the owner may prefer to continue to feed the restricted diet but it may be possible to identify specific causative foodstuffs by doing a provocation test. In this way, a more extensive list of ingredients that the dog can eat is built up and this ultimately may help to improve long-term owner compliance. A provocation test is performed by continuing to feed the restriction diet but introducing sequentially, one at a time, former dietary components or individual proteins and carbohydrates, at 7- to 14-day intervals, to determine whether that component results in an increase in pruritus.

Possible outcomes of a diet trial

- A marked reduction (>50%) or complete resolution of pruritus during, or by the end of, the diet period (up to 12 weeks), followed by increased pruritus on challenge and further improvement with re-institution of the restricted diet. Confirms a diagnosis of an adverse food reaction. With a case that shows only a partial response to the diet, suspect a concurrent pruritic disease such as atopic dermatitis.
- A reduction in pruritus, with no increase on challenge. Does not confirm an adverse food reaction. The dog improved for some other reason than the diet such as concurrent antiparasitic or antimicrobial therapy, a seasonal effect or just a spontaneous resolution in pruritus.
- No response at all to the diet trial – suspect a concurrent disease (e.g. atopic dermatitis) or poor compliance.

In this case, at the second visit and after the resolution of the secondary infections, a food trial was started. A hydrolysed commercial diet based on soy and chicken proteins was fed for 6 weeks at the first instance. The pruritus gradually reduced and ultimately resolved during this period. At the end of 6 weeks (Fig. 11.6), the dog

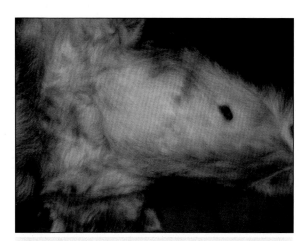

Figure 11.6 Ventral chest and abdomen after 6 weeks on a diet trial.

was challenged with the original diet, which resulted in increased erythema and pruritus around the ears within 3 days. The dog was switched back to the hydrolysed diet again and remission was once again obtained. To further confirm the diagnosis, the challenge was repeated and again resulted in increased pruritus and then resolution with feeding the hydrolysed diet.

The possibility of doing provocation tests was discussed with the owner at this point but was declined. The owner wished to find a limited ingredient hypoallergenic commercial selected protein diet to feed the dog long term and in this case the dog was maintained successfully on a turkey- and rice-based kibble.

DIAGNOSIS

The history, clinical signs, and result of the diet trial and subsequent challenges confirmed the diagnosis of an adverse food reaction in this case.

PROGNOSIS

The prognosis for an adverse food reaction is very good provided the owners are vigilant and avoid the offending foods for the life of the animal. Occasional flares of pruritus due to pyoderma, *Malassezia* dermatitis or possibly ectoparasitic disease should be expected and treated promptly.

AETIOLOGY AND PATHOGENESIS

Despite the amount written about cutaneous adverse food reactions in recent years, the exact mechanisms by which ingestion of a food can result in pruritus are still poorly understood. However, adverse reactions to food are classified according to the possible pathogenesis. True food allergy (food hypersensitivity) has a proven immunological basis, whereas food intolerance is non-immunologically mediated. Food intolerance includes: food idiosyncrasy, a reaction resembling food allergy but without immunological involvement; pharmacological reactions to substances in food such as reactions to vasoactive amines in chocolate, fish or cheese; toxic reactions to foods or substances in foods, such as pathogenic bacteria, mycotoxins, preservatives, colouring agents and antioxidants; and lastly, metabolic reactions such as lactose intolerance in humans. Hence we now talk about cutaneous adverse food reactions (CAFRs) rather than food allergy, although some adverse food reactions in dogs will be true hypersensitivities. Clinically it is not possible to differentiate between immunological and non-immunological reactions to ingested foods, or food additives, and most of the time in veterinary dermatology we do not know what type of pathomechanism is involved.

In the limited numbers of studies which have investigated CAFRs in dogs, most have demonstrated that dogs tend to react to more that one food. In one study of 25 dogs, the average was 2.4; in another study one dog reacted to nine different foodstuffs. Beef, dairy products, wheat, chicken, lamb, eggs and soy have been implicated in adverse food reactions in dogs. In cats, milk, beef, fish, egg, chicken and, in some studies, 'commercial food' are all reported as potential causes.

Food allergy

The major food allergens in people are glycoproteins with a molecular weight of 10–70 kDa. The molecular weight of food allergens in cats and dogs is not known. The role of cross-reactions between environmental allergens, such as pollens, and dietary proteins is not known in animals; however, exacerbation of clinical signs, due to cross-reactivity between environmental and dietary allergens, has been reported in humans. Examples of this include: apple and birch pollen; celery and mugwort pollen; and melon, banana and ragweed pollen. One dog was reported that was sensitized to cedar pollen and also showed a reaction when fed tomato. It is possible that there may be shared epitopes between foods, for example between different species of poultry, that could result in cross-reactions.

Overall, the pathomechanism of food allergy is not well understood in the domestic species but is likely to be mainly IgE or T-cell mediated, and there may also be a role for IgG-mediated reactions. Type I hypersensitivity is probably at least partially responsible for pruritus via cross-linkage of food allergen-specific IgE on sensitized mast cells in the gut and skin, and subsequent release of proinflammatory and pruritogenic mediators. However, pruritus could arise from any number of other potential pathways. There is evidence from experimental models that type 1 hypersensitivity reactions are seen in dogs with cutaneous manifestations of food allergy.

With regard to the immunological responses to foods, there are mechanisms preventing exposure of potential food allergens to the immune system, including:
1. Breakdown of large, potentially allergenic protein molecules by gastric acids, pancreatic enzymes and intestinal cell lysozymes.
2. Movement of food through the GIT by peristalsis.
3. The mechanical barrier provided by tight junctions between enterocytes and the mucous layer lining the intestinal epithelial cells.
4. Binding of allergenic molecules by secretory IgA in the mucous layer and lamina propria of the gastrointestinal tract.

In order for food allergens to be presented to the immune system and generate an inappropriate immunological response, it is likely that there has to be a combination of events involving damage to the protective mechanisms within the GIT along with concurrent ingestion of allergens. The following are situations in which it is speculated that this set of circumstances may arise.

- It has been demonstrated that infants and very young animals tend to absorb many more peptides and glycoproteins in comparison to adults and the feeding of a wide variety of different foodstuffs at this stage may overload the mechanisms which result in antigenic tolerance.
- It is possible that viral GIT infections and endoparasite infestation may damage the gut wall and contribute to the absorption of antigenic material.
- The presence of a heavy endoparasite burden has been shown to encourage the formation of IgE antibodies, although it is also considered that an endoparasite burden may reduce the likelihood of developing hypersensitivity responses in some individuals.
- There is likely to be a genetic component involved in the development of hypersensitivity responses to food allergens.

In healthy humans, up to 2% of all ingested food is absorbed intact across the enterocyte barrier and is presented to the immune system. As a result, food-specific, circulating IgG and IgE antibodies have been shown to be a normal phenomenon in man and are seen in the majority of dogs. Although there is evidence that type 1 hypersensitivity reactions are seen in dogs with food allergy, oral provocation to known dietary allergens in dogs not only increases allergen-specific IgE to these allergenic proteins, but also to other dietary components to which the individual may have been sensitized. Thus, from a practical point of view this limits the value of the serum allergy testing for dietary hypersensitivity, because food-specific IgE and IgG antibodies are seen in healthy animals. For these reasons, the measurement of allergen-specific serum IgE has not been proven to have a useful degree of sensitivity or specificity in individual cases for the diagnosis of food allergy and cannot currently be recommended.

EPIDEMIOLOGY

The true incidence of cutaneous adverse food reactions in dogs is not known, but is reported as being anything from 1% to 5% of all dermatological conditions and up to 30% of allergic dermatoses. Provided the offending food is fed on a regular basis, the clinical signs are non-seasonal and almost continuous. However, in those dogs that are only fed the offending diet intermittently, recurrent intermittent pruritus may be seen.

The condition is seen at any age from weaning to aged animals although young dogs may be at increased risk. It may occur concurrently with other allergic diseases such as atopic dermatitis, and some authors suggest that a distinction between food allergy and atopic dermatitis is artificial and that atopic dermatitis may be exacerbated by either environmental and/or dietary allergens. Most studies have not identified a breed predilection for adverse food reactions. However, in other studies a number of breeds are reported to be predisposed. Interestingly, these tend to be the breeds that are predisposed to atopic dermatitis. Recurrent otitis externa and/or media are reported in up to 80% of dogs with an adverse food reaction.

TREATMENT

Prior to starting a diet trial, ectoparasitic disease and any secondary pyoderma or *Malassezia* dermatitis should have been resolved to establish a baseline level of pruritus. During the diet trial, it is often necessary to control pruritus and this may be done with the intermittent use of short-term glucocorticoid therapy. The treatment used by one of the authors (P.F.) is prednisolone 0.5–1 mg/kg s.i.d. for 3 days, repeated as required during the trial. The owner is instructed to give a course of treatment whenever the pet becomes uncomfortably pruritic. The benefit of this approach is that controlling pruritus helps to improve client compliance but the dosage regime does not mask the response to the diet trial. Nevertheless, for this reason, it is advisable to ensure the owner does not give glucocorticoids for the 2 weeks prior to final clinical assessment of the response to the diet trial.

NURSING ASPECTS

Although there are no specific nursing issues in dogs with adverse food reactions, nurses can advise and monitor the individual during the trial period. If giving advice, nurses should be aware of the implications of a diet trial, what food the animal is being fed, the importance of avoiding all other foodstuffs and what treats may or may not be allowed (for example, fresh food, consisting of the same protein and carbohydrate sources as those of the proprietary diet are usually permissible). Certainly, nurses can be a great help in improving owner compliance by regular phone contact and encouragement during the course of the diet trial. Owners may have an expectation that the diet is going to rapidly result in a miraculous improvement of their pet's skin problem and it is important to manage their expectations and reinforce that this is a diagnostic test that is important to complete but which may or may not ultimately make a difference.

CLINICAL TIPS

- Adverse reactions to food can occur at any age.
- The history and clinical signs of adverse food reactions share many features with allergic and parasitic dermatoses, and therefore to reach a diagnosis requires ruling out infectious and parasitic diseases before a diet trial is started.
- Get the client on your side at the outset by explaining the reasons for and against adverse food reactions and why a diet trial should be performed.
- Explain to the client that adverse food reactions are easy to manage and worth investigating for this reason alone. A diagnosis of an adverse food reaction may mean their pet will not require long-term drug therapy, some of which may have harmful side-effects.
- During the trial period dogs will have to be prevented from scavenging and consideration should be given to keeping cats indoors.
- In a multi-pet household, the animal under investigation should, ideally, be fed separately from the others. It is best to point out these

issues to the owner, rather than to assume that they understand all the implications of a diet trial.

- Select a diet that will maximize the likelihood of good compliance. Many owners will not ultimately comply with home-cooked diets even if they appear enthusiastic at the outset.
- Give written instructions on the dos and don'ts of the diet trial.
- When necessary, pruritus should be managed in any pet undertaking a diet trial to improve owner compliance.
- Ensure thorough flea control is continued, and pyoderma and *Malassezia* infections are controlled, during the course of the diet trial.
- Do not rely on positive or negative serum allergy tests for food allergens.
- Ask the client to report any adverse effects as soon as they occur.
- For continuity the client should see the same vet at each visit.

FOLLOW-UP

Six months later the dog had not shown signs of pruritus, all through a hot summer period, further supporting the diagnosis of an adverse food reaction in this case.

SECTION 2

SCALE AND CRUST WITHOUT PRURITUS

12 Introduction to crusting and scaling

The outermost layer of the skin, the epidermis, is made up of multiple layers of cells (Fig. 12.1). The predominant cell type is the keratinocyte, and the epidermis is divided into basal, spinous, granular (variably present in dogs and cats) and cornified layers depending on the morphological features keratinocytes assume as they undergo progressive differentiation to form the stratum corneum.

Under normal circumstances, the epidermis is replaced every 3–4 weeks. The process of keratinocyte migration and differentiation is complex and carefully controlled. Daughter keratinocytes produced by stem cells of the basal layer of the epidermis travel up through the various layers of the epidermis and undergo a process of maturation and differentiation. The end products of this process are fully keratinized corneocytes, the cells that make up the stratum corneum. The cornified cell is packed with filamentous proteins; it normally does not have a nucleus and is imperceptibly shed from the surface of the stratum corneum, either as an individual cell or as small clusters of cells not visible to the naked eye. This desquamation process is the result of enzymatic breakdown of both the desmosomes (the small connections that bind the cells together) and the intercellular lipid 'glue' (present in the stratum corneum).

SCALING

Scaling is the visible accumulation of flakes of stratum corneum on the skin surface or in the hair coat, and can occur for many different reasons. Scale varies in colour and consistency, and may be white, silver, yellow or brown to grey. Scale may be branny, fine, powdery, flaky, greasy, dry, loose, adherent or 'nit-like'. Scaling may be focal, multifocal or diffuse in distribution.

Many diseases affect the normal maturation, differentiation and desquamation processes, and can result in scaling. The appearance and distribution of the scale varies depending on the causative disease. Diffuse dorsal scaling is seen in association with pruritus as a result of cheyletiellosis (see Chapter 5). Another common cause of scaling with a multifocal distribution is as a result of epidermal collarette formation. These are circular rims of scale that are the remains of pustules after they have ruptured (Fig. 12.2). Diseases associated with epidermal collarettes include pyoderma, demodicosis, dermatophytosis and pemphigus foliaceus. Multifocal patches of scaling evident over the dorsal trunk commonly arise from sites of pyoderma and are due to the formation of epidermal collarettes. Tightly adherent patches of scale which are difficult to remove are seen in some forms of ichthyosis, a rare, congenital disorder occurring mainly in young dogs associated with a failure of breakdown of intercorneocyte adhesion (Fig. 12.3). Follicular casts, nit-like accumulations of scale surrounding hair shafts, are representative of hair follicle pathology and are seen in follicular diseases such as sebaceous adenitis and vitamin A-responsive dermatitis (Fig. 12.4).

After an insult, one of the defence and repair mechanisms of the skin is to increase the rate of production of keratinocytes, so that all the layers of the epidermis become thicker. There may then be increased and abnormal desquamation of larger clusters of corneocytes that become visible to the naked eye as scale. In this altered process of keratinization the corneocytes may retain their nuclei. This is known as parakeratosis, a more primitive pattern of cornification (the initial stratum corneum in foetal skin is parakeratotic). Some metabolic diseases, including zinc-responsive dermatosis, necrolytic migratory erythema and lethal acrodermatitis of bull terriers, result in thickening of the stratum corneum with marked confluent layers of parakeratotic corneocytes (parakeratotic hyperkeratosis) and resultant visible adherent scale.

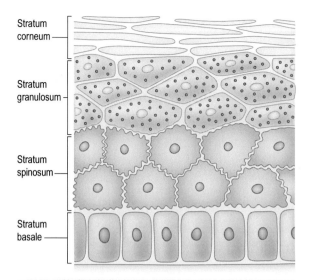

Figure 12.1 Layers of the epidermis.

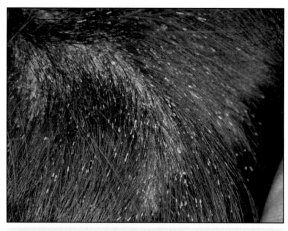

Figure 12.4 Follicular casts and scaling in a case of sebaceous adenitis in a Bernese mountain dog.

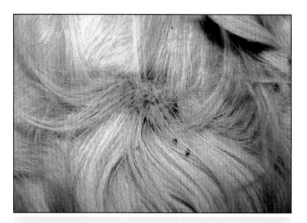

Figure 12.2 Epidermal collarette resulting from pyoderma in a golden retriever.

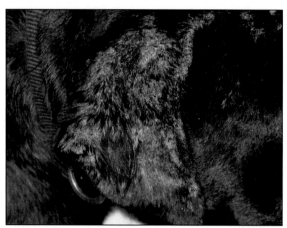

Figure 12.5 Crusting over the pinna of a boxer with scabies.

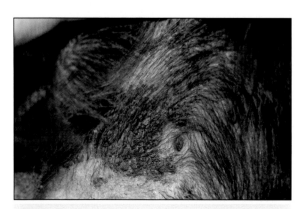

Figure 12.3 Tightly adherent scale in a case of ichthyosis in a Gordon setter.

CRUST

Crust is formed from the accumulation of dried serum, pus or haemorrhage, along with hair, cells and sometimes medication, on the skin surface. Crust is representative of a breach of epithelial integrity and there are many diseases that can result in its formation, including vesicular, pustular, erosive or ulcerative disorders. Serous crusts tend to be yellow or honey coloured and may be seen in excoriation due to self-trauma and in scabies (Fig. 12.5). Crust formed from pus tends to be yellow to brown, or green, in colour. Pustular diseases such as pyoderma and pemphigus foliaceus produce focal, often

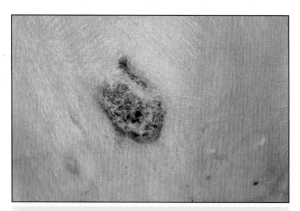

Figure 12.6 Large pustule and crust resulting from pustule rupture in a dog being treated with immunosuppressive doses of glucocorticoids.

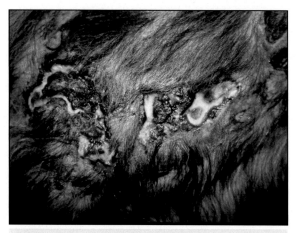

Figure 12.9 Haemorrhagic crusts in a case of vasculitis.

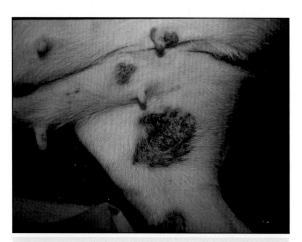

Figure 12.7 Focal crusting in a case of pemphigus foliaceus.

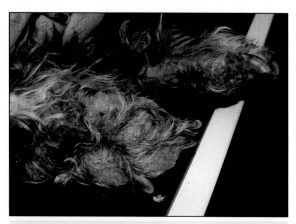

Figure 12.10 Crusting in a case of hepatocutaneous syndrome.

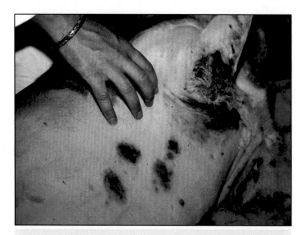

Figure 12.8 Haemorrhagic crusts in a case of German shepherd pyoderma.

circular, crusts, the crust forming from the pustule contents after it ruptures (Figs 12.6 and 12.7). Dark brown- or red-coloured crusts tend to have a large component of blood within them and would be indicative of deeper tissue damage. German shepherd pyoderma (Fig. 12.8), a particularly severe form of deep pyoderma, and vasculitis (Fig. 12.9) are examples of diseases that may result in the formation of haemorrhagic crusts. Tightly adherent crusts are characteristic of zinc-responsive dermatosis and necrolytic migratory erythema (Fig. 12.10).

Sebaceous adenitis

INITIAL PRESENTATION

Alopecia, scaling and follicular casts.

INTRODUCTION

Sebaceous adenitis is a scaling, variably pruritic skin disorder of uncertain aetiology. The disease results in the inflammation and destruction of sebaceous glands, follicular hyperkeratosis and commonly, secondary pyoderma. Grossly, the disease results in a scaling skin disorder associated with follicular cast formation and variable alopecia.

CASE PRESENTING SIGNS

A 7-year-old, neutered male Bichon Frise was presented with scaling and alopecia.

CASE HISTORY

There are marked breed variations in the way sebaceous adenitis presents, but typically the owner will report a gradual onset of skin lesions with variable scaling, alopecia and pruritus. The head and pinnae are often the first areas to be affected. The earlier signs of the disease may go relatively unnoticed and the dog may be presented with more severe lesions due to secondary pyoderma. There are no systemic signs associated with the disease.

The relevant history in this case was as follows:

- A 2-month history of scaling and partial alopecia over the dorsal trunk, and also scaling over the concave aspects of the pinnae.
- Papules and plaques had been noted over the muzzle and periocular regions.

- The dog had been moderately pruritic, particularly in association with the development of the papular lesions over the face.
- There had been no signs suggestive of systemic involvement.
- There was one other dog in the house, a sibling that had not been affected.
- There was no history suggestive of zoonosis.
- The dog was fed a good quality, complete dried fish and potato diet with occasional packeted wet food and fresh chicken, and given only water to drink.
- Routine flea control consisted of monthly applications of selamectin to both dogs.
- Recent treatment had consisted of borage oil-based essential fatty acid supplementation.

CLINICAL EXAMINATION

There are substantial variations in the clinical appearance of sebaceous adenitis between breeds.

Longer-haired dogs present with variable scaling, alopecia and usually marked follicular cast formation (Fig. 12.4), and a fine silvery scale on the inner aspects of the pinnae is commonly seen in springer spaniels. Lesions can progress to large patches of broken hairs and tightly adherent scale. The pinnae, trunk, temporal region and tail tend to be affected in the early stages, but severe disease can result in generalized involvement.

In short-haired dogs such as the Hungarian viszla, lesions consist of focal, coalescing, annular plaques of scaling and partial alopecia.

Feline sebaceous adenitis is a rare disease characterized by multifocal annular areas of alopecia, scaling, crusting and follicular casts. Pruritus can be absent to marked, and tends to be more severe if there is secondary pyoderma.

The physical examination was within normal limits. Examination of the skin revealed:

- Well-demarcated areas of alopecia, slight erythema and hyperpigmentation over the periocular skin, bridge of the nose and muzzle (Fig. 13.1).
- Generalized partial truncal alopecia with fine adherent scaling and yellow-coloured follicular casts involving groups of adjacent hair shafts (Figs 13.2 and 13.3).
- Prominent follicular casts over the medial pinnae and in areas over the trunk and tail.

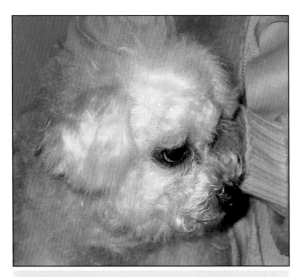

Figure 13.1 Sebaceous adenitis. Alopecia over the periorbital skin and adjacent to the nasal planum.

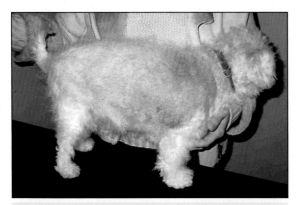

Figure 13.2 Generalized partial alopecia as a result of sebaceous adenitis.

DIFFERENTIAL DIAGNOSES

This was a diffuse, partial alopecia involving scaling and follicular cast formation. Follicular casts are made up of keratosebaceous material, and are literally a cast of the hair follicle lumen that forms a collar around the hair shaft and is extruded from the hair follicle as the hair grows (see Chapter 12). They represent follicular pathology, in particular follicular hyperkeratosis.

There are several diseases that can result in follicular cast formation and alopecia, including:

- Sebaceous adenitis
- Demodicosis
- Dermatophytosis
- Pyoderma
- Staphylococcus folliculitis
- Follicular dysplasia
- Sterile pyogranulomatous disease
- Hypothyroidism
- Hyperadrenocorticism
- Cutaneous lymphoma.

CASE WORK-UP

The definitive diagnosis of sebaceous adenitis is made on histopathological examination, but skin scrapes, fungal culture and trichographic examination were also indicated.

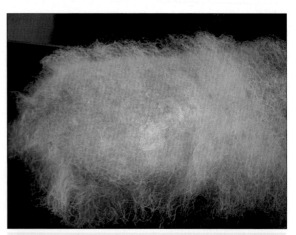

Figure 13.3 Sebaceous adenitis resulting in partial alopecia and discolouration due to follicular cast formation.

The following diagnostic tests were performed:
- Multiple skin scrapes, which showed no evidence of ectoparasitism.
- Fungal cultures of material taken using the MacKenzie brush technique. No dermatophytes were grown from this material.
- Trichographic examination revealed many follicular casts (see Fig. 2.9). There was a mix of anagen and telogen hair follicles.
- Four skin samples, from areas of alopecia on the trunk, were harvested by means of a 6-mm biopsy punch under sedation and local anaesthesia. Histopathological findings included marked orthokeratotic hyperkeratosis and a mixed, but predominantly mononuclear, nodular dermatitis in the mid dermis, with the nodules situated adjacent to hair follicles and corresponding to the sites of sebaceous glands. Sebaceous gland remnants could be seen within the foci of inflammation.

DIAGNOSIS

The history, clinical signs and histopathological examination were consistent with a diagnosis of sebaceous adenitis.

PROGNOSIS

Sebaceous adenitis is an incurable disease that is likely to require lifelong management. In most cases, the symptoms can be satisfactorily controlled. Although dogs experience pruritus that can affect quality of life, there is no systemic involvement. The disease does have a tendency to wax and wane, and interpretation of any apparent response to treatment should be made with this in mind.

ANATOMY AND PHYSIOLOGY REFRESHER

Sebaceous glands are alveolar glands that open and secrete their contents into the hair follicle infundibulum by way of the pilosebaceous duct (Fig. 13.4). They secrete a mixture of lipids, known as sebum, into the follicular lumen. This mixture coats the hair shaft and exits from the opening of the follicle onto the stratum corneum, where it comprises the most abundant lipids present on the skin surface. Sebum forms a surface emulsion with secretions from atrichial sweat glands that spreads over the skin surface, keeping it soft and pliable. It also spreads

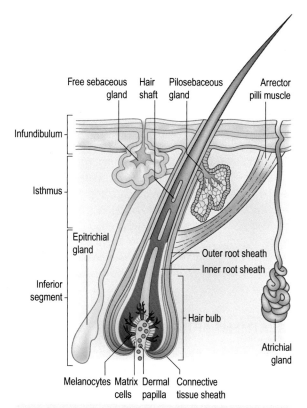

Figure 13.4 Diagram of hair follicle and associated adnexae. (Source: Anita Patel.)

over hair shafts and gives the hair coat a glossy sheen. The fact that the pilosebaceous duct opens into the hair follicle at the base of the infundibulum (rather than near the surface of the skin) suggests that sebum may also have a role within the hair follicle, as well as on the surface of the epidermis. Diseases in which sebaceous glands are absent are associated with keratin plugging of the follicular infundibulum. In dogs with sebaceous adenitis, the lack of lubrication results in infundibular cornified material becoming attached to the exiting hair shaft, thus forming the distinctive follicular cast.

It has been suggested that sebaceous adenitis is the result of an immune-mediated pathogenesis resulting in inflammation and destruction of sebaceous glands. However, other possible causes include a hereditary and developmental inflammatory destruction of sebaceous glands, a cornification abnormality leading to sebaceous duct and sebaceous gland inflammation and atrophy, and an anatomical defect in sebaceous glands leading to lipid leakage and a resulting foreign body response. Indeed, the variable clinical appearance between breeds could suggest differing underlying aetiologies.

EPIDEMIOLOGY

There are strong breed predilections for sebaceous adenitis in the standard poodle, Hungarian viszla, Japanese akita, samoyed and English springer spaniel. This suggests a genetic basis for the disease, and an autosomal recessive mode of inheritance has been proposed in the standard poodle. Interestingly, sebaceous adenitis seems to be commonly recognized in the English springer spaniel in the UK but not in the USA. The disease is most frequently seen in young adults, but there are no sex predilections.

TREATMENT OPTIONS

Therapy is aimed at treating pyoderma, minimizing the inflammatory response directed towards the sebaceous glands, rehydration of the skin and reduction of scaling. The response to therapy tends to vary between breeds, and perhaps depends on the severity and duration of the disease. As already stated, the tendency for the symptoms to spontaneously wax and wane further complicates the assessment of efficacy.

A number of different treatments have been reported to be of value in sebaceous adenitis.

Antibacterial therapy: If there is evidence of pyoderma, a minimum of 3 weeks of systemic antibacterial therapy is indicated, which may result in significant clinical improvement.

Topical therapy: Shampoos containing sulphur and/or salicylic acid help to reduce scaling. Initially, treatments should be two or three times weekly, reducing to once weekly for maintenance therapy. The shampoo should be followed by thorough rinsing in clean water and a final humectant rinse. Humectants moisturize the stratum corneum by absorbing water. Propylene glycol has both antiseborrhoeic and humectant properties. There are commercially available preparations containing propylene glycol that can be applied as a final rinse following shampoo treatment, or as a spray that may be applied daily to the skin.

Essential fatty acid supplements: Essential fatty acid (EFA) supplementation of omega-6 and omega-3 fatty acids has been reported to be of variable value in the treatment of sebaceous adenitis; it is usually combined with the use of topical therapy. The mode of action is unclear, but EFAs have mild anti-inflammatory actions and they may also be of benefit in the replacement of fatty acids in the skin and hair coat. The author's preferred initial treatment for sebaceous adenitis is to start topical treatment as described above in conjunction with EFA supplementation.

Vitamin A and retinoids: Vitamin A and synthetic retinoids regulate the growth and differentiation of epithelial tissues and have effects on keratinocytes. They have antiproliferative, anti-inflammatory and immunomodulatory properties, and have been shown to be useful in the treatment of sebaceous adenitis.

Reported dosages for vitamin A are somewhat empirical, but it is most commonly used at a dosage of 1000 IU/kg q24 h. A dose rate of 10 000 IU b.i.d. per dog has also been used and this was increased to 20–30 000 IU b.i.d. in cases that did not respond satisfactorily. Reported response rates were that 80% of dogs showed an improvement within 3 months.

Isotretinoin is a synthetic retinoid and is effective for the treatment of some cases of canine sebaceous adenitis at a dosage of 1–3 mg/kg q24 h. Around 50% of cases can be expected to benefit with reduced scaling and hair regrowth. One drawback in the use of synthetic retinoids is their expense.

Vitamin A and synthetic retinoids have numerous side-effects in man, including teratogenicity, cheilitis, inflammation and xerosis of the skin, decreased tear production, hepatotoxicity and hyperlipidaemia. The incidence of side-effects in the dog appears to be low, but routine biochemistry including triglycerides, and a Schirmer tear test, should be performed prior to starting therapy. Biochemistry should be repeated 1 and 2 months after starting treatment, and tear production should be monitored monthly for the first 6 months. These tests should then be repeated every 6–12 months. Both high-dose vitamin A and isotretinoin are highly teratogenic and their use should be avoided in any dogs intended for breeding, because as well as being teratogenic, they can also result in decreased spermatogenesis. Clients should be warned of the risk of accidental ingestion of these drugs and, clearly, great care must be taken by women of child-bearing age in the handling of synthetic retinoids.

Corticosteroids: Some texts have reported that corticosteroids are of no value in the treatment of sebaceous adenitis, but the author's experience is that at anti-inflammatory doses of 0.5–1.0 mg/kg they can be helpful in the management of some cases.

Ciclosporin: Ciclosporin at a dosage of 5 mg/kg has been a useful therapy for the treatment of canine and feline sebaceous adenitis. Treatment in dogs was associated with apparent regeneration of sebaceous glands. In the UK this is an unlicensed use for this drug, and in view of its expense and potent immunosuppressive effects, it should not be considered a first-line treatment. The efficacy of ciclosporin probably stems from the fact that, as well as its anti-inflammatory and immunomodulatory effects, it also stimulates hair growth by inducing anagen.

Treatment in this case: Initial treatment consisted of clindamycin at a dosage of 10 mg/kg b.i.d. for 3 weeks, supplemented with daily essential fatty acid supplements, three times weekly salicylic acid shampoos and daily propylene glycol sprays. The essential fatty acid supplements and topical therapies were continued for 3 months.

Re-examination after 3 months of topical therapy revealed further hair loss and the persistence of scaling and follicular cast formation over the pinnal margins, face and tail. At this point, systemic vitamin A therapy was introduced at a dosage of 1000 IU/kg q24 h. Prior to starting the treatment, a Schirmer tear test and full haematological and biochemical examinations were performed.

After 12 weeks of vitamin A therapy there was reduction in scaling and some hair regrowth over the tail. A repeat Schirmer tear test showed a marked decrease in tear production and the vitamin A therapy was discontinued. The tear production subsequently recovered to pretreatment levels.

After discussion with the owner, the dog was started on ciclosporin therapy at a dosage of 5 mg/kg s.i.d. The essential fatty acid supplements, salicylic acid shampoos and propylene glycol sprays were continued.

Six months after starting the ciclosporin therapy, there was excellent regrowth of hair over all previously affected areas (Fig. 13.5).

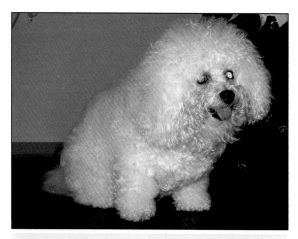

Figure 13.5 The same dog as in Fig. 13.3 following 6 months of ciclosporin therapy.

CLINICAL TIPS

As with all histopathological examination, it is important to take sufficient samples so that many adnexal structures may be observed. If the histopathologist is able to observe inflammation directly targeting the sebaceous gland, then the diagnosis is straightforward. However, in longer-standing cases, there may be a complete absence of sebaceous glands without inflammation in most sections, and many sections need to be examined to confirm that the absence of glands is widespread before being able to confirm the diagnosis. Thus, it is advisable to submit four or five punch biopsy samples from different areas of skin, even if the lesions in different areas appear similar.

When applied as a spray or mist, large volumes of propylene glycol are required to treat large-breed dogs with sebaceous adenitis. Propylene glycol is available in bulk quantities from veterinary wholesalers, and this product may be safely used diluted 50:50 with water and applied to the dog using a plant hand sprayer.

FOLLOW-UP

Ciclosporin was continued, but the frequency of administration of ciclosporin was gradually reduced to 50 mg every fourth day. The dog has been maintained on this dosage for 3 years, with no recurrence of disease. Although it was discussed, the owner was reluctant to withdraw therapy altogether in case of recrudescence.

Exfoliative dermatitis with thymoma

14

INITIAL PRESENTATION

Scaling, crusting, erythema and alopecia.

INTRODUCTION

Exfoliative dermatitis has been described in association with thymoma, both in people and in cats. A number of well-recognized paraneoplastic syndromes, such as cachexia, leucocytosis, hypercalcaemia and hyperglycaemia, are due to the systemic effects of hormones and/or other factors produced by the tumour, or its metastases, rather than the direct effect of the neoplastic invasion itself. In rare cases paraneoplastic signs such as exfoliative dermatitis, erythema multiforme, myasthenia gravis, myositis and myocarditis have been associated with thymoma.

In some of these cases, the paraneoplastic syndrome can be more life threatening than the tumour. Early recognition of such syndromes and appropriate treatment can lead to resolution of the clinical signs, and improve the quality of life and the survival time of the patient. This chapter describes the cutaneous clinical presentation in a cat with a thymoma.

CASE PRESENTING SIGNS

An 8-year-old, spayed British short-haired cat, weighing 3.35 kg, from a multi-cat household, was referred with a history of a severe exfoliative and crusting dermatitis.

CASE HISTORY

Most cats with thymoma present with a history of dyspnoea, coughing, lethargy and anorexia, which are often associated with the presence of a large space-occupying mass in the cranial mediastinum. The onset of cutaneous signs is usually sudden, with no previous history of dermatological disease. As most affected cats are old, owners often relate some of the signs, such as lethargy or changed demeanour, to age. The appetite in most cases is unaffected.

The relevant history in this case was:
- The cat's general health had been unaffected.
- The cat was reported to have a normal appetite and was fed on a variety of proprietary diets.
- The onset of dermatological signs was sudden and only 3 weeks before presentation.
- The initial signs were non-pruritic profuse scaling and crusting on the dorsum and mild bilateral conjunctivitis.
- Skin scrapings and fungal culture were negative for ectoparasites and dermatophytes.
- There was no history of a cough or any other respiratory signs.
- Trial treatments with selamectin and chloramphenicol eye ointment were prescribed.
- The condition did not appear to be contagious to the other cats in the household, or zoonotic.

CLINICAL EXAMINATION

This condition is characterized by moderate to severe exfoliation, erythema and alopecia, affecting mainly the face and the pinnae. The lesions may progress to the dorsum and the legs, and may eventually involve the whole body. Secondary bacterial and *Malassezia* infections can further complicate the disease.

The relevant findings of a physical and dermatological examination were:

- The body and coat condition were poor (Fig. 14.1).
- The heart rate was 130 beats per minute, temperature 39.5°C and bilateral thoracic auscultation was unremarkable. The peripheral lymph nodes were marginally enlarged.
- Oral examination revealed a small lingual ulcer, dental calculus and plaque.
- The hair was easily epilated.
- There was generalized erythema with crusting and scaling on the trunk (Fig. 14.2).

- Alopecia, erythema, focal crusting, comedones, hyperpigmentation and a brown waxy exudate were evident on the perianal area, extending to the ventral aspects of the abdomen and the medial aspects of the thighs (Fig. 14.3).
- There was scaling and crusting on the medial aspect of the elbows (Fig. 14.4).
- Mild scaling was evident on the pads of all four feet (Fig. 14.5).

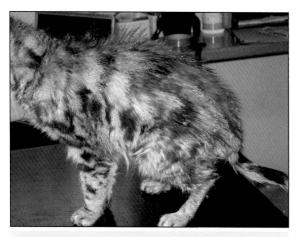

Figure 14.1 Poor body and coat condition.

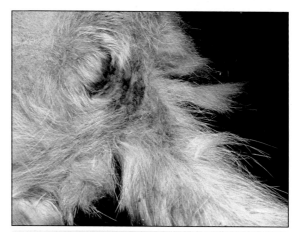

Figure 14.3 Erythema, crusting, hyperigmented macules and alopecia on the perineum.

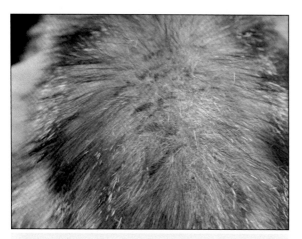

Figure 14.2 Crusting, scaling and hypotrichosis on the dorsum.

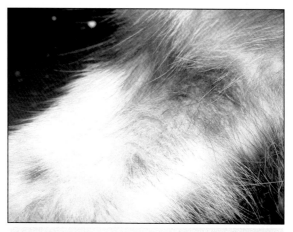

Figure 14.4 Scaling and alopecia on the medial aspects of the elbow.

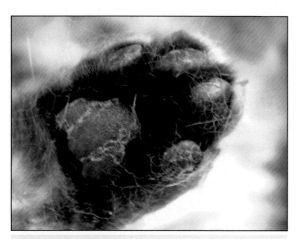

Figure 14.5 Scaling on the footpad.

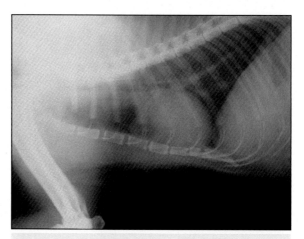

Figure 14.6 A smoothly outlined, round soft-tissue opacity just cranial to the cardiac silhouette at the level of the fourth costochondral junction.

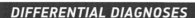

DIFFERENTIAL DIAGNOSES

Based on the history and clinical signs, the differential diagnoses included:

- Paraneoplastic exfoliative dermatosis associated with a thymoma
- Cutaneous epitheliotropic lymphoma
- Pemphigus foliaceus
- Systemic lupus erythematosus
- Demodicosis
- Feline sebaceous adenitis
- Cheyletiellosis
- Dermatophytosis.

CASE WORK-UP

Demodicosis and cheyletiellosis were ruled out on repeated multiple skin scrapes and in the case of the latter, lack of response to the previous antiparasitic treatment. Microscopic examination of hair plucks failed to reveal any evidence of fungal infection. As an earlier fungal culture had been negative, it was not repeated in this case (N.B. if further case work-up had failed to confirm a specific diagnosis it could have been repeated).

Haematology and biochemistry were mainly unremarkable, which is normal in these cases. Serological tests for FIV and FeLV were negative.

Thoracic radiography revealed a circumscribed spherical soft tissue or fluid opacity just cranial to the heart (Fig. 14.6).

Histology was required to confirm or exclude the other differential diagnoses and five skin biopsies were performed. Histological examination revealed surface epidermal changes of exudation, orthokeratotic hyperkeratosis and large numbers of surface coccoid bacteria. Very few apoptotic cells were present in the lower epidermis and an interface pattern was not obvious. Most sections of the biopsies did not, in this case, show the typical changes seen with this condition.

Normally, one would expect to see changes that are consistent with an interface dermatitis, with orthokeratotic hyperkeratosis affecting the epidermis and follicular epithelium, and with sebaceous glands often being absent. Hydropic degeneration of keratinocytes, at the basal and spinous levels, is also frequently evident, although at times it may be subtle. Apoptotic cells are normally present, in varying numbers, in all the epidermal layers. Mild to moderate mononuclear infiltrate may be seen at the dermoepidermal junction.

As with all disease processes, some histological changes in cases of thymoma-associated exfoliative dermatitis can be subtle and they vary considerably from case to case.

DIAGNOSIS

The putative diagnosis of paraneoplastic exfoliative dermatosis was based on the history, clinical signs, thoracic radiography and the histopathological examination of skin biopsies. Ultimately the diagnosis was confirmed on response to surgery.

PROGNOSIS

The prognosis depends on the successful removal of the tumour and postoperative care and recovery. It also depends on whether the neoplasm is benign or malignant. Once the tumour is removed, the cutaneous signs resolve within a short period; however, if it has metastasized to a distant site the prognosis is poor.

ANATOMY AND PHYSIOLOGY REFRESHER

The thymus gland is located in the anterior mediastinum where it lies on the sternum between the two lung lobes. The thymus is at its maximum size at puberty, after which it involutes. It is generally not visible in adult animals. The thymus consists of lobules which are divided by septae formed of connective tissue and are packed with epithelial cells. The outer parts of the lobules form the cortex, which is densely populated with lymphocytes. The inner part forms the medulla, with fewer lymphocytes but more antigen-presenting cells.

Naive T cells, produced by the bone marrow, are transported to the thymus where they undergo maturation. It is in the thymus where the T cells undergo positive and negative selection. Those cells that are not selected undergo apoptosis. The T cells that are released by the thymus are able to mount an immune response to foreign antigens. If a small number of cells that have not undergone the selection process escape into circulation they may also mount an immune response to self-antigens, which can result in autoimmunity.

The pathogenesis of the cutaneous lesions is not understood but it is thought to be a graft-versus-host type reaction where the cytotoxic T cells mount an attack on the epidermis, resulting in interface dermatitis with apoptosis. A feline study where CD3+ lymphocytes were demonstrated in five cats with exfoliative dermatitis suggested that the process is likely to be T-cell mediated. The exact pathophysiology is not known but there is a direct link between the presence of the thymoma and the skin disease, as successful surgical removal of the tumour reverses the cutaneous signs and improves both the quality and the longevity of the patient's life.

EPIDEMIOLOGY

Exfoliative dermatitis associated with thymoma is an uncommon to rare condition seen mainly in older cats (>10 years). Sex and breed predilections are not known.

TREATMENT

The treatment of choice involves surgical excision of the tumour mass, which is usually benign and well demarcated, and does not involve the lymphatic system or other surrounding tissue. Chemotherapy may be required in malignant cases and follow-up radiographic monitoring is advisable. For any of these procedures, referral to a surgical oncologist is recommended.

Treatment in this case

In this case a small, well-circumscribed mass of about 2 cm in diameter was removed from the pericardium via a cranial median sternotomy (Fig. 14.7), by a specialist soft-tissue surgeon. An incisional biopsy was taken from tissue surrounding the cranial vena cava, a right-side chest drain was inserted and the sternotomy closed. The drain was removed the following day.

Immediate postoperative recovery was uneventful and the sutures were removed 10 days later, at which point the skin was no longer erythematous and the hair

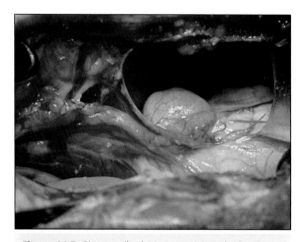

Figure 14.7 Circumscribed mass anterior to the heart. (From Withrow S, Vail D (2007): Withrow and MacEwen's Small Animal Clinical Oncology, 4th Edition. Saunders, Oxford, with permission of Elsevier.)

shedding had markedly reduced. Within a few days following surgery the cat developed an upper respiratory infection that responded to antimicrobial treatment with 50 mg of amoxicillin/clavulanate every 12 hours.

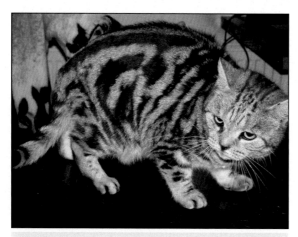

Figure 14.8 Normal coat and body condition at 12 months after surgery.

NURSING ASPECTS

Intensive care nursing will be required post-surgery.

CLINICAL TIPS

- This is an unusual condition with an acute onset. Usually, pruritus is not reported in early stages.
- The scaling and crusting are very marked and almost resemble the skin of a 'rabbit with cheyletiellosis'.
- The condition can be treated successfully, when there is early recognition.
- The owners need to be warned that even though most thymic tumours are benign, the exact nature of the neoplasm can only be determined after surgical excision.
- Fine-needle aspirate biopsies obtained by ultrasound guidance may aid in the preoperative diagnosis of the nature of the tumour, but malignancy can be missed.

FOLLOW-UP

The cat progressively improved and, 12 months later, it had a full hair coat with normal skin (Fig. 14.8) and weighed 4.6 kg. Subsequent chest X-rays did not reveal any abnormalities. Two years after thymectomy the cat was in good health with only an occasional upper respiratory tract infection reported.

15 Epitheliotropic lymphoma

INITIAL PRESENTATION

Scaling, crusting, hypopigmentation and alopecia.

INTRODUCTION

Cutaneous lymphoma is subdivided histologically into epitheliotropic and non-epitheliotropic forms. Cutaneous epitheliotropic lymphoma is an uncommon condition, characterized by infiltration of neoplastic T lymphocytes into the epidermis and the follicular epithelium. The condition mainly occurs in dogs, but it has also been reported in cats, ferrets, hamsters, rats and mice. In humans, epitheliotropic lymphoma is commonly referred to as mycosis fungoides and this term is often loosely used for the disease in animals. An advanced form of mycosis fungoides in man, the 'Sezary syndrome', is characterized by generalized, exfoliating erythroderma, pruritus, peripheral lymphadenopathy and large number of circulating malignant lymphocytes. The d'emblée form of epitheliotropic lymphoma in man refers to a rapidly progressive form of the disease. A subclassification of mycosis fungoides is Pagetoid reticulosis, where histologically there is striking epidermotropism. In dogs these terms are not always useful, as the clinical signs and the progression of the disease vary from that in humans, but are nevertheless used in histological classification. Canine epithelioptropic lymphoma is progressive and often poorly responsive to treatment.

CASE PRESENTING SIGNS

A 10-year-old, neutered male golden retriever presented with generalized truncal scaling and nasal depigmentation.

CASE HISTORY

A common observation in cases of canine epitheliotropic lymphoma is failure to respond to any particular treatment and an associated progression of symptoms, but the deterioration rate varies between individuals. Some dogs may be pruritic. Most do not exhibit signs of systemic disease unless there is internal metastasis but lethargy may be reported. Some dogs may have a history of allergic skin disease that had previously been relatively well managed.

The relevant case history in this dog was:
- The first signs of scaling and nasal depigmentation had started about 9 months prior to presentation and progressively worsened.
- There had been intermittent pruritus.
- Other than a long-standing history of intermittent otitis externa, there had been no history of dermatological disease prior to onset of scaling and nasal depigmentation.
- Concurrent medication included meloxicam for the management of pain, caused by osteoarthritis of the hip joints.
- Previous treatments included cefalexin and prednisolone to which there had been no response.
- The dog had been recently treated with three applications of selamectin at fortnightly intervals.
- The dog was fed a variety of commercial diets and there was a very long-standing history of intermittent diarrhoea, which had been assumed to be a dietary intolerance.
- The animal was exercise intolerant.

- There was no evidence of zoonosis and there were no other pets in the household.

CLINICAL EXAMINATION

There are four clinical presentations of epitheliotropic lymphoma commonly described in the dog:
- Generalized erythema and scaling (exfoliative erythroderma)
- Mucocutaneous erythema, depigmentation, crusting and ulceration
- Solitary or multiple plaques and nodules
- Infiltrative oral mucosal disease.

As the disease progresses all four clinical entities may be present, as demonstrated in this case. The significant findings on examination of this golden retriever were:
- Oral erosions and ulceration were present on the gingival mucosa above the upper molars and the canines.
- Depigmentation of the nasal planum, lip margins, muzzle, eyelids (Figs 15.1 and 15.2) and the margins of the footpads (Fig. 15.3).
- In places, loss of the cobblestone appearance of the nasal planum.
- Generalized scaling affecting the trunk (Fig. 15.4).
- The physical examination was unremarkable with no peripheral lymph node enlargement.

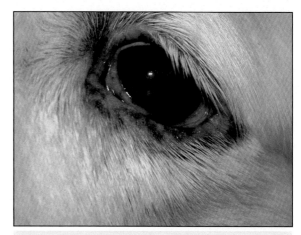

Figure 15.2 Depigmentation on the eyelids.

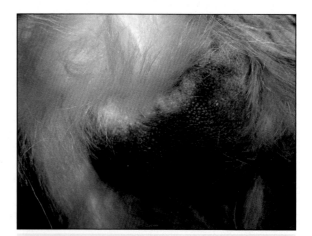

Figure 15.3 Depigmentation on the edges of the footpad.

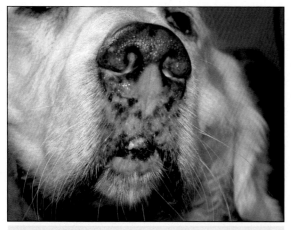

Figure 15.1 Depigmentation on the nasal planum.

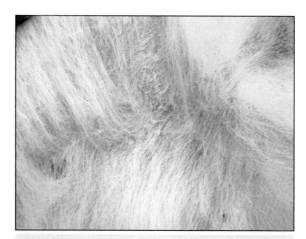

Figure 15.4 Scaling in haired skin on the trunk.

DIFFERENTIAL DIAGNOSES

Depending on the stage and clinical signs of the disease at the time of presentation, a number of different differential diagnoses have to be considered. In this case, given the generalized scaling, together with the crusting, mucocutaneous and oral lesions, the following were considered:

- Cutaneous epitheliotropic lymphoma
- Cutaneous adverse drug reaction
- Cutaneous lupus erythematosus
- Pemphigus complex
- Bullous pemphigoid
- Secondary superficial staphylococcal pyoderma
- Vitiligo
- Cheyletiellosis
- Hypothyroidism
- Sarcoptic mange.

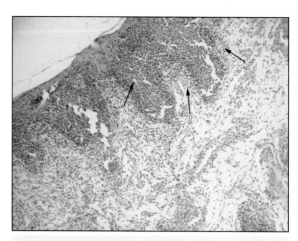

Figure 15.5 Histological section showing infiltration of neoplastic cells into the epidermis.

CASE WORK-UP

The history and the clinical signs were suggestive of epitheliotropic lymphoma, but the diagnosis should be confirmed by histology. Likewise, cutaneous adverse drug reactions, cutaneous lupus erythematosus and conditions in the pemphigus complex are also confirmed by the relevant histological changes for each particular condition.

The following diagnostic tests were performed:

- Four skin samples were obtained by punch biopsy under general anaesthesia. General anaesthesia was required in order to biopsy the nasal planum, where local anaesthesia is not feasible. The significant findings on histological examination were mild to moderate orthokeratotic and parakeratotic hyperkeratosis, with moderate epidermal hyperplasia and infiltration of the epidermal and follicular epithelium with neoplastic lymphocytes (Fig. 15.5). In addition, small aggregates of intraepidermal lymphocytes, referred to as Pautrier's abscesses, were seen. These findings were diagnostic for epitheliotropic lymphoma.
- Coat brushings, skin scrapings and tape-strip preparations were used to rule out sarcoptic mange and cheyletiellosis.
- Haematological and biochemical examinations were unremarkable, and there was no evidence of abnormal circulating lymphocytes (Sezary cells).
- Thyroid function tests (total T4, free T4, cTSH) and a thyroglobulin autoantibody test were within reference ranges.
- Survey thoracic radiographs did not reveal any evidence of pulmonary metastasis.

DIAGNOSIS

A diagnosis of cutaneous epitheliotropic lymphoma was made based on the histological findings. Although there was no evidence of pulmonary metastasis, other organ involvement could not be ruled out without further investigations, which the owner declined to have done in this case.

PROGNOSIS

The prognosis for epitheliotropic lymphoma is grave. Reported survival times from the time of diagnosis range from a few weeks to up to 2 years.

AETIOPATHOGENESIS OF CUTANEOUS LYMPHOMA

The aetiology in dogs is not known. Whether the disease starts as a reactive process or as a neoplastic one is not clear. In humans there is a suggestion that persistent antigenic stimulation or abnormalities of Langerhans' cells may be involved in the clonal proliferation of T cells. In affected cats, tumour DNA, amplified by PCR, has shown FeLV proviral DNA, although the cats were FeLV negative on serological testing.

Canine epitheliotropic lymphoma is of T-cell origin and studies have shown that they express CD3 and CD45 with mostly CD8 cell surface molecules. A few may express CD4 and, rarely, are CD4/CD8 negative. In contrast, human cases express CD4 cell surface molecules. It is likely that the tropism for the epithelium is due to the tumour cells expressing adhesion molecules that are able to bind to specific ligands on keratinocytes.

EPIDEMIOLOGY

About 1% of all canine tumours are cutaneous lymphoma; however, the precise incidence of epitheliotropic lymphoma is not known, as this statistic includes both the epitheliotropic and non-epitheliotropic forms. It does, though, seem to be diagnosed with increasing frequency. It is mainly seen in older dogs and the average age is about 10 years. There are no breed or sex predispositions.

TREATMENT OPTIONS

Several treatment modalities have been reported for the condition. They include topical therapies, systemic therapies, radiation therapy and surgical excision in cases of solitary lesions.

Topical therapies: Topical treatment with methchlorethamine has been reported to be successful in the patch-plaque stage in dogs and in people; however, this is a potent sensitizing agent with health and safety concerns for clients applying it, which limits its use. Furthermore, most dogs present with advanced disease and therefore its use is limited. The use of topical glucocorticoids, carmustine and retinoids has been reported in people, but not yet in dogs. Bathing the dog with a keratolytic and keratoplastic shampoo helps to reduce scale and control secondary infections.

Systemic therapies: Chemotherapy for cutaneous lymphoma does not alter its clinical progression or improve the survival time, but does in some cases improve the quality of life. Most cases are eventually euthanized, because of poor quality of life or secondary complications. Prednisolone (1–2 mg/kg s.i.d.), isotretinoin (1–3 mg/kg s.i.d.) and acetretin (0.5–1.5 mg/kg s.i.d.) are of some value in improving quality of life. Neither isotretinoin nor acetretin are licensed for veterinary use and, because of numerous side-effects in humans, written informed consent should be obtained (see Chapter 13). More recently, the use of lomustine (CCNU) has been reported to be beneficial in more than 75% of dogs treated. The drug was administered orally at a dose range between 50 and 100 mg/m^2 and was reported to be well tolerated. Adverse effects included myelosuppression and hepatic toxicity. Improvement in clinical signs was limited to between 75 and 182 days in the majority of cases; however, 17% of dogs had complete remission, with the duration exceeding 500 days. CCNU may therefore be an option to improve both quality of life and survival time in some individuals.

Other treatment options include: use of feline recombinant interferon omega; and chemotherapy with cyclophosphamide; doxorubicin, vincristine and prednisolone in combination or singly.

Because of the health and safety requirements associated with the use of some of these drugs, both treatment and post-therapy monitoring are best done at a specialist cancer treatment centre.

Concurrent secondary infections are common in many cases and should be treated with antibiotics. The choice of the appropriate antibiotic therapy should be based on cytology and/or culture and sensitivity testing.

Treatment in this case

In this case, after a discussion on the options available, the cost of each option and their potential adverse effects, the owner opted to just use prednisolone monotherapy at a dosage of 1 mg/kg once daily to alleviate some of the inflammation and improve the dog's quality of life. Higher doses of prednisolone resulted in unacceptable polyuria, polydipsia and polyphagia.

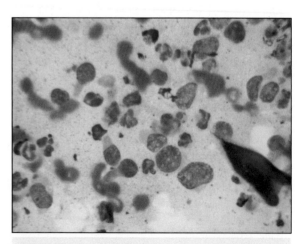

Figure 15.6 Lymphocytes showing anisocytosis and anisokaryosis and neutrophils on an impression smear.

CLINICAL TIPS

Occasionally, if ulcerated lesions are present, an impression smear from the surface may reveal malignant lymphocytes, which can be an early clue (Fig. 15.6). These lymphocytes are not, however, present in all cases.

Bathing the dog to remove the crust and scale aids in alleviation of pruritus and helps to improve quality of life.

FOLLOW-UP

The dog was euthanized about 2 months later because it developed severe gastrointestinal disease.

16 Cheyletiellosis in a rabbit

INITIAL PRESENTATION

Minimally pruritic, dorsal scaling predominantly between the shoulders.

INTRODUCTION

Ectoparasite infestation is a common problem in rabbit veterinary practice, with the most common parasites, *Cheyletiella* sp. and *Leporacarus* sp., both being referred to as rabbit fur mites. With cheyletiellosis, affected individuals usually have *Cheyletiella parasitovorax*, although *C. takahasii*, *C. ochotonae* and *C. johnsoni* have also been reported.

Cheyletiella is an obligate non-burrowing mite that feeds on the keratin layer of the epidermis, creating pseudo-tunnels through the scale and debris on the skin surface. The mite may also pierce the skin with its needle-like mouth parts to feed on tissue fluids. Transmission is by direct contact. The entire life cycle of *Cheyletiella* takes place on the host and is completed in 14–35 days. Despite preferring to remain on the host, adult females can survive off the rabbit host for approximately 10 days.

Clinical signs of cheyletiellosis are variable. Many rabbits will harbour the mite with no overt signs of skin disease but, where present, clinical signs are usually confined to mild pruritus with large soft white flakes of scale, with occasional alopecia, in the interscapular region or other dorsal body surfaces. Mites are just about visible to the naked eye and in moderate to severe infestations rabbits may appear to have 'walking dandruff'. The disease is more common in young or immunosuppressed individuals and in animals suffering from an underlying condition that prevents grooming.

Diagnosis is via microscopic examination of acetate tape strips, or coat brushings, and treatment is fairly straightforward unless there is a more serious underlying disease.

Another common ectoparasite of rabbits is the other rabbit fur mite, *Leporacarus gibbus* (formerly named *Listrophorus gibbus*). It is also found in the fur of rabbits and infestations are often asymptomatic. If clinical signs are present they might include alopecia, seborrhoea and scaling. As with cheyletiellosis, an infestation severe enough to cause clinical signs is usually associated with an underlying disease process. The diagnosis and treatment of *Leporacarus* sp. is the same as for *Cheyletiella* sp.

CASE PRESENTING SIGNS

A 3-year-old, female neutered Dutch rabbit (*Oryctolagus cuniculus*), weighing 2.3 kg, was presented with a 10-day history of minimally pruritic, dorsal scaling predominantly between the shoulders.

CASE HISTORY

Complete and thorough history taking is very important. Much of the information obtained may not initially seem related to skin disease or the clinical presentation. However, over 75% of problems seen in rabbits and other small mammal pets are due to improper housing, diet, environment and general poor husbandry. This in turn will lead to general ill thrift, immunocompromise and increased susceptibility to ectoparasite infestation. The presenting signs may simply be the consequence of a more serious underlying disease such as dental problems or osteoarthritis (as discussed in the 'Anatomy and physiology refresher' section).

The relevant case history in this case was:

- The rabbit had been acquired at 6 weeks of age and was kept with another male, neutered rabbit from the same litter.
- Both pets were free-ranging house rabbits, with regular access to the garden each day.
- Vaccinations against myxomatosis and viral haemorrhagic disease were carried out every 6 and 12 months respectively, but no other preventative healthcare such as flea treatment or blowfly strike prevention was used.
- Their diet consisted of a commercial pelleted rabbit food fed twice daily, as much as they would consume in 10–15 minutes. Alongside this, a wide selection of vegetables and ad lib hay was offered and eaten.
- There were no other general health problems; appetite, urination and defecation were all normal.
- The owner had noticed the presence of a significant area of white flakes between the shoulder blades of one of the rabbits 10 days prior to presentation. This was thought to be associated with mild pruritus.
- The in-contact rabbit and owner were not affected with any lesions or pruritus.

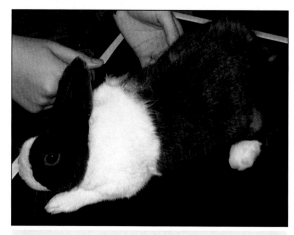

Figure 16.1 Dorsal scale in a rabbit.

CLINICAL EXAMINATION

Prior to focusing on the dermatological problems, a full physical examination should be carried out to evaluate for any concurrent disease or additional abnormalities. In this case, the general physical examination was unremarkable, with only dermatological abnormalities noted. Examination also included otoscopic dental examination to evaluate the teeth, which was unremarkable, although not entirely reliable (see 'Clinical tips' section). Oral pain associated with dental problems is very common in pet rabbits. This pain will reduce grooming and can be an underlying cause for a dermatological problem.

The dermatological examination in this case confirmed an area of marked scaling dorsally between the scapulae, although there was also mild scaling extending caudally along the dorsal midline of the back (Figs 16.1 and 16.2). The skin in these areas was mildly erythematous and there was thinning of the coat in the worst affected area.

The clinical signs of cheyletiellosis can be variable and are generally not severe. Many rabbits can harbour the mite asymptomatically, with no detectable signs of skin disease. In individuals that develop lesions, they are initially often subtle and may lead to a delay in seeking veterinary advice.

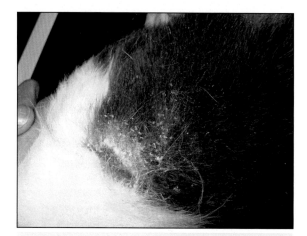

Figure 16.2 Close-up of dorsal scale in a rabbit.

When these patients are eventually presented to a veterinary surgeon, the clinical signs are usually confined to large soft white flakes of scale in the interscapular region. There may occasionally be mild pruritus, but this is not a consistent feature. The mites can often just about be seen with the naked eye as they move about in the loose scale, giving rise to the descriptive term of 'walking dandruff'. Depending on the duration and severity of the infestation, crusting may also be present, with alopecia and moderate to marked pruritus.

Ectoparasite infestation is more common in young or immunosuppressed rabbits, or those suffering from an underlying condition that reduces or prevents grooming (see 'Anatomy and physiology refresher' section).

The differential diagnoses in this case were:
- Cheyletiellosis
- *Leporacarus* sp. infestation
- Pediculosis
- Flea infestation
- Harvest mite infestation
- Demodicosis
- Zinc deficiency
- Dermatophytosis
- Keratinization defect.

CASE WORK-UP

Ectoparasites are a very common cause of dorsal scurf in rabbits, so microscopic examination of the scurf is indicated. As previously mentioned, it is possible to visualize *Cheyletiella* sp. with the naked eye, but this should not be relied upon for a definitive diagnosis.

Acetate tape strips: The rabbit was gently restrained and two acetate tape strips were taken from the area of dorsal scale. These were mounted on a microscope slide and examined under the low-power objective (×40 magnification). Mites are found in greatest numbers over the scapulae, but may also be encountered on the back of the head, the neck and rarely on the caudal abdomen. *Cheyletiella* mites are typically saddle shaped with hook-shaped mouth parts and are easily seen using the described technique (Figs 16.3 and 16.4). Specific identification of the mite is not required in practice, and the vast majority found on rabbits will be *C. parasitovorax*.

It is useful to repeat the acetate tape strips in different affected areas to increase the likelihood of finding parasites. The sample should also be evaluated for other parasites such as *Leporacarus* sp., lice and fleas.

Cheyletiella mites were found in this case and further examination of the tape strips did not reveal any other ectoparasites. A negative result on acetate tape strips may have prompted further diagnostic tests.

Coat brushings: Examinations of coat brushings, or collections of scale, mounted on a slide might be equally useful in diagnosing cheyletiellosis. The scale should be collected and placed on a slide with liquid paraffin, then covered with a coverslip. The slide should be examined under low power, as with the acetate tape strips.

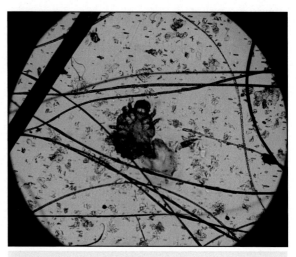

Figure 16.3 *Cheyletiella parasitovorax*.

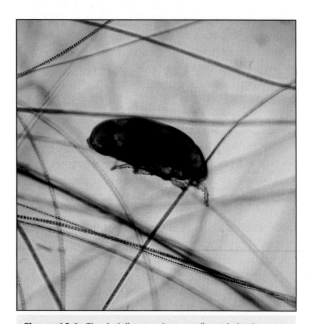

Figure 16.4 *Cheyletiella parasitovorax* (lateral view).

Skin scrapes: Occasionally, superficial skin scrapes may be required to demonstrate *Cheyletiella* sp. Skin scrape samples would also need to be obtained to evaluate for burrowing mites such as *Sarcoptes* sp. or follicular mites such as *Demodex* sp., since these are less likely to be found in the scale.

Dermatophyte culture: Dermatophyte culture may be carried out if multiple evaluations for ectoparasites were negative. *Trichophyton mentagrophytes* is common in outdoor rabbits, whereas *Microsporum canis* and *M. gypseum* are more common in pet and house rabbits. The presenting signs and the demonstration of *Cheyletiella* mites in the scurf made dermatophytosis unlikely in this case.

Blood sampling: Since cheyletiellosis may be associated with immunosuppression or an underlying disease, samples may be obtained for haematology and biochemistry (see 'Clinical tips' for help with blood sampling). This will provide the clinician with an overview of the patient's health status. Serology for *Encephalitozooan cuniculi* would also be useful in cases that are complicated or refractory to treatment. Routine haematology and biochemistry were unremarkable in this case. *Encephalitozooan cuniculi* serology was negative.

Radiography: Since underlying disease is common, radiography of the thorax, abdomen and skull (for dental disease) would be indicated in complicated cases or those unresponsive to treatment.

DIAGNOSIS

The positive finding of *Cheyletiella parasitovorax* on acetate strip examination of the scurf, with no evidence of other parasites, was adequate to reach a diagnosis of cheyletiellosis. Further investigation via blood work did not reveal any other abnormalities. Treatment for cheyletiellosis was initiated in this case, but no underlying cause for the cheyletiellosis was established.

PROGNOSIS

The prognosis for cheyletiellosis in the rabbit is often very good. However, in some cases, the presence of a serious underlying problem may alter the prognosis.

If the initial treatment course does not solve the problem, asymptomatic carriers (including dogs, cats and other rabbits) or survival of parasites off the host must be suspected. It is common for only certain individuals in a group to be clinically affected at any one time and transmission occurs via close contact. Therefore, concurrent treatment of in-contact rabbits, and even in-contact dogs and cats, should be carried out.

ANATOMY AND PHYSIOLOGY REFRESHER

Parasitology: *Cheyletiella* belongs to the class arachnida and the order Acarina (mites), and is the commonest cause of ectoparasitic disease in rabbits. Arachnida differ from insects in that there is no differentiation into head, thorax and abdomen. Either there is differentiation into cephalothorax and abdomen (spiders) or the body is completely fused (ticks and some mites).There are four pairs of legs, chelicerae which are pincer shaped or modified for piercing, the palps or pedipalps, which are leg-like in appearance and, with the epistome and hypostome, make up the principal structure of the mouth parts. There are no wings and the abdomen has no appendages, only the opening of the anus and ventral genital opening. There is a wide variety of forms, depending on the hosts' lifestyle. They are mostly oviparous and the larva resembles the adult, except that it has three pairs of legs and no genital organs. The larval stage is followed by three nymphal stages before sexual maturity is reached.

Cheyletiella are medium-sized mites, with the female measuring 450×200 µm and the smaller male measuring 320×160 µm. They are very active with a yellow–white body, making visualization difficult on albino animals. The short sturdy limbs lack a tarsal claw, but carry a distinctive comb-like row of hairs. The palpi are short and broad, with a prominent claw curving inwards, giving a pincer-like appearance.

Skin anatomy: The basic skin structure and function in rabbits is essentially the same as found in other pet mammals, and also man. In fact, the skin of rabbits is frequently used in studies of human skin disease.

In rabbits, hairs arise singly or in multiples from hair follicles, creating the characteristic dense coat found in most rabbits. (*Interesting fact*: Chinchillas have the densest coat of all the small mammals due to an impressive 60 hairs per follicle.)

In most regions the skin is covered with a dense fur that consists of a soft undercoat and stiff guard hairs. Some breeds, such as the Rex, have no primary hairs, leaving the dense covering of secondary hairs exposed. The absence of the coarser primary hairs gives them their characteristic soft feeling. Unfortunately, this soft fine coat offers little protection to the hocks and predisposes this breed to ulcerative pododermatitis in that region. Primary hairs in other mammals are associated with sweat glands. However, rabbits only have sweat glands in the lips and cannot pant effectively, making them highly susceptible to overheating.

Rabbits become covered with soft hair just a few days after birth. This baby coat is then replaced by an intermediate coat at 5–6 weeks old. This intermediate coat does not contain moulting hairs and is the coat that is used in the rabbit fur industry.

Seasonal moulting patterns are more obvious in rabbits than other small mammals, especially those housed outdoors. There are often two complete coat changes per year. During the moult there are distinct areas of fur in various stages of growth. The moult usually begins on the head, works down the neck and back, with the abdomen being last to shed. Nutrition and environmental stimulus will influence the moulting process. Temperature also has an effect; the summer coat is shorter than the winter coat and may even be a slightly different colour. Some breeds with fluffier coats (e.g. dwarf lop and miniature lop) develop patches of alopecia during moulting.

Rabbits require dietary essential amino acids despite synthesis in the caecum. Keratin contains large amounts of cystine, synthesized from the essential amino acid methionine. Lysine is also important in keratin formation, as well as fibrin and collagen. In general, cereals are deficient in lysine and methionine, whereas green vegetables are not. Sulphur amino acid deficiency can be reflected in poor coat quality in rabbits that are unwell or fed predominantly on cereal. Selective feeding from mixed rations is very common and results in over-consumption of cereals at the expense of the more nutritious aspects of the diet.

Certain colour point breeds like Californian or Siamese Sable may show black hair regrowth in previously shaved areas. This is likely to be a temperature-dependent change, as seen in Siamese cats.

Grooming

Many skin diseases, including cheyletiellosis, are associated with an underlying disease process that affects the animal's ability to groom effectively. A healthy rabbit will spend a significant portion of its time grooming, and rabbits kept together will also spend time grooming each other. Any circumstance or illness that prevents a rabbit from licking and grooming properly will reduce the removal of parasites from the fur and lead to a dull coat, full of dead hair and skin debris, which in turn will contribute to skin disease. In the case of cheyletiellosis, it will provide increased food material for the mites and a better environment for their survival and proliferation on the host.

Some of the underlying problems that will interfere with grooming in rabbits include:

Breed: Coat texture can affect the ability to groom properly. For example, the fine fluffy coat of angoras can be impossible for the rabbit to lick and groom effectively.

Dental disease: Rabbit teeth are open rooted, meaning that in healthy rabbits they continue to erupt throughout their entire life. The occlusal surface and correct crown length are maintained by *attrition* (grinding of the opposing teeth in the absence of food) and *abrasion* (from fibrous material in the diet). This means that the *duration* of feed intake is likely to be more important than the hardness of the food, in terms of maintaining healthy teeth. Until recently, dental disease in rabbits was assumed to be congenital, but now other factors are known to be involved. Acquired dental disease is a progressive problem comprising crown and root elongation, deterioration in tooth quality, loss of alveolar bone and tooth support, lingual and buccal spikes damaging oral soft tissues, and tooth root abscessation. These processes result in significant dental pain, which makes the rabbit reluctant to groom properly, thereby predisposing it to skin disease.

Contributing factors to dental disease include metabolic bone disease (from inadequate dietary calcium absorption), poor diet and lack of dental wear. Dental disease typically occurs in rabbits housed indoors or in a hutch, fed on mixed cereal rations, with occasional vegetables and sporadic access to the lawn. Wild rabbits and pet rabbits that are allowed unrestricted outdoor grazing rarely develop this disease. Housed rabbits that consume diets rich in grass, hay and vegetables, and are regularly allowed outside, are less likely to be affected.

Diet: Rabbits will selectively feed if given the opportunity. Mixed cereal rations allow selection of the most palatable portions of the food, such as flaked peas, biscuit and maize, which are high in energy and deficient in calcium. The pellet part of the ration, which contains the vitamins and minerals, is often left uneaten and discarded. The rabbit quickly fulfils its energy requirements and spends little time eating other roughage such as vegetables and hay. This selective feeding will lead to dental disease (due to lack of fibre and calcium), vitamin, mineral and amino acid deficiencies (see above), and obesity, all of which can affect coat quality and the ability to groom.

One method of preventing this selective feeding is to offer a complete pelleted rabbit food, where each pellet eaten is nutritionally complete. When this is fed twice daily (in small quantities that are consumed over 20 minutes), along with fresh vegetables and ad lib grass and hay, many of the above problems are avoided. The success of wild rabbits is testament to the fact that grass is a balanced source of vitamins, minerals, digestible and indigestible fibre for rabbits.

Obesity: If a rabbit is permitted to selectively feed on carbohydrate-rich mixed rations and gets little exercise, then it will become overweight. Obesity will make grooming certain areas more difficult, predisposing it to skin disease.

Spinal disease and osteoarthritis: Any problem that reduces a rabbit's range of motion will interfere with self-grooming.

Other medical problems: Whilst dental disease, inadequate diet, obesity and spinal problems are often causes of poor grooming, any illness that results in debilitation will obviously reduce a rabbit's ability to groom effectively. Therefore, in cases that are severe or do not respond to initial treatment, a thorough investigation for an underlying cause is important.

EPIDEMIOLOGY

There is little or no published data on the epidemiology of cheyletiellosis. One study has shown that in six laboratory rabbit colonies, each group had subclinical infestations with *Cheyletiella parasitovorax*. The range of infested individuals ranged from 15% to 60% within the colonies, with an overall infestation rate of 43.2%. Other studies have shown the prevalence of infestation to be as high as 70%, but not necessarily associated with any clinical signs. There is no reported genetic link to infestations.

Cheyletiellosis is zoonotic in 30% of cases, resulting in a focal to multifocal dermatitis. Papules are usually present on the forearms and neck, but lesions on the waist and legs have also been described. The mite does not reproduce on the human host; therefore, infestations are self-limiting, provided re-infestation is not occurring. Once affected rabbits are treated, the human lesions tend to regress over 24 hours. Rabbit owners should limit contact with infested rabbits during the treatment period, and gloves should be worn if contact is essential.

TREATMENT OPTIONS

Several treatments have been recommended for ectoparasite control in rabbits, but most are not licensed in the UK.

Ivermectin: Ivermectin is currently the treatment of choice for cheyletiellosis and can be given parenterally,

orally or topically. If used topically, good absorption is achieved by diluting the aqueous solution in propylene glycol at a ratio of 1:10 ivermectin:propylene glycol. At a dose rate of 0.2–0.4 mg/kg for two to three treatments 14 days apart, ivermectin is widely found to be effective against *Cheyletiella*, despite the fact that the mites do not appear to feed on blood. If a group of animals needs treatment, such as a breeding colony of rabbits, then a larger volume of ivermectin in propylene glycol can be made up. This can then be administered to the whole group topically from a spray bottle, at a dose of 0.2–0.4 mg/kg based on the body weight of the group as a whole. More recently, a company has marketed a product containing ivermectin (Xeno450; Genitrix), for *the prevention and treatment of common internal and external parasites of rabbits, guinea-pigs and ferrets.* This is not licensed in the same way as other drugs, but has received a veterinary medicine marketing authorization in accordance with the Small Animal Exemption Scheme (SAES). With respect to the use of medicines according to the veterinary cascade, the legal position is somewhat vague. The SAES does not fall within the confines of the veterinary cascade. Therefore, strictly speaking, we should use ivermectin products licensed in other species for treatment of cheyletiellosis in rabbits. However, this product is specifically marketed for rabbits and may be preferred by some vets and owners. In this author's (SS) opinion, use of either product is acceptable and justifiable, but we should not be misled into thinking that we must use the SAES product. The treatment dose is one tube (0.45 mg ivermectin) per kg, repeated 2 and 4 weeks later. Ivermectin should be avoided in pregnant or lactating animals.

Selamectin: Selamectin is also anecdotally safe and effective at treating mites and lice, and is recommended topically at 6–18 mg/kg, but is not licensed in small mammals. A small dog or cat pipette can be decanted into a syringe and an accurate dose administered. Then the owner can take the remainder home for subsequent dosing. In this author's experience, a single repeated dose after 2–4 weeks has been effective in the majority of cases, but there are no published studies supporting this dosing interval.

Permethrin: Permethrin is another drug marked under the SAES (see above) for the control of flies, fleas, ticks and lice in small mammals. However, studies funded by the manufacturer show it may also be effective against *Cheyletiella*.

Fipronil: Fipronil *has a specific licensed contraindication for use in rabbits.* Interestingly, it is reported to be effective against mites in rabbits and has been used by one author with no adverse effects. However, the therapeutic index is narrow and, due to several reports of suspected adverse reactions, the product is absolutely contraindicated in rabbits. There have been debates about the true cause of mortality following fipronil spray use in rabbits. There may be an idiosyncratic reaction; it may be due to the pungent odour of the alcohol carrier or the effects of chilling if not kept in a warm environment post-application. Given the effectiveness of other treatments for cheyletiellosis in rabbits, treatment with fipronil has no justification.

Shampoos: Removing excess scale can markedly improve the clinical signs of cheyletiellosis in rabbits. Washing the rabbit once or twice weekly with selenium sulphide shampoo is useful in removing the keratin that the mites feed on. It also has reported insecticidal properties but bathing rabbits can be difficult due to their dense fur and the risk of chilling. The stress associated with bathing may also be unacceptable and there are reports of shock and death in rabbits following the use of baths. No medicated shampoos are licensed for use in rabbits.

Lime dips: Weekly lime sulphur dips are very effective against *Cheyletiella* when used for 3–6 weeks.

Imidacloprid: Imidacloprid is one of the few licensed topical ectoparasiticides for use in rabbits. It is used for the treatment of fleas, but is ineffective against *Cheyletiella*. It is reported to be effective for lice but not licensed for that purpose.

Environmental control: Whilst lice live entirely on the host, eggs and adult female *Cheyletiella* can live off the host for up to 10 days in cool conditions; therefore, environmental control is required to eliminate infection. This control can be carried out with most of the household flea sprays currently available. The environment must be well ventilated before replacing the rabbit.

Underlying problems: It is important to remember that any detected underlying cause should also be addressed to reduce the likelihood of recurrence.

TREATMENT

In this case, the rabbit was treated with 0.4 mg/kg ivermectin subcutaneously, every 14 days for three treatments. The in-contact rabbit was also treated in the same way. Whilst the other rabbit showed no clinical signs of disease, it is important to treat in-contact animals in case they act as a reservoir for re-infestation. The owner was advised to thoroughly clean the house and use an environmental insecticide.

There was a marked reduction in the amount of dorsal scurf when presented for the second treatment, and the rabbit continued to appear healthy. By the third treatment the clinical signs had almost completely resolved. There was no recurrence after cessation of treatment.

NURSING ASPECTS

Clipping

Rabbits' skin is thinner than that of dogs and cats, and can therefore be easily torn and traumatized. Patience, good light and not rushing are important when clipping away fur; sometimes sharp scissors are preferable to clippers. The fine fur of rabbits easily becomes trapped in the clipper blades, preventing them from cutting effectively. Stretching the skin out in front of the blades and moving the clippers slowly over the skin will reduce trauma and facilitate effective hair removal. Good quality, well-maintained sharp clippers are essential for rabbits, and preferably a separate pair should be kept solely for use in rabbit patients. Mats in the coat can be gently pulled apart and the dead hair teased out before combing through the rest of the coat. Care is required, since it is possible to rip the skin when trying to pull out mats.

Handling

Most rabbits are used to human contact, and are amenable to being picked up and examined. A gentle but firm approach is required, whilst being ready to restrain the patient more firmly should the need arise. Unhandled rabbits can be sensitive and jumpy in unfamiliar surrounds. If not adequately prepared, the rabbit can easily leap high off the table in front of a horrified owner. Rabbits very rarely bite, although serious scratches can be received by the powerful hind feet.

Lifting

Rabbits can be lifted from a carrier with a hand around each side of the chest, like with cats. If the patient seems nervous, then it can be lifted by the scruff with the other hand supporting the hind legs. Alternatively, rabbits can be wrapped in a towel and lifted from their box. *It is no longer acceptable to lift rabbits by their ears.*

Trancing

Otherwise referred to as hypnosis or tonic immobility, trancing is a transitory, involuntary and reversible state of immobility that can be induced in rabbits by physical restraint on their backs. The animal initially struggles and tries to escape, followed by a period of immobility, which may persist without further restraint. Trancing is ended when the rabbit regains its righting reflux and may occur spontaneously or from external stimulation. It is widely accepted that this is a *terminal defence mechanism*, perhaps reducing the chance of being eaten if caught by a predator; therefore, it is likely to be associated with fear and distress. A recent study showed that during trancing there were increases in respiratory and heart rates, increases in plasma corticosterone levels, fear and struggling during induction, and hiding and displacement activities post-trancing. This suggests that this technique is stressful in rabbits and, although useful for restraint, it is unlikely to be beneficial or pleasurable for the rabbits. Trancing may be referred to as hypnosis, leading to the incorrect belief that the rabbit is happy and relaxed, and it *must not* be used to carry out painful procedures as an alternative to analgesia or anaesthesia.

CLINICAL TIPS

During the initial consultation, a significant portion of time is spent on obtaining a thorough history about all aspects of the rabbit's care. This incorporates lots of information which may not be directly related to a dermatological problem, but is none the less very important. *Three-quarters of problems seen in rabbits and other small mammal pets are due to inadequate husbandry, often resulting from lack of client education.*

Remember that ectoparasitic infestations may be secondary to a more serious underlying disease. If response to treatment is poor, the signs are severe or the rabbit appears to have other problems, then a full diagnostic investigation is indicated.

Dental exam

It is very important to consider dental disease as a contributing factor to, or even primary cause of, cheyletiellosis. Therefore, part of the clinical examination should include dental examination. Rabbits have a small opening to their mouth, the oral cavity is long and their lips are very sensitive to touch, making examination of the teeth more difficult than in dogs and cats. It is fairly straightforward to gently place an otoscope into the oral cavity and examine the teeth, but the veterinary surgeon must appreciate and account for the limitations associated with this technique. Significant dental pathology is easily overlooked, especially of the caudal cheek teeth. Therefore, finding a lesion confirms that treatment is required, but if no abnormalities are detected and the rabbit has potential signs of dental disease, a more thorough examination is required. This is best carried out under general anaesthesia or heavy sedation, using specialist rabbit mouth gags and cheek dilators.

Visualization

Whilst *Cheyletiella* are visible with the naked eye, they are fairly small and easily missed on the animal. Using a hand lens makes visualizing them far easier, although examination of scale under the microscope is preferable.

Blood sampling

Blood may be collected from the marginal ear vein, jugular vein, cephalic vein or saphenous vein depending on the size of the patient. The central ear *artery* should not be used, since this can lead to pinna necrosis if sufficiently damaged. Application of local anaesthetic (EMLA cream) is likely to make sampling easier. Safe blood volumes to take are 7–10 ml/kg, allowing adequate sample collection in most sized rabbits.

17 Pemphigus foliaceus in a cat

INITIAL PRESENTATION

Crusting skin disease.

INTRODUCTION

Pemphigus foliaceus is an uncommon, sterile pustular, autoimmune skin disease that is recognized in both dogs and cats. The pustules quickly rupture, resulting in the formation of extensive crusting of affected areas. The degree of crusting is one of the diagnostic features of this disease. The definitive diagnosis is confirmed by cytology and histopathological examination.

CASE PRESENTING SIGNS

An 11-year-old female, spayed, black and white domestic short hair was presented with a 2-month history of severe crusting skin lesions.

CASE HISTORY

Typically, pemphigus foliaceus presents with a history of crusting skin lesions that most commonly start over the pinnae and face, with later involvement of the trunk and limbs. Paronychia is a common finding in cats. Pruritus may be absent to severe, and many cases show intermittent depression, pyrexia and anorexia. Quite frequently, when questioned, owners may have recognized a waxing and waning of the symptoms over time.

The relevant history in this case was:
- A 3-month history of crusting lesions initially involving the right pinna with later involvement of the left pinna, face, nasal planum and dorsal trunk. She had also developed a purulent and crusting paronychia. There had been no obvious evidence of pruritus or pain.
- The cat also had a 5-year history of glucocorticoid-responsive, summer seasonal ventral pruritus and symmetrical alopecia over the limbs and tail. Pruritus had persisted despite thorough flea control, but the symptoms had been responsive to corticosteroids. However, corticosteroid therapy had precipitated the onset of diabetes mellitus the previous year and treatment had been withdrawn. The symptoms of diabetes mellitus had resolved on treatment withdrawal.
- She had been anorectic and very lethargic for the past 48 hours.
- There was one other cat in the household, a male sibling, that was unaffected.
- There was no evidence of zoonosis.
- The patient had access to the garden area.
- The cat was fed a diet of various proprietary tinned cat foods.
- She had received routine immunization for feline calici virus, rhinotracheitis and leukaemia 8 months previously. She received regular worming treatment, although not for 2 months prior to the onset of the skin lesions. She received monthly applications of fipronil spot-on.
- At the time of examination, the cat had been treated with enrofloxacin at a dosage of 6 mg/kg s.i.d. with no clinical improvement.
- There had been no response to twice daily applications of a triamcinolone-containing cream to the pinnae.
- Previous histopathological examination had shown a non-specific, superficial inflammatory skin disease.

CLINICAL EXAMINATION

- Rectal temperature was 104.2°F.
- There was moderate peripheral lymphadenopathy.

- There was extensive crusting over the pinnae (Fig. 17.1), bridge of the nose (Fig. 17.2), the pre-auricular skin and one focal crusted lesion over the mid dorsum. Removal of the crust revealed shallow, exudative, erosions.
- There was a purulent paronychia affecting some of the digits on all four feet (Fig. 17.3).

DIFFERENTIAL DIAGNOSES

Crusting is caused by leakage of pus, serum or blood onto the skin surface. In this case the colour of the crust was not consistent with haemorrhage but suggested a purulent discharge. One possible origin of such crusts is from a pustular skin disease.

The combined presence of focal crusting lesions affecting the pinnae and bridge of the nose, along with a purulent paronychia, was highly suggestive of pemphigus foliaceus.

Alternative, but less likely, crusting and erosive skin diseases included:

- Pyoderma
- Dermatophytosis
- Cutaneous or systemic lupus erythematosus
- Vasculopathy or vasculitis
- Cutaneous drug reaction
- Squamous cell carcinoma.

CASE WORK-UP

Cytology is an essential diagnostic tool where there is an exudative discharge. Fungal culture was also indicated to rule out any involvement of dermatophytosis.

The following diagnostic tests were performed:

- Cytology of pus from beneath crusted lesions and from the nail folds, which showed numerous neutrophils and acantholytic keratinocytes (Fig. 17.4).
- Cytology of pus from the nail folds also revealed small numbers of cocci and rods.
- Fungal culture of material taken using a toothbrush technique, which did not grow dermatophytes.
- Histopathological examination of four samples from representative skin lesions, harvested using a 6-mm biopsy punch. There was a mixed superficial perivascular dermatitis, mild to moderate irregular epidermal

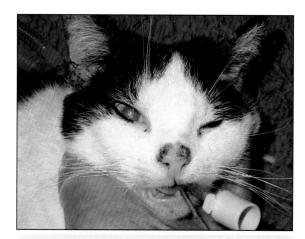

Figure 17.2 Crusting over the bridge of the nose and pinnae.

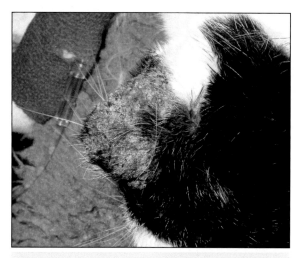

Figure 17.1 Severe crusting on the pinnae.

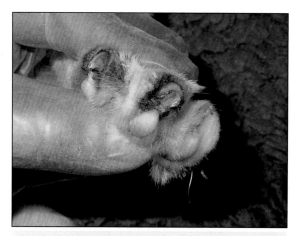

Figure 17.3 Purulent and crusting paronychia.

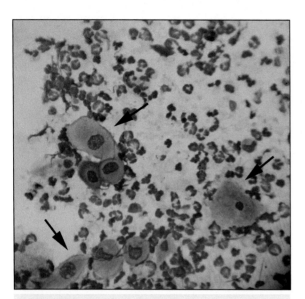

Figure 17.4 Neutrophils and acantholytic keratinocytes (arrowed) on cytology preparation from a cat with pemphigus foliaceus. ×1000 original magnification. Diff Quik® stain.

hyperplasia, and subcorneal pustules/crusts containing mainly non-degenerate polymorphonuclear cells and numerous acantholytic keratinocytes. There was no evidence of bacteria, mites and dermatophytes in the sections examined.

- A blood sample was taken. Routine haematological and biochemical examinations were unremarkable, and FeLV and FIV serology were negative.

DIAGNOSIS

The history, clinical signs, cytological and histopathological examinations, and the negative fungal culture, were consistent with a diagnosis of pemphigus foliaceus.

PROGNOSIS

The prognosis for feline and canine pemphigus foliaceus is very variable. Mildly affected cases with localized lesions may respond to topical medications. At the other end of the spectrum, there are very severe cases that may be refractory to therapy or that may develop life-threatening side-effects to treatment. In young animals, permanent resolution may follow successful medical therapy; in other cases, ongoing therapy is required to prevent recrudescence.

AETIOLOGICAL AND PATHOPHYSIOLOGICAL ASPECTS OF PEMPHIGUS FOLIACEUS

Pemphigus foliaceus is currently considered a heterogeneous autoimmune skin disease, resulting from the formation of predominantly IgG1 and IgG4 autoantibodies that target the intercellular spaces of the stratum spinosum and stratum granulosum of the epidermis. The precise target(s) (autoantigens) of these antibodies remain(s) unclear. There have been no studies reporting the nature of the specific autoantigen in cats, but a considerable amount of work has been done in looking for the autoantigen in canine pemphigus foliaceus. It was originally thought that the major autoantigen was desmoglein-1, a component of the desmosomes, which are responsible for keratinocyte–keratinocyte adhesion in the epidermis of the skin and hair follicles, but recent work has shown that this is an antigen of minor importance in canine pemphigus foliaceus, highlighting the heterogeneous nature of this disease.

Pustule formation: The exact mechanism of pustule formation in association with antibody formation is complex and incompletely elucidated. However, antibody binding to desmosomal structures leads to the release of plasminogen by keratinocytes that results in activation of plasmin, a protease that destroys desmosomal structures, leading to acantholysis and the separation of keratinocytes in the stratum spinosum. The clefts thus formed are filled by neutrophils migrating into the epidermis from the circulation to form pustules. Acantholytic keratinocytes, cells that have become detached from the stratum spinosum as a result of the acantholytic process, are also present within the pustules. These cells are nucleated, as opposed to the fully differentiated cells of the stratum corneum that have lost their nuclei. They tend to have a rounded appearance and have basophilic staining characteristics. The cytological finding of acantholytic keratinocytes combined with a neutrophilic infiltrate is consistent with pemphigus foliaceus, but may also be found in cases of bacterial pyoderma and also dermatophytosis, particularly in cases of infection with *Trichophyton* spp.

Trigger factors

Drug induced: Most cases of pemphigus foliaceus in both cats and dogs appear spontaneously. However, a subset of cases may be drug induced and, in these cases, the disease should resolve when the drug is discontinued. Drug-related pemphigus foliaceus has been reported following administration of cefalexin and trimethoprim-potentiated sulphonamides in dogs, and ampicillin and methimazole in cats.

Chronic skin disease: Anecdotally, dermatologists report cases of canine pemphigus foliaceus that occur in association with a history of chronic skin disease. Typically, these cases have a history of chronic inflammatory, pruritic skin disease and then suddenly develop a more severe disease associated with pustules and crusting, diagnosed as pemphigus foliaceus. Whether there is a cause and effect association with the chronic skin disease is not clear. There is the possibility that some of these cases may be a cutaneous drug reaction associated with drugs used to treat the chronic skin disease.

Sunlight: There is some evidence that sunlight exposure may be a triggering factor for pemphigus foliaceus, particularly in lesions affecting the face. Some experimental work has found that UVB exposure of non-lesional skin from a dog with facial pemphigus foliaceus led to acantholysis.

EPIDEMIOLOGY

There is little epidemiological information on the incidence of either canine or feline pemphigus foliaceus; however, this is an uncommon condition, with a reported incidence in one referral hospital population of only 0.3% of patients referred for skin disease. It does, however, account for around one-third of canine autoimmune skin diseases, and in the authors' experience is the most common autoimmune skin disease in cats.

No definitive breed predisposition has been reported in the cat. Some studies have shown a familial incidence of canine pemphigus foliaceus in the Japanese akita, Dobermann, Finnish spitz, schipperke, bearded collie, Newfoundland, dachshund, English cocker spaniel, chow-chow and Shar Pei. There appears to be no age or sex predisposition in either cats or dogs.

TREATMENT OPTIONS

Glucocorticoids

Glucocorticoids are the mainstay of treatment for pemphigus foliaceus. Mild focal lesions may be responsive to topical therapy, but more severely affected cases require immunosuppressive doses of corticosteroids to achieve remission.

General guidelines: It is beneficial to use the highest recommended dosage until clinical signs abate, because this usually results in the quickest clinical response and, ultimately, a lower total cumulative glucocorticoid dosage. Short-acting glucocorticoids such as prednisolone or methylprednisolone are the drugs of choice. Cats generally require higher dosages than dogs to achieve the same clinical effect; one reason for this is they have fewer glucocorticoid receptors. Treatment is administered until complete remission of clinical signs and then the dosage is very gradually tapered down over a period of months to maintenance levels. If there is a poor response to prednisolone or methylprednisolone, then triamcinolone, betamethasone or dexamethasone may be administered.

Immunosuppressive glucocorticoid dosages for induction and maintenance:
Prednisolone
- Induction: *dogs*, 2–4 mg/kg/day divided twice daily; *cats*, 4–6 mg/kg/day divided twice daily.
- Maintenance: *dogs*, 0.5–2 mg/kg on alternate days; *cats*, 1–4 mg/kg on alternate days.

Methylprednisolone
- Induction: *dogs*, 1.5–3 mg/kg/day divided twice daily; *cats*, 3–5 mg/kg/day divided twice daily.
- Maintenance: *dogs*, 0.4–1.5 mg/kg on alternate days; *cats*, 0.8–2.5 mg/kg on alternate days.

Dexamethasone/betamethasone
- Induction: *dogs*, 0.3–0.6 mg/kg s.i.d.; *cats*, 0.4–1 mg/kg s.i.d.
- Maintenance: *dogs*, 0.05–0.1 mg/kg every 2–3 days; *cats*, 0.1–0.2 mg/kg every 2–3 days.

Adverse effects of glucocorticoids: Glucocorticoids, particularly at these dosages, will commonly result in adverse effects. In general, cats are more resistant to the side-effects of glucocorticoids than dogs. Short-term side-effects of glucocorticoids in dogs and cats can include polyuria, polydipsia, polyphagia, panting, mood alteration including aggression, and diarrhoea. Long-term side-effects include the signs of iatrogenic hyperadrenocorticism: weight gain, redistribution of body fat and muscle atrophy leading to a pot-bellied appearance, hepatomegaly, alopecia, comedone formation, calcinosis cutis (dogs only), pyoderma and demodicosis. Urinary tract infections, diabetes mellitus, pancreatitis and gastrointestinal ulceration are other potential complications. Skin fragility is a rare but serious side-effect in cats treated with glucocorticoids. Recently, congestive cardiac failure has been reported in cats, particularly following long-acting glucocorticoid injections. Sudden withdrawal of glucocorticoids, following prolonged administration, can lead to an Addisonian crisis.

Chlorambucil

The alkylating agent chlorambucil is commonly used, in addition to systemic glucocorticoids, at a dosage of 0.1–0.2 mg/kg q24 h/48 h for the management of pemphigus foliaceus in small dogs and cats. A 2-mg tablet is the smallest tablet size available in the UK, and to avoid the necessity of the owner having to break the tablets, a 2-mg tablet is generally administered on alternate days to treat cats weighing between 4 and 6 kg. Chlorambucil is not licensed for use in animals in the UK. Alkylating agents are slow acting and a case treated solely with chlorambucil could take up to 8 weeks to respond, which is why these drugs are generally administered with glucocorticoids. However, in the longer term, their use can reduce the cumulative dose of glucocorticoids required to achieve and maintain remission of the disease.

The adverse effects of chlorambucil include gradual bone marrow suppression, including neutropenia and thrombocytopenia, alopecia and gastrointestinal disturbance. Cerebellar toxicity has been reported when administered at very high doses.

Azathioprine

The purine synthesis inhibitor, azathioprine, is another treatment option that may be considered in addition to glucocorticoid therapy for the treatment of canine pemphigus foliaceus. **However, there is a high risk of irreversible bone marrow suppression with the use of azathioprine in cats and the drug should not be used in this species.**

Azathioprine is metabolized in the liver to 6-mercaptopurine, the active metabolite, which affects the formation of nucleic acids. The primary effect of the drug is inhibition of T cell lymphocyte function and T cell-dependent antibody synthesis with little effect on B cells. Azathioprine has a slow onset of action and frequently takes 4–6 weeks to be effective. In view of the slow onset, it is usually initially administered along with glucocorticoids. Ultimately, in long-term control of the disease, azathioprine may have a glucocorticoid-sparing effect or it may be possible to withdraw glucocorticoid therapy altogether. The dosage in dogs is usually given at 2 mg/kg s.i.d. (1.2–2.5 mg/kg). If there is no clinical response and no evidence of lymphopenia after 4–6 weeks, the dosage may be increased. Once remission is achieved, it may be possible to reduce to alternate-day therapy.

There are two main pathways for metabolism of 6-mercaptopurine. Firstly, thiopurine methyl transferase (TPMT) activity results in methylation and oxidation and, secondly, xanthine oxidase, present in the liver, metabolizes azathioprine to 6-thiouric acid, an inactive compound. Low levels of erythrocyte TPMT activity are associated with increased drug toxicity in man and low TPMT has also been demonstrated in some dogs.

The principal toxic effect of azathioprine is bone marrow suppression with thrombocytopenia and anaemia. In general, this develops gradually. Lymphopenia is a frequent finding and appears to correlate with a favourable therapeutic response. Other adverse effects include diarrhoea, which may be haemorrhagic; hepatotoxicity; and acute pancreatitis – possibly due to decreased pancreatic secretion.

Close patient monitoring is advisable when using azathioprine and should initially include haematology (including platelets) and biochemistry every 2 weeks. After the disease has been controlled and dosages are being tapered, monitoring may be reduced to every 2–3 months.

Ciclosporin and tacrolimus

Both ciclosporin and tacrolimus are immunosuppressive agents that have the potential to treat autoimmune disease. These drugs block regulatory proteins that up-regulate activation genes of T helper lymphocytes, particularly interleukin-2, a cytokine responsible for lymphocyte proliferation. However, up to the time of writing, there has been no published evidence as to the efficacy of ciclosporin in the treatment of pemphigus foliaceus in cats. A small-scale study using ciclosporin to treat canine pemphigus foliaceus showed a very poor response rate, although this may have been a reflection of inadequate dosage. Tacrolimus was reported to be helpful in the treatment of canine pemphigus erythematosus, but this is a localized disease, and tacrolimus has the potential for severe toxicity if administered systemically and so was not an option for the treatment of the generalized disease in this cat.

Chrysotherapy

Gold has immune-modulating effects, but its exact mode of action is unknown. Aurothioglucose was reported to be effective for the treatment of pemphigus in cats, but it is no longer available. The only preparation now available is sodium aurothiomalate, but there are no reports on its use for the treatment of feline pemphigus foliaceus. Toxic reactions to gold therapy in cats and dogs include bone marrow suppression, oral ulceration and glomerulonephropathy. One drawback to using gold injections is that they have to be given by painful deep intramuscular injection. Routine monitoring when using gold should include a complete blood count every 2–3 weeks, and full serum biochemical examination and urinalysis every 4–6 weeks for the first few months of therapy. These tests should be repeated every 3–6 months thereafter.

Treatment in this case

The extent and severity of the lesions in this case were an indication to use a treatment which was going to be both effective and produce a rapid therapeutic effect.

The decision was made to start treatment with a combination of prednisolone at a dosage of 4 mg/kg divided b.i.d. and chlorambucil (2 mg on alternate days). The owner understood that there was a significant risk of inducing diabetes mellitus with this treatment.

Within 3 weeks, there had been an improvement in the appearance of the lesions with resolution of pinnal crusting and paronychia, although the dorsal crusting lesions persisted, but after 6 weeks of treatment all crusting lesions had resolved (Figs 17.5, 17.6 and 17.7).

Glycosuria and hyperglycaemia were evident on repeat haematological and biochemical examinations after 2 weeks of glucocorticoid therapy, and so insulin therapy was initiated.

The treatment of an autoimmune skin disease is a balance between giving sufficiently high dosages of medication to achieve remission and yet not inducing serious adverse effects. On occasions, this can be a difficult balance to achieve. Drug dosages vary from patient to patient and depend on the response to treatment, the severity of adverse effects monitored clinically, and on the results of haematological and biochemical parameters. Once remission has been achieved, it is important to taper drug dosages as slowly as possible; rapid dose reductions can result in earlier and more severe recrudescence of disease. Drug dosages should be tapered to the level at which the disease is just observed to recur. This is the only way to establish the lowest drug dosages required for long-term control of disease.

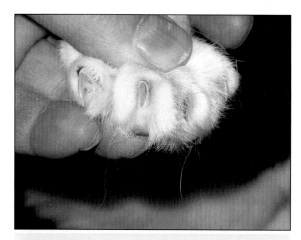

Figure 17.6 Resolution of skin lesions following treatment with prednisolone and chlorambucil.

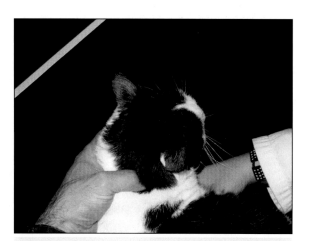

Figure 17.5 Resolution of skin lesions following treatment with prednisolone and chlorambucil.

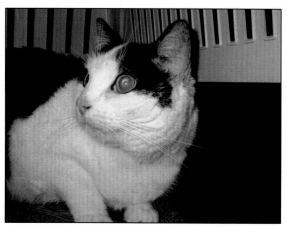

Figure 17.7 Resolution of skin lesions following treatment with prednisolone and chlorambucil.

NURSING ASPECTS

In severe cases of pemphigus foliaceus in both cats and dogs, gentle bathing to remove the crust will speed resolution of the disease and be soothing to the animal. A whirlpool bath is the best way to accomplish this, but soaks in a warm bath or gentle use of a shower head will have a similar beneficial effect. Plain water should be used rather than shampoos or detergent-based products.

Nurses should be familiar with the side-effects of glucocorticoid and other immunosuppressive therapies.

FOLLOW-UP

Over a 4-month period, the dosage of prednisolone was gradually reduced (Table 17.1). Routine haematology and biochemistry were initially performed fortnightly and urinalysis weekly, as shown in Table 17.1. Insulin therapy was required until the prednisolone dosage was reduced to 1 mg daily, at which point it could be discontinued without glycosuria or hyperglycaemia. Alternate-day chlorambucil therapy was maintained throughout the treatment course. The owner noted recurrence of erythema and scaling over the pinnae when the alternate-day prednisolone dosage was reduced to 1 mg on alternate days, which resolved when increased to 1.5 mg on alternate days. At the time of writing, the cat has been maintained on prednisolone (1.5 mg) alternating with chlorambucil (2 mg) for the past 8 months without recurrence of the skin lesions.

Table 17.1 Example of prednisolone and chlorambucil (values in parentheses) drug dosage reductions for treatment of pemphigus foliaceus*

Week	Day 1 A.m.	Day 1 P.m.	Day 2 A.m.	Day 2 P.m.	Day 3 A.m.	Day 3 P.m.	Day 4 A.m.	Day 4 P.m.	Day 5 A.m.	Day 5 P.m.	Day 6 A.m.	Day 6 P.m.	Day 7 A.m.	Day 7 P.m.
1	10	10	10	10 (2)	10	10	10	10 (2)	10	10	10	10 (2)	10	10
2 (CBC/B)	7.5	7.5 (2)	7.5	7.5	7.5	7.5 (2)	7.5	7.5	7.5	7.5 (2)	7.5	7.5	7.5	7.5 (2)
3	7.5	7.5	7.5	7.5 (2)	7.5	7.5	7.5	7.5 (2)	7.5	7.5	7.5	7.5 (2)	7.5	7.5
4 (CBC/B)	5.0	5.0 (2)	5.0	5.0	5.0	5.0 (2)	5.0	5.0	5.0	5.0 (2)	5.0	5.0	5.0	5.0 (2)
5	5.0	5.0	5.0	5.0 (2)	5.0	5.0	5.0	5.0 (2)	5.0	5.0	5.0	5.0 (2)	5.0	5.0
6 (CBC/B)	5.0	2.5 (2)	5.0	2.5	5.0	2.5 (2)	5.0	2.5	5.0	2.5 (2)	5.0	2.5	5.0	2.5 (2)
7	5.0	2.5	5.0	2.5 (2)	5.0	2.5	5.0	2.5 (2)	5.0	2.5	5.0	2.5 (2)	5.0	2.5
8	5.0	(2)			5.0	(2)	5.0			(2)	5.0		5.0	(2)
9	4.0		5.0				4.0	(2)	4.0		4.0	(2)	4.0	
10 (CBC/B)	3.0	(2)	3.0		3.0	(2)	3.0		3.0	(2)	3.0		3.0	(2)
11	2.5		2.5	(2)	2.5		2.5	(2)	2.5		2.5	(2)	2.5	
12	2.0	(2)	2.0		2.0	(2)	2.0		2.0	(2)	2.0		2.0	(2)
13	1.5		1.5	(2)	1.5		1.5	(2)	1.5		1.5	(2)	1.5	
14	1.0	(2)	1.0		1.0	(2)	1.0		1.0	(2)	1.0		1.0	(2)
15	2.0		0	(2)	2.0		0	(2)	2.0		0	(2)	2.0	
16 (CBC/B)	0	(2)	2.0		0	(2)	2.0		0	(2)	2.0		0	(2)
17	1.5		0	(2)	1.5		0	(2)	1.5		0	(2)	1.5	
18	0	(2)	1.5		0	(2)	1.5		0	(2)	1.5		0	(2)
19	1.0		0	(2)	1.0		0	(2)	1.0		0	(2)	1.0	
20	0	(2)	1.0		0	(2)	1.0		0	(2)	1.0		0	(2)
21	1.5		0	(2)	1.5		0	(2)	1.5		0	(2)	1.5	

*Dosages shown in mg. B, biochemistry; CBC, complete blood count.

CLINICAL TIPS

The diagnosis of pemphigus foliaceus is based on a combination of clinical signs, and cytological and histopathological examinations.

Clinical signs in cats

In contrast to canine pemphigus foliaceus, feline lesions tend to be milder, and feline pustules are very fragile and quickly rupture and form crusts. A purulent, sometimes caseous, paronychia affecting the majority of the digits is a frequent finding in cats with pemphigus foliaceus.

Clinical signs in dogs

Intact pustules are more likely to be seen in canine pemphigus foliaceus; they tend to be large and may span multiple hair follicles.

Lesion distribution

Although the disease can be generalized in both cats and dogs, predilection sites include the medial aspects of the pinnae, the bridge of the nose, footpads and the nasal planum. The presence of pustules or focal crusted macules over the medial aspects of the pinnae is strongly suggestive of pemphigus foliaceus.

Sampling

The diagnosis of pemphigus foliaceus is based on cytology and histopathology. An intact pustule is the best lesion to sample both for cytology and for histopathology, but they are fragile transient lesions and rapidly rupture to form crusts. Furthermore, the disease waxes and wanes and pustules may be formed for only a few hours to days, followed by a long period of crusting. Thus, in many cases, there may be no pustules when the animal is presented and, in this situation, direct impressions for cytological evaluation may be made from the underside of crust. Similarly, crusted erosions may be sampled for histopathological examination. In these situations, the diagnosis of pemphigus foliaceus is made by examination of the crust and it is important to include the crust in the submission, particularly if it becomes detached from the underlying skin during the biopsy process.

Antibacterials

The diagnosis of pemphigus foliaceus should not be based solely on finding neutrophils and acantholytic keratinocytes on cytology, because the latter cells may be seen in cases of pyoderma and dermatophytosis. Thus, it is advisable to perform fungal cultures and start systemic antibacterial therapy while waiting on the results of the histopathological examination. Some of these cases of apparent pemphigus foliaceus respond completely to antibacterials.

18 Metabolic epidermal necrosis

INITIAL PRESENTATION

Erythema, crusting, exudation and fissuring associated with hepatic disease in a dog.

INTRODUCTION

Metabolic epidermal necrosis (MEN), also known as superficial necrolytic dermatitis, necrolytic migratory erythema and hepatocutaneous syndrome, is a cutaneous reaction pattern associated with systemic disease. In dogs it has been associated with hepatic disease (cirrhosis, neoplasia and hepatitis), glucagon-secreting pancreatic tumours, with antiepileptic drugs such as phenytoin and phenobarbitone, and with mycotoxins. In humans, it is mostly associated with glucagon-secreting pancreatic tumours, although it may also be found in patients with liver cirrhosis or celiac disease. Recently, MEN has been subdivided into those cases associated with hepatic dysfunction and without a pancreatic tumour (MEN-HS), cases associated with a glucagon-secreting pancreatic syndrome (MEN-GS), and cases where there are raised liver enzymes, but the presence of a pancreatic tumour is not conclusively ruled out (MEN-ND).

CASE PRESENTING SIGNS

An 11-and-a-half-year-old, spayed cross-breed was presented with facial and pedal dermatitis and lameness.

CASE HISTORY

Duration of the condition at presentation is usually a few days to a few weeks. Most cases present with progressive skin lesions consisting of erythema, crusting and scaling over pressure areas and, frequently, lameness. These symptoms are poorly responsive to any treatment although there may be temporary improvement with antimicrobial therapy. There may be a history suggestive of systemic involvement with lethargy and perhaps anorexia. There may be gastrointestinal signs associated with hepatic dysfunction and many dogs develop concurrent diabetes mellitus resulting in polyuria and polydipsia. Pruritus is uncommon, but owners may report that the dog is foot licking.

The relevant history in this case was:
- The dog was in pain and was reluctant to walk.
- There was a poor response to non-steroidal analgesia (carprofen) and antibiotic treatment.
- The dog showed reduced appetite.
- Polydipsia without polyuria was observed.
- Pedal lesions had developed rapidly, and consisted of erythema, crusting and exudation on the plantar aspects of the feet, associated lameness and a reluctance to walk. Similar changes had developed over the elbows and the lip margins within a few weeks of the onset of the foot lesions.
- The dog had been fed on proprietary commercial canned and dried food since puppyhood. The food was stored in a dry environment and there had been no signs of mould growth on the food.
- The in-contact dogs were not affected.

CLINICAL EXAMINATION

General examination may reveal hepatic enlargement and abdominal pain, or may be unremarkable. A cutaneous examination usually reveals symmetrical facial and pedal distribution of lesions. Other areas of friction are commonly affected, and in some cases lesions on the ventral abdomen and other mucocutaneous sites may develop as the condition advances. Lesions usually consist of thick adherent crusts, erythema, exudation, erosions, ulceration and fissuring. The footpads are almost always involved, with lesions ranging from mild to severe hyperkeratosis, erosions and fissuring. Lesions on the ventral abdomen resemble target lesions, with a central area of hyperpigmentation surrounded by crusts and scale which can progressively coalesce to involve large areas. Often, secondary bacterial and *Malassezia* colonization is also reported.

In this case the relevant findings on clinical examination were:

- Anterior abdominal discomfort was noted during a general examination.
- There was a symmetrical distribution of lesions affecting the commissures of the lips, lateral aspects of the elbows and the feet.
- Detailed examination revealed marked erythema and exudation of the plantar skin, mild crusting on the margins of the pads, and erosion and fissuring of the pads themselves (Fig. 18.1).
- Paronychia was evident on some of the digits (Fig. 18.2).
- Crusting and scaling lesions were also present on the elbows (Fig. 18.3) and the lip commissures.

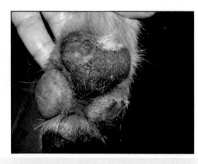

Figure 18.1 Erythema, fissuring, depigmentation, crusting and exudation on the foot.

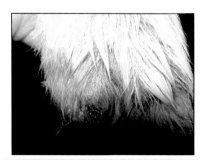

Figure 18.2 Pus, erythema and swelling on the digit.

DIFFERENTIAL DIAGNOSES

There are a number of diseases which affect the footpads and the differential diagnosis included:

- Metabolic epidermal necrosis
- Erythema multiforme
- Adverse drug reaction
- Sterile neutrophilic dermatitis (resembling Sweet's syndrome)
- Pemphigus foliaceus
- Vasculitis
- Systemic lupus erythematosus
- Zinc-responsive dermatosis
- Generic food dermatosis
- Contact allergic or irritant dermatitis.

Some of the conditions, like zinc-responsive dermatosis and generic food dermatosis, were unlikely because of the subject's age, breed and the dietary history. However, a systematic case work-up is always required to confirm the diagnosis.

CASE WORK-UP

Haematology and biochemistry are indicated in these cases. Abormalities are seen in dogs with MEN-HS, but not necessarily in dogs with MEN-GS. Elevated liver enzymes (alkaline phosphatase, alanine aminotransferase, aspartate aminotransferase) are a very common finding in cases of MEN-HS.

Serum amino acid assays may document hypoaminoacidaemia but this is not generally performed in practice.

A glucagon assay can be performed and may help to determine whether a glucagon-secreting tumour is responsible for the cutaneous signs. However, this assay

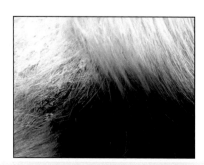

Figure 18.3 Scaling and hyperkeratosis on the elbow.

has special sampling and transport requirements because glucagon is an unstable hormone. Furthermore, both the test and the cost of transport to the laboratory are expensive.

Histology is indicated with this presentation and most of the conditions on the differential list may be diagnosed on histopathological examination. Metabolic epidermal necrosis has characteristic histological changes, including parakeratotic hyperkeratosis, intracellular oedema of keratinocytes and superficial perivascular to interstitial dermal inflammation.

Ultrasonagraphy is a useful non-invasive diagnostic tool to assess and differentiate between MEN-GS and MEN-HS.

Surgical exploration: Gross examination of the liver via a laparotomy and liver biopsy could be considered for a further evaluation.

The following diagnostic tests were performed:
- Cytology. Tape-strip preparations from the feet revealed keratinocytes and coccoid bacteria.
- Haematology and biochemistry. In this case, alanine aminotransferase (625 U/l; normal reference range 10–100 U/L) and alkaline phosphatase (440 U/l; normal reference range 20–200 U/L) were markedly raised. Blood glucose (5.4 mmol/l) and haematological parameters were within reference ranges. Pre- and postprandial bile acid levels were within normal limits. Urinalysis was unremarkable.
- Histopathology. In this case several skin samples were obtained by punch biopsy under general anaesthesia. Samples were taken from the edge of the footpads, other crusted lesions, the ventral interdigital skin and elbow. They revealed orthokeratotic and parakeratotic hyperkeratosis, intracellular oedema of epidermal keratinocytes, epidermal hyperplasia with the formation of rete ridges and a mixture of inflammatory cells in the superficial dermis. This has been described as the 'pink, white and blue zones' when sections are examined under low-power magnification (Fig. 18.4). Apoptosis and hydropic changes of the basal epidermis and interface dermatitis were absent. These findings supported the diagnosis of metabolic epidermal necrosis.
- In this case, an abdominal ultrasound examination revealed a grossly abnormal liver with a nodular appearance of hepatic lobes (Fig. 18.5). A fine-needle aspirate biopsy was obtained during this procedure, which revealed a mixture of inflammatory cells in the

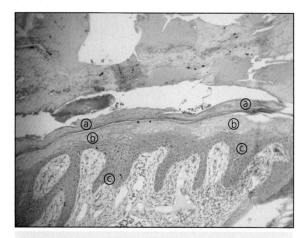

Figure 18.4 Pink (a), white (b) and blue (c) zones on a histological section showing parakeratosis, intracellular oedema of the spinous layer and epidermal hyperplasia respectively. This is considered pathognomic for metabolic epidermal necrosis.

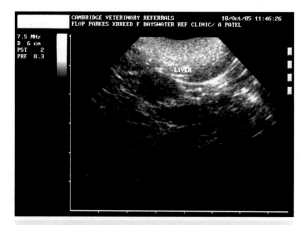

Figure 18.5 Abdominal ultrasound showing hypoechoeic changes throughout the liver parenchyma. (Courtesy of P. Mannion.)

aspirate, but a conclusive diagnosis was not possible by this method. Other abdominal organs, including the pancreas, were of normal appearance. Ultrasound-guided fine-needle aspirates of the liver have their limitations, as the exact changes in liver architecture cannot be determined and the aspirate sample may have cells that are not representative of the pathological change.

The owner in this case declined the exploratory laparotomy because of the poor overall prognosis.

DIAGNOSIS

A diagnosis of metabolic epidermal necrosis associated with hepatic dysfunction and secondary skin infection was made.

PROGNOSIS

The prognosis is poor, but the quality of life can be improved in some cases with supportive treatment.

PATHOPHYSIOLOGY

Most canine cases are associated with hepatic disease; however, the condition is also associated with glucagon-secreting pancreatic tumours.

MEN-HS

Hepatic abnormalities are documented in dogs with MEN-HS, by abnormally raised liver enzymes, through dynamic function tests and/or by ultrasound examination. Individuals with liver cirrhosis, hepatic neoplasia, and presumed hepatotoxicity due to mycotoxins and anticonvulsant drugs are included in this group. A recent study demonstrated that serum amino acid concentration in dogs diagnosed with MEN was significantly lower than in normal dogs and in those with acute or chronic hepatitis. It has been suggested that increased amino acid catabolism, because of a hepatopathy, explains the resulting hypoaminoacidaemia. This depletion results in epidermal necrosis, but the pathway that leads to the necrosis is not known.

MEN-GS

A direct link between removal of a glucagon-secreting pancreatic tumour and the resolution of the skin lesions has been demonstrated in people. MEN-GS has been reported in only a very small number of dogs. Elevated glucagon levels have been documented in some canine cases; however, this test has its limitations in general practice (see 'Case work-up' section). Hypoaminoacidaemia, due to the catabolic effects of excessive glucagon, is thought to be responsible for the skin lesions. It has been postulated that the epidermis is particularly susceptible, because its constant growth requires a continuous supply of proteins and amino acids. Depletion of this supply may lead to epidermal necrosis. It has also been suggested that an aberrant zinc and/or fatty acid metabolism may be involved in the pathogenesis.

EPIDEMIOLOGY

This is an uncommon condition seen in older dogs with an average age of onset of 10 years. It can occur in any breed, but small breeds such as West Highland white terriers, Shetland sheepdogs, cocker spaniels and Scottish terriers are over-represented in the literature. Studies have shown that male dogs are also over-represented.

TREATMENT

There are a number of documented options to improve the quality of life for the animal. They involve:
- Nutritional support
- Antimicrobial treatment
- Supplements
- Antifibrotics
- Surgery.

Nutritional support

Good quality protein and commercial diets, specifically for liver disease, are recommended in all cases. Daily supplementation of egg yolks (four per day) are recommended for long-term support. Hypoaminoacidaemia is responsible for the cutaneous lesions and reversing this has shown to help some dogs. Amino acids can be administered orally or intravenously. An amino acid supplementation may be given orally in the form of a powder (ProMod®; Abbott) added to the food. This is a cost-effective supplementation available on prescription. Intravenous amino acids infused through a central vein slowly over 6–8 hours can produce a dramatic clinical improvement in some cases for variable periods of time. This treatment is repeated weekly. Suitable intravenous amino acid preparations are available in both the UK and USA. However, problems associated with the intravenous infusion of hypertonic solutions can occur (see 'Nursing aspects').

Antimicrobial treatment

Antimicrobial therapy for secondary infections is recommended. Systemic antibacterial therapy is indicated if there is significant bacterial infection but if malasseziosis is present, topical treatment is recommended at the first instance with resort to systemic antifungal therapy if there is a poor response. Note that many of the systemic antifungals can result in raised liver enzymes and can cause gastrointestinal disturbances in some cases.

Supplements

Essential fatty acid supplementation is reported to help some dogs, possibly because it helps maintain epidermal function. Additionally, vitamins K and B, and zinc sulphate (10 mg/kg s.i.d.), zinc gluconate (5 mg/kg s.i.d.) or zinc picolinate (1.5 mg/kg s.i.d.) should be supplemented to the diet of dogs with MEN.

Antifibrotics

Colchicine, an antifibrotic agent used for inhibiting progression of cirrhosis, given at 0.3 mg/kg/day, helped one dog and lengthened its life. Confirmation of fibrotic changes associated with liver cirrhosis is necessary before prescribing colchicine, which may require a laparotomy to take liver biopsies. Colchicine is unlicensed for veterinary use and written informed consent is needed for its use in an animal.

Surgery

The surgical excision of a glucagon-secreting tumour can reverse the clinical signs in people. This effect has also been reported in dogs, but postoperative complications of pancreatitis and biliary obstruction have also been reported. Surgical excision is not an option if the tumour has metastasized.

Treatment in this case

In this case amoxicillin/clavulanate (12.5 mg/kg b.i.d.) was prescribed for the secondary bacterial infection. Antifungals were not indicated. Egg yolks, ProMod® (Abbott) and Hills canine l/d were given to the dog. Essential fatty acid at the manufacturer's recommended dose was also administered. Zinc supplementation was not deemed to be necessary as the dog was being fed a prescription diet with a high zinc content.

NURSING ASPECTS

- Bathing exudative and ulcerated lesions with chlorhexidine to remove crusts may make the dog more comfortable.
- Nursing care is essential if intravenous amino acids are supplemented. These are better administered through a central vein, because the risk of thrombophlebitis increases with administration through a peripheral vein. Other side-effects of a hypertonic solution include oedema and cellulitis.

CLINICAL TIPS

- Histology is necessary to confirm the diagnosis of the cutaneous lesions, but identifying the systemic cause can sometimes prove challenging.
- Abdominal ultrasound is best performed by an experienced person, or referred to a specialist, as some of the changes can be subtle.
- Management of the condition is potentially costly and it is best to give the owner a realistic picture of all potential outcomes prior to commencing therapy. Some owners prefer to opt for euthanasia and in some cases this is the most humane course of action.

FOLLOW-UP

The dog was euthanized after 4 weeks of treatment, because of anorexia and cachexia.

Zinc-responsive dermatosis

Crusting and scaling over pressure points.

INTRODUCTION

There are various canine nutrient-responsive dermatoses described, including vitamin A- and zinc-responsive dermatoses and essential fatty acid deficiency. These conditions may be associated with dietary deficiencies or imbalances, or genetic defects resulting in an inability to absorb nutrients. With the ready availability of good quality diets over the last two decades, conditions resulting from dietary deficiency are uncommon to rare but can still occur. This report describes a case of zinc-responsive dermatosis associated with the feeding of a poor quality, predominantly cereal-based diet.

CASE PRESENTING SIGNS

A 3-year-old, entire male Border collie was presented with crusting and pruritus.

CASE HISTORY

The history in zinc-responsive dermatoses will tend to vary depending on the breed of dog affected (see 'Aetiopathogenesis' section). Syndrome II zinc-responsive dermatosis most commonly affects puppies fed zinc-deficient diets but a change of diet or gastro-intestinal disease can result in symptoms in an adult dog. One study from North America showed that most Northern breed dogs developed lesions during the winter months. Initial lesions tend to be erythematous, with subsequently alopecia, crusting and scaling over pressure point areas and areas of skin trauma. Affected dogs are variably pruritic.

The history in this case was as follows:
- The dog had been acquired by the owner as a puppy at 2 months of age.
- There was no previous history of skin disease.
- A few months previously, prior to the onset of skin lesions, the patient had developed persistent diarrhoea which had resolved with a change from tinned dog food to a cereal-based diet.
- Within a few weeks of the change of diet, the dog had developed a pruritic, crusting scrotal dermatitis. In addition, crusting lesions had developed around the eyes and lips.
- The dog was slightly depressed, although appetite and thirst were unaffected.
- Antibacterial therapy using cefalexin at a dosage of 20 mg/kg b.i.d. had resulted in no improvement.
- There were no other pets in the household.
- There was no evidence of zoonosis.

CLINICAL EXAMINATION

Zinc-responsive dermatosis predominantly affects areas of the skin subject to 'microtrauma', such as the perioral and periocular skin, the elbows, hocks and footpads. The nasal planum may be affected. Early lesions are erythematous with subsequent alopecia, crusting and scaling. Erosions underlie the crust.

In this case:
- The patient was afebrile.
- There were well-demarcated, focal areas of crusting and partial alopecia over the perioral (Fig. 19.1) and periocular skin. The crusts were grey in colour.
- Nail folds, interdigital areas (Fig. 19.2) and the caudal aspects of both hock joints (Fig. 19.3) were similarly

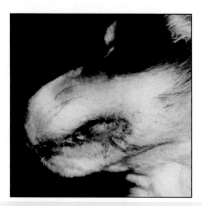

Figure 19.1 Perioral crusting.

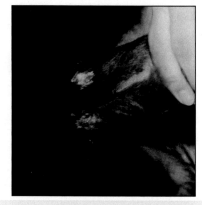

Figure 19.3 Crusting and scaling over the hocks.

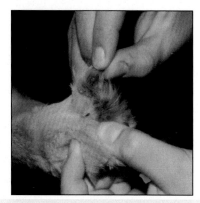

Figure 19.2 Crusting and scaling over the interdigital skin.

affected. Elevation of crusts revealed erosions and exudation (Fig. 19.4).
- There was mild footpad hyperkeratosis.
- There were thick, black-coloured crusts adherent to the skin over the scrotum.

DIFFERENTIAL DIAGNOSES

This was a crusting dermatosis affecting primarily pressure point areas. The lesions, in association with a history of being fed a high cereal diet, were suggestive of a zinc-responsive dermatosis, but other possible differentials included:
- Demodicosis
- Sarcoptic mange
- Dermatophytosis
- Pyoderma
- *Malassezia* dermatitis
- Metabolic epidermal necrosis
- Pemphigus foliaceus.

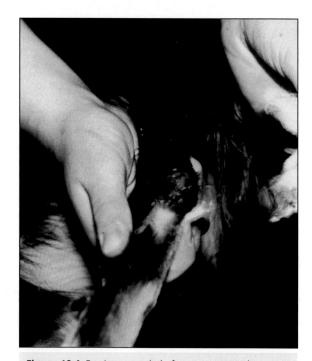

Figure 19.4 Erosions revealed after crust removal.

CASE WORK-UP

The diagnosis of zinc-responsive dermatitis is based on a combination of history, clinical signs and histopathological examination. It is important to rule out the involvement of demodicosis and dermatophytosis where there is evidence of alopecia or scaling. Cytology will help to confirm the presence of secondary staphylococcal pyoderma and parakeratotic keratinocytes. Serum or hair zinc levels may be abnormal in both syndrome I and II cases, but there is considerable overlap between

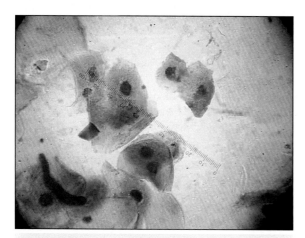

Figure 19.5 Parakeratotic corneocytes from a case of zinc-responsive dermatosis. ×400 original magnification. Diff Quik® stain.

affected and healthy animals, and therefore this test is of limited diagnostic value. Additionally, the measurement of zinc concentration is fraught with difficulty because it is a ubiquitous environmental mineral, and contamination from glass tubes, rubber stoppers and so on will tend to result in spuriously high results. Blood levels of zinc in man are known to fluctuate rapidly following infections, injury and stressful stimuli, resulting in redistribution of zinc from the blood to other body compartments, and blood level measured during these events may not accurately reflect total zinc nutrition status. Hair zinc concentration only reflects long-term zinc status.

The following diagnostic tests were performed:
- Multiple deep skin scrapings from affected areas, which showed no evidence of ectoparasitism.
- Cytology on impression smears from the underside of removed crust and eroded surfaces revealed neutrophils, occasional macrophages and clusters of parakeratotic corneocytes (Fig. 19.5).
- Fungal culture of crusts and hair plucks from lesional sites, which were negative.
- Four samples of skin from the hock joints and perioral region were harvested using a 6-mm biopsy punch and submitted for histopathological examination. The examination revealed dense parakeratotic crusting on the skin surface, extending down into the hair follicles. There was marked acanthosis. There was a superficial perivascular, predominantly plasmacytic,

infiltrate. No *Demodex* mites, bacteria or fungi were evident.

DIAGNOSIS

The history, clinical signs and results of the histopathological examination were consistent with a diagnosis of zinc-responsive dermatosis.

PROGNOSIS

The prognosis for zinc-responsive dermatosis in syndrome II cases is usually good. Correction of the diet alone should result in resolution of skin lesions within 4–6 weeks, and the addition of zinc supplementation should hasten the clinical response. Zinc supplementation may be withdrawn in syndrome II cases once the lesions have resolved. Lifelong zinc supplementation is required in 75% of syndrome I cases. In some cases, the response to zinc supplementation has been poor; concurrent low-dose prednisolone therapy has been shown to improve the clinical response in these cases.

AETIOPATHOGENESIS OF ZINC-RESPONSIVE DERMATOSIS

Zinc is an essential nutrient, and is important in metabolism, immunological function and epidermal integrity. In the human body it is present in over 200 metalloenzymes, and a zinc-deficient state can result in cutaneous, gastrointestinal, neurological and growth defects, as well as inducing immunosuppression. In the skin, zinc is concentrated within the epidermis. Despite body stores, zinc deprivation will result in a zinc-deficient state within a few days.

Three different syndromes have been described. Lethal acrodermatitis of bull terriers is an inherited autosomal recessive trait caused by an inability to absorb sufficient zinc that closely resembles acrodermatitis enteropathica in humans. The disease results in growth defects, skin disease, neurological abnormalities and immunosuppression in puppies and young dogs, very few of which survive to adulthood. Historically, the two other presentations of zinc deficiency have been classed as syndromes I and II. Syndrome I affects predominantly Siberian huskies and malamutes that are being fed well-balanced diets. Although occasionally other breeds of dog have been affected, the incidence supports a genetic linkage. It is thought that the condition arises because of an inability to effectively absorb zinc from the gastro-intestinal tract and, indeed, this has been demonstrated in some malamutes. Syndrome II is seen predominantly in dogs that are fed either cereal-based diets containing high levels of plant phytates that bind zinc and prevent absorption, a commercial diet that is deficient in zinc, or imbalanced home-prepared diets. Most commonly, syndrome II is seen in rapidly growing puppies when zinc demand is greatest, but adult dogs, as in this case, may also be affected.

Anecdotally, there are dermatologists who believe that the division into syndrome I and syndrome II is somewhat misleading, and that all these dogs have some inability to absorb zinc, which is exacerbated by the feeding of dried food diets with high cereal content.

Zinc deficiency clearly affects the differentiation and maturation process within the epidermis. In the normal process of epidermopoiesis, daughter cells are produced by the keratinocytes of the stratum basale that travel up through the epidermis, undergoing a complex maturation process and are eventually shed from the surface of the stratum corneum as terminally differentiated corneocytes. Corneocytes (or squames) are fully keratinized, flattened cells that have lost their nuclei. The zinc-deficient state associated with zinc-responsive dermatosis (or lethal acrodermatitis of bull terriers) affects the normal maturation process and results in parakeratotic hyperkeratosis. Parakeratotic corneocytes are cells that have retained their nuclei and hyperkeratosis refers to a thickening of the stratum corneum. Parakeratotic hyperkeratosis is one of the diagnostic features of zinc-responsive dermatoses, but may also be seen in metabolic epidermal necrosis, vitamin A-responsive dermatosis, *Malassezia* dermatitis, hereditary nasal hyperkeratosis of Labrador retrievers and a number of other inflammatory skin diseases.

EPIDEMIOLOGY

Zinc deficiency is an uncommon to rare cause of skin disease in the dog, mainly seen in Alaskan malamutes and Siberian huskies, but may be seen in any breed fed a diet deficient in zinc. Young to middle-aged dogs are most commonly affected, but the age range in one study was from 2 months to 11 years. There is no sex predilection for the disease.

TREATMENT OPTIONS

Treatment is based on correction of dietary imbalances, treatment of secondary bacterial and yeast infections, and zinc supplementation.

Topical therapy consisting of warm water soaks helps to loosen and remove the crusts. The application of emollient ointments may be beneficial in some cases. Systemic and topical antibacterial and antifungal therapy would be indicated if there is pyoderma and/or a *Malassezia* dermatitis.

An initial daily dosage of zinc supplement of 1.0 mg of elemental zinc per kg body weight was recommended although, in a more recent study, doses of up to 11 mg/kg were required to resolve lesions. Suitable preparations include zinc sulphate (10 mg/kg q24), zinc gluconate (5 mg/kg q24) or zinc picolinate (1.5 mg/kg q24). It is suggested that therapy should be continued for 1 month before assessing the response and the daily dosage should be increased by 50% if the initial dosage is not effective. Most cases show an improvement within 6 weeks of starting zinc supplementation. Zinc sulphate is a gastric irritant and, to decrease the incidence of vomiting, tablets should be crushed and mixed with food.

Intravenous zinc supplementation has been reported to be of benefit in syndrome I cases that do not respond well to oral supplementation, although there is a risk of cardiac arrhythmia when using this form of therapy. It has also been shown that low anti-inflammatory doses of prednisolone (0.5 mg/kg) have been helpful in aiding resolution of skin lesions, particularly in Siberian huskies refractory to treatment with zinc supplementation alone. The prednisolone may improve absorption of zinc from the gut, or it may be that it merely aids in resolution of the skin lesions. An improved clinical response has also been seen when the diet was supplemented with omega-6/omega-3 fatty acids.

Treatment in this case: The dog was already receiving antibacterial therapy and treatment was continued for a further 2 weeks, using cefalexin (20 mg/kg b.i.d.).

Zinc supplementation was administered in the form of an amino acid chelated preparation at a dosage of 1.5 mg/kg s.i.d.

Daily warm water soaks of crusted lesions were advised.

The diet was switched to a good quality proprietary, pelleted lamb and rice kibble.

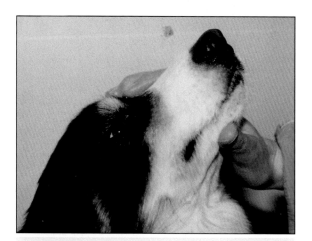

Figure 19.6 Resolution of perioral crusting following change of diet and zinc supplementation.

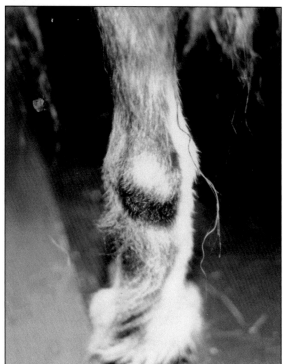

Figure 19.7 Resolution of hock lesions following change of diet and zinc supplementation.

CLINICAL TIPS

Nucleated (parakeratotic) squames were evident on cytological examination of lesions (Fig. 19.5). These are cells from the stratum corneum that have retained their nuclei. Parakeratotic corneocytes are seen in many inflammatory skin disorders and are in effect produced as the result of a repair mechanism. Very large numbers of these cells are seen in certain metabolic diseases, such as zinc-responsive dermatoses and metabolic epidermal necrosis. There is a danger that these cells may be confused with the acantholytic keratinocytes seen in pemphigus foliaceus (see Chapter 17), but in fact they have different features. Whereas these cells are obviously flattened, somewhat translucent and angular in appearance, acantholytic keratinocytes are rounded and much darker staining.

FOLLOW-UP

Reinspection after 3 weeks of therapy revealed that all the crusting lesions had resolved (Figs 19.6 and 19.7). This result confirmed the diagnosis of zinc-responsive dermatosis. The good quality diet was continued, but zinc supplementation withdrawn after a further 2 weeks. Four months later, the patient was still lesion free and there had been no evidence of diarrhoea.

SECTION 3

ALOPECIA

20 Introduction to alopecia

HAIR FOLLICLE ANATOMY AND PHYSIOLOGY

Hair, a characteristic of mammals, serves several important functions including thermal insulation, a barrier to physical, chemical, thermal and microbial insults, photoprotection and as a visual stimulus for sexual attraction in some cases. Hair follicles also serve as a site for re-epithelialization during wound healing.

The hair follicle unit consists of the hair follicle itself, the sebaceous gland, sweat gland and an arrector pili muscle (Fig. 20.1). Anatomically the hair follicle is divided into three segments: the infundibulum, the isthmus and the hair bulb (see Chapter 13, Fig. 13.5). The hair follicle consists of inner and outer tubes, the inner and outer root sheaths. The inner root sheath and the hair shaft itself arise from and are produced by a swelling at the base of the hair follicle called the hair bulb.

Carnivores (dogs, cats, etc.) have compound follicles, which means that hairs produced by multiple hair follicles exit from the same infundibulum at the skin surface. Some of these hairs are large-diameter 'primary' hair shafts and the remainder are small 'secondary' undercoat hairs.

The hair growth cycle

Hair growth occurs in a cyclical manner comprising an active growth phase, a transitional phase and a resting, involutory phase.

The active growth phase is termed anagen, and is followed by a transitional period, catagen, and a resting phase, telogen (Fig. 20.2a–c). The duration of each phase varies according to age, body region, breed and sex, as well as intrinsic, extrinsic and external factors. Breed has a dramatic effect on the hair cycle, with some dogs having an anagen- or a telogen-dominated hair cycle. Breeds such as poodles and Bichon Frise have anagen-dominated cycles. Essentially, this is where hair

follicles are in anagen for long periods of time. These are breeds that require hair cuts. Plush-coated breeds such as the chow-chow, Malamutes and Pomeranians have telogen-dominated hair cycles. This is where the hair follicle spends long periods of time in telogen with a retained telogen hair shaft. Presumably, evolutionarily speaking this is advantageous in a cold climate when hair growth requires protein and energy.

Hair in dogs is replaced in a mosaic pattern, which means that over the same area of skin there will be hair follicles at all three stages of the hair cycle at the same time, in contrast to mice, where the hair cycle occurs in waves starting at the head. In dogs and cats there are peaks of hair growth in spring and autumn; however, this pattern is further influenced by the photoperiod, temperature and nutritional status.

Factors controlling the hair growth cycle

The control of hair growth is complex and still relatively poorly understood. There are many factors controlling hair growth that can be summarized as intrinsic, extrinsic and external factors (mainly identified from research into the murine hair growth cycle).

Intrinsic factors are produced by epithelial and mesenchymal cells in and around the hair follicle and include:
- Cytokines/growth factors
- Hormones (paracrine/autocrine)
- Neuropeptides
- Adhesion molecules
- Oncogenes and tumour suppressor genes.

Extrinsic factors are produced by organs other than the skin and include:
- Hormones (thyroid hormones, sex hormones, cortisol, melatonin, prolactin)
  - Stimulators of anagen – include thyroid hormones and ACTH

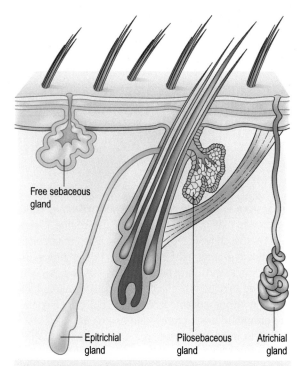

Figure 20.1 The hair follicle and sweat glands. Free sebaceous glands and atrichial glands open directly to the skin surface; pilosebaceous and epitrichial glands open into the hair follicle lumen.

Labels: Free sebaceous gland; Epitrichial gland; Pilosebaceous gland; Atrichial gland

- Inhibitors of anagen – include glucocorticoids and oestrogen
- Neural – neuropeptides, catecholamines
- Immunological – mast cells, macrophages
- Genetics
- Nutritional status
- Disease states.

External factors affecting hair growth and hair loss include:
- Photoperiod
- Temperature
- Friction
- Drug therapy.

Sebaceous glands: The sebaceous glands are simple alveolar glands, with ducts opening into the infundibulum (pilosebaceous gland) or directly onto the skin surface via the epidermis (free sebaceous glands). The latter are found around the lip margin, anus, external ear canal and the eyelid (Meibomian gland and the glands of Zeis). The frequency and size of the glands vary at different points on the body. They are most abundant adjacent to the mucocutaneous junctions, in the interdigital spaces, at the dorsal neck, rump and on the chin; they are not found on the nasal planum or footpads. Sebum is the lipid-rich secretion produced by the sebaceous glands, and its formation is strongly influenced by endocrine and other extrinsic factors such as age, nutritional status and disease. Sebum has both protective and behavioural roles. When combined with sweat it forms a waxy emulsion, which provides protection against microbial organisms. Sebum is rich in wax esters that coat the hair shaft, providing it with a protective barrier and gloss. In recent years, the sebaceous gland has been used in modulating the distribution of topical treatments, such as flea products. Conditions affecting the sebaceous gland are likely to affect the hair quality, e.g. alopecia due to sebaceous adenitis, an immune-mediated condition.

Sweat glands: There are two types of sweat glands (Fig. 20.1): epitrichial (ducts that open into the hair follicle) and atrichial or eccrine (ducts open onto the epidermal surface). Sweat glands in general are widely dispersed in the skin, but are not present in all skin. Most atrichial glands are found in glabrous skin, but a few are dispersed throughout hirsute areas. The largest and most numerous epitrichial glands are found at the mucocutaneous junctions, dorsal neck, rump and interdigital areas. Atrichial glands are found in the nasal planum and in the footpads. Specialized sweat glands are found in the ear canal (ceruminous glands) and in the eyelids (Moll's glands).

Sweat is formed by a combination of cell death and secretion, and is composed of inorganic ions, water, immunoglobulins, amino acids and waste products, such as urea and lactic acid. Sweat forms an emulsion with sebum to play a role in skin protection and in scent production.

ALOPECIA

Alopecia is defined as the absence of hair from areas where it is normally present. Alopecia may be localized, multifocal, symmetrical or generalized.

Alopecia can be due to:
- Self-trauma from pruritus caused by ectoparasitic disease, microbial infections and hypersensitivities. Pruritic skin disease and associated self-trauma is probably the most common cause of alopecia.

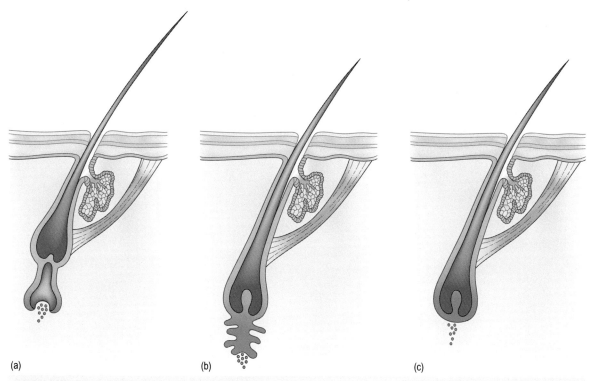

Figure 20.2

(a) Anagen hair – new hair being formed below a telogen.

(b) Catagen phase – transitional period between the anagen and telogen hair.

(c) Telogen hair – resting phase.

- Folliculitis as a result of staphylococcal infections, dermatophytosis, demodicosis or autoimmune folliculitides.
- Failure of the hair growth cycle, i.e. due to an endocrinopathy.
  - Endocrine abnormalities can affect the hair growth cycle either directly or indirectly, resulting in growth arrest and alopecia. Oestradiol, testosterone and adrenal steroids delay the onset of anagen, whereas thyroid hormone initiates anagen.
- Dysplastic disorders of the hair follicle. Follicular dysplasias are characterized by abnormally, or incompletely, formed hair follicles or hair shafts. Follicular dysplasia can be divided into a group affecting the hair cycle (cyclical recurrent flank alopecia and alopecia X) and those affecting the process of melanization during the formation of the hair (colour dilution alopecia and black hair follicle dysplasia).
- Destruction of hair follicles as a result of scarring or neoplastic infiltration.

Clinical approach to alopecia

As with most diseases in dermatology, a thorough history is essential and should give the clinician a good idea of the nature of the disease process (see Chapter 1). Important factors include age of onset, the presence or absence of pruritus and whether or not the alopecia developed as a result of or prior to the onset of pruritus, and whether there have been other skin lesions in addition to the alopecia. The presence or absence of systemic signs is of paramount importance in cases where an endocrinopathy might be involved.

Clinical presentations: The clinical examination can yield useful information as to the cause of the alopecia. Multifocal, roughly circular, asymmetrical, spreading patches of alopecia usually indicate the presence of a folliculitis. Symmetrical, non-pruritic and non-inflammatory alopecia over the trunk would be suggestive of an endocrinopathy or follicular dysplasia.

Diagnostic tests: Skin scrapes are mandatory in all cases of alopecia to rule out the involvement of demodicosis. Similarly, examination for fungi should be performed if there is evidence of inflammation or scaling. Histopathology may be helpful in establishing the cause of the disease. It is advisable to treat secondary pyoderma prior to taking samples for histopathology. In most cases of alopecia, 6- or 8-mm biopsy punch samples are adequate. Multiple samples should be taken in cases of alopecia, starting at the centre and radiating outwards into the unaffected areas of skin.

This section of the book describes cases where alopecia is the predominant presenting clinical sign and is divided according to presentation, into symmetrical, multifocal and focal alopecia, and alopecia associated with systemic disease. The selection of cases includes endocrinopathies and follicular dysplasias affecting the hair growth cyce or hair shafts, and infectious, parasitic or immune-mediated diseases affecting the hair follicle.

21 Feline symmetrical alopecia

INITIAL PRESENTATION

Non-inflammatory, symmetrical hair loss.

INTRODUCTION

Symmetrical alopecia is a common presentation in the cat. Historically, the alopecia was thought to be due to an endocrinopathy because of the lack of any apparent inflammation in many cases. It is now known that the majority of cases of symmetrical alopecia are due to pruritus. There are many causes for symmetrical alopecia, including parasitic and allergic disease, and a thorough and systematic investigation is indicated in recurrent disease to try to identify and correct the underlying cause.

CASE PRESENTING SIGNS

A 4-year-old, neutered male cat was presented with a history of persistent ventral alopecia.

CASE HISTORY

As in all dermatology cases, a thorough history (see Chapter 1) is essential in making an accurate diagnosis. Frequently, in cases of symmetrical alopecia, the client may be unaware that the cat is actually overgrooming.

The history in this case was as follows:

- There was an 8-month history of progressive alopecia affecting the ventral trunk.
- The owner had seen the cat overgrooming the ventral trunk and was aware that the alopecia was self-induced.

- The use of an Elizabethan collar for 3–4 weeks had resulted in regrowth of hair, but the alopecia recurred on removal of the collar.
- There had been a good response to glucocorticoid therapy, with regrowth of hair over the affected area, but treatment resulted in an excessive appetite and weight gain.
- There was one other cat and a dog in the same household. Neither of these animals had developed any skin lesions.
- Fleas had been seen on both cats following a stay in a cattery, prior to the onset of the alopecia. Since then, all animals in the household had been treated with monthly applications of fipronil spot-on and the house environment had been treated with a permethrin and methoprene spray.
- During a 4-week period a commercial, pelleted, chicken hydrolysate diet was fed to both cats, but no change in hair growth was noted during this time.
- There was no evidence of zoonosis.

CLINICAL EXAMINATION

Feline symmetrical alopecia usually presents as non-inflammatory hair loss, although there may be evidence of focal excoriations. The most frequently affected areas include the neck, forelimbs, groin and flanks.

Examination revealed:

- A body condition score of 5/9 and weight 5.6 kg (slightly obese)
- Bilateral systolic heart murmur

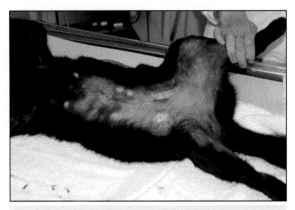

Figure 21.1 Self-induced, symmetrical alopecia over the ventrum in a cat with atopic dermatitis.

- Examination of the skin revealed non-inflammatory, partial to complete alopecia over the axillae, ventral chest, groin and medial thighs (Fig. 21.1).

DIFFERENTIAL DIAGNOSES

There are four main categories of disease that result in pruritus in cats: parasites; infections; hypersensitivity disorders; and a diverse fourth group which includes some infectious, autoimmune, metabolic and neoplastic diseases amongst others. When drawing up a list of differential diagnoses with a view to further investigation, it is important to initially rule out/ treat parasitic infestations before considering the infectious and allergic causes of pruritus. Pruritus is often multifactorial and a methodical approach, following a series of sequential diagnostic rule-outs, will maximize the chances of making a diagnosis and instituting successful treatment and management.

In this case, there was a history of flea exposure, but thorough flea control had been instituted with no improvement, so flea allergy dermatitis, as a sole cause of the pruritus, was unlikely. Nevertheless, flea allergy dermatitis could still be involved and thorough flea control would need to be maintained. A limited antigen diet trial had been tried, but only for 4 weeks, and this is too short a period to be able to thoroughly exclude a cutaneous adverse food reaction. Ideally, a diet trial should be continued for a minimum of 6 weeks and on occasion for as long as 3 months.

There was no history of an anxiety-inducing situation, but psychogenic alopecia should be considered where there is symmetrical alopecia.

The principal differential diagnoses in this case were:
- Flea allergy dermatitis
- Cheyletiellosis
- Harvest mite infestation
- Demodicosis
- Dermatophytosis
- Atopic dermatitis
- Cutaneous adverse food reaction
- Psychogenic alopecia.

CASE WORK-UP

The initial diagnostic tests taken at the first examination were to investigate the possible involvement of ectoparasitism and to rule out the involvement of dermatophytosis.

The following diagnostic tests were undertaken:
- Trichographic examination revealed fractured hair shafts from affected areas (see Fig. 2.6, Chapter 2). There was no evidence of ectoparasitism on microscopic examination of scale and skin scrapes from the dorsal trunk, and no evidence of *Demodex* mites on skin scrapes from the areas of alopecia over the ventrum.
- There was no evidence of dermatophytes on Wood's lamp examination. No dermatophytes were grown from material collected from the hair coat using the MacKenzie brush technique.

The first stage in the investigation of feline pruritus, whatever the presentation, is to rule out the involvement of ectoparasitism, particularly fleas. Visual examination for evidence of flea infestation, and microscopic examination of scale and skin scrapes for the detection of ectoparasites, are insensitive methods and thorough treatment of the patient, all in-contact animals and the household (and possibly car) environments is always indicated in these cases. If there has been no response to thorough ectoparasitic therapy, a diet trial and possibly intradermal and/or an ELISA environmental panel are indicated. Thus, the following further investigations were conducted:

Trial ectoparasitic treatment: Good flea control was already in place, but in order to be confident about ruling out the involvement of cheyletiellosis, all animals were treated with fortnightly applications of selamectin for a period of 4 weeks. There was no response to this and the cat continued to overgroom. Monthly applications of fipronil were continued after the trial selamectin therapy.

Diet trial: An extended, 10-week, restricted antigen diet trial was conducted, feeding a proprietary capelin and tapioca food. To give relief from pruritus, for the first 4 weeks of the trial the patient was treated with prednisolone (10 mg s.i.d. for 1 week then 5 mg s.i.d. for 1 week then 5 mg every other day). Re-examination after 4 weeks showed a marked improvement, with resolution of overgrooming and some hair regrowth over affected areas, but marked polyphagia had been evident and the cat had gained weight. After a further 6 weeks, there was recrudescence of overgrooming and alopecia.

Intradermal testing: An intradermal test was performed on completion of the diet trial, which gave positive reactions to the house dust mite *Dermatophagoides farinae*, the storage mites *Acarus siro* and *Tyrophagus putrescentiae*, as well as sheep epithelia, mixed feathers, couch grass, orchard grass, lambs quarter and alder.

Note that intradermal and serological allergy testing are less reliable and can be harder to interpret in the cat compared to the dog; nevertheless, some cats will produce strong positive reactions to one or both tests. The main reason to conduct these tests is for selection of allergens for immunotherapy.

DIAGNOSIS

The history, clinical signs, lack of response to thorough ectoparasitic therapy, and the extended diet trial and the positive intradermal test all supported and confirmed a diagnosis of atopic dermatitis. As with any investigation of pruritus, a positive intradermal test (or ELISA panel) alone would not support the diagnosis of atopic dermatitis, as healthy animals are frequently positive on these tests and a positive test does not rule out the involvement of the other differentials.

PROGNOSIS

Although atopic dermatitis is a lifelong, incurable condition, the prognosis for effective control of symptoms and

Table 21.1 Causes of symmetrical alopecia in cats

Flea allergy dermatitis
Pediculosis
Cheyletiellosis
Ectopic otodectic mange
Demodicosis
Trombiculidiasis
Dermatophytosis
Atopic dermatitis
Cutaneous adverse food reaction
Paraneoplastic alopecia
Hyperthyroidism
Epitheliotrophic lymphoma
Psychogenic alopecia

a good quality of life is good in the majority of cases, although some cases can be challenging to manage.

AETIOPATHOGENESIS OF SYMMETRICAL ALOPECIA

The non-inflammatory nature of most cases of symmetrical alopecia in cats, and the response to 'hormonal' therapies such as megestrol acetate, initially led to the misconception that feline symmetrical alopecia was a hair growth cycle disorder, possibly an endocrinopathy. It is now known that, in the majority of cases, the alopecia is due to pruritus and the resulting self-trauma. There are, however, some rarer causes of symmetrical alopecia that are due to causes other than pruritus (see Chapter 28). Table 21.1 lists the common and some less common causes of symmetrical alopecia in cats.

Feline cutaneous reaction patterns

There are three other frequently encountered manifestations of feline pruritus: head and neck pruritus, miliary dermatitis, and lesions of the eosinophilic granuloma complex. These three presentations, along with symmetrical alopecia, have been termed the feline cutaneous reaction patterns. Cats may present with more than one reaction pattern at any one time. The recognition of one of the feline reaction patterns does not constitute a diagnosis, and although initial symptomatic therapy may be quite appropriate, further investigation is indicated for cats with recurrent disease, in order to try and establish the underlying cause of the pruritus and institute specific therapy for it. It is common for cats presenting with any of the feline cutaneous reaction patterns to have multiple diseases, including atopic dermatitis, flea allergy dermatitis and a cutaneous adverse food reaction.

Because of the diverse nature of the possible differential diagnoses, a systematic approach to the diagnosis is required. The work-up of such a case can be protracted and challenging, and it is important that the client understands from the outset the nature of such an investigation. The client must be committed and good communication is vital for a successful outcome. Cats can be very uncooperative with respect to diagnostic procedures and, at times, the necessity to treat symptoms to prevent further suffering can hinder diagnostic procedures.

EPIDEMIOLOGY

Symmetrical alopecia is a frequent clinical presentation and many of the underlying causes are encountered on a daily basis. The alopecia in this case was due to atopic dermatitis. The incidence of atopic dermatitis in cats is controversial. Most reports would suggest that this is a common disease and may perhaps be the most common feline allergic skin disease in geographical areas where the prevalence of fleas is low. An inherited predisposition has not been documented, although there are reports of familial involvement that do suggest a genetic component. No breed or sex predilections have been demonstrated, but young cats appear to be predisposed.

TREATMENT OPTIONS

Prior to starting treatment, the clinician should spend time discussing with the client the various options for treatment, their efficacy, cost and likely side-effects. The treatment choices available are essentially similar to those detailed in Chapter 6 for the treatment of canine atopic dermatitis, and include allergen avoidance and the use of antihistamines, essential fatty acid supplementation, glucocorticosteroids, ciclosporin and allergen-specific immunotherapy.

Antihistamines and essential fatty acid supplementation: Antihistamine therapy and/or essential fatty acid supplementation may be of benefit in the management of feline symmetrical alopecia due to atopic dermatitis. Antihistamine therapy in cats seems to be a more effective therapy for pruritus in comparison to dogs. Chlorphenamine (chlorpheniramine) is considered

the antihistamine of choice when treating feline atopic dermatitis. The use of concurrent antihistamine and essential fatty acid supplementation gave an improved response in one study.

The following antihistamines may be of benefit:
- Chlorphenamine (chlorpheniramine), 0.4 mg/kg b.i.d.
- Hydroxyzine, 10 mg/cat q b.i.d.
- Clemastine, 0.5 mg/cat b.i.d.
- Cyproheptadine, 2 mg/cat b.i.d.

Glucocorticoids: In general, the long-term use of glucocorticoids should be avoided, but because of their high good efficacy and low cost, glucocorticoids are commonly used for the management of feline allergic skin disease. Certainly, when there are financial constraints, they are probably the most appropriate treatment. Additionally, there is an argument for the use of glucocorticoids in cats with seasonal hypersensitivities where treatment is only required for a few months of the year.

Alternate-day therapy allows the hypothalamic–adrenal–pituitary axis time for recovery and makes the long-term use of glucocorticoids safer than daily treatment. Thus, the shorter-acting glucocorticoids, prednisolone or methylprednisolone, are the most appropriate drugs for the management of feline atopic dermatitis.

Although the use of short-acting glucocorticoids is preferred, it may be necessary to use longer-acting injectable products when it is not possible for owners to administer oral therapy to cats.

In general, cats are more resistant to, and develop fewer side-effects to, glucocorticoids in comparison to dogs. However, polyphagia, excessive weight gain, diabetes mellitus and, in rare cases, skin fragility syndrome are all potential side-effects. In addition, the onset of congestive heart failure has been documented in cats following glucocorticoid administration, in particular following treatment with methylprednisolone acetate.

Prednisolone dosage and administration:
- *Induction*: 1–2 mg/kg given once or divided twice daily (lesions of the eosinophilic granuloma complex may require higher dosages to achieve remission).
- *Maintenance*: 1 mg/kg on alternate days, gradually reducing to the lowest dosage that just controls the pruritus.

Ciclosporin: Although an unlicensed product in the UK, clinical experience and a limited number of studies have shown ciclosporin to be a beneficial treatment for feline atopic dermatitis. It seems to be effective at an initial dosage of 5–7 mg/kg s.i.d. and in some cases it may be possible to reduce to alternate-day or twice-weekly therapy following a good response to daily dosage. Several weeks of therapy may be required before maximal response is seen. Side-effects may include gastrointestinal disturbance and gingival hyperplasia. Ciclosporin is a potent, immunosuppressive drug. There is at least one report of fatal toxoplasmosis in cats being treated with ciclosporin, and it is recommended to assess FIV, FeLV and toxoplasma serology prior to commencing therapy. It may be inadvisable to treat cats that are positive on toxoplasma serology.

Allergen-specific immunotherapy (ASIT): Immunotherapy is an option for treatment in cases where specific causative allergens have been identified. Many studies have demonstrated efficacy of immunotherapy for the treatment of feline atopic dermatitis. Reported response rates to immunotherapy vary between 50% and 75%. Certainly, in the authors' experience this is a safe and in some cases highly beneficial therapy for the management of feline atopic dermatitis. One concern about the use of immunotherapy is the length of time it can take for any improvement to become apparent. The treatment should be continued for up to 1 year before being discontinued on the grounds of lack of efficacy.

Treatment in this case

When selecting treatment, consideration must be given to the severity of the case and the expectations and requirements of the owner. In this case, the patient was experiencing ongoing pruritus that required effective management.

- Thorough flea control was maintained.
- Allergen-specific immunotherapy using alum-precipitated allergens was initiated. The results of the intradermal test were used to formulate the vaccine.
- Because of the current severity of pruritus and the weight gain associated with glucocorticoid therapy, the decision was made to start therapy with ciclosporin at a dosage of 6 mg/kg s.i.d. Routine haematology and biochemistry, and FeLV, FIV and toxoplasma serology were performed prior to starting treatment. No abnormalities were detected on these tests.

CLINICAL TIPS

Pruritus

As already stated, in some cases the owner may be unaware that the cat with symmetrical alopecia is pruritic. The following points may be helpful when documenting the pruritus:

- Is there excessive grooming, licking, biting or scratching? Does the cat suffer from hairballs, constipation, or is hair frequently seen in the faeces?
- Look for stubby broken hairs. Are there inflammatory skin lesions (erythema, scale, crusts) in addition to overt alopecia?
- In self-induced trauma, the distal end of almost all the hairs will be broken instead of the normal tapered appearance on trichographic examination.
- As a last resort, application of an Elizabethan collar will lead to partial regrowth of hair in cases of self-induced alopecia.

Elizabethan collars

Some dermatologists recommend the use an Elizabethan collar following application of spot-on flea treatments to cats that are excessively overgrooming. There is a concern that the cat licks off and ingests the product, leading to apparent treatment failure. The collar is used for up to 48 hours following application.

Diet trials

Diet trials in cats are fraught with difficulty. Cats scavenge and will often obtain food from waste bins or be fed by well-meaning neighbours, and it is possible that many cases of food reactions in cats go undiagnosed for this reason. Consideration should be given to confining cats indoors for the duration of a diet trial, but the clinician should be aware that confinement might lead to overgrooming, as a result of boredom or stress. Cats can be fussy eaters and in the authors' experience, they are more likely to eat a proprietary food than a home-cooked diet. Cyproheptadine, as well as having antihistaminic therapy, is also an appetite stimulant in cats and has been used to encourage cats to eat a restriction diet.

It is often necessary to control pruritus during a diet trial to prevent severe self-trauma. Glucocorticoid therapy should be used in these cases. A useful side-effect of this may be stimulation of the appetite, resulting in the cat eating the novel diet. Glucocorticoids should be withdrawn at least 2 weeks before completion of the restriction diet in order to be able to assess response. If the pruritus does not recur within a few days, continue the restricted diet for another month before provocative challenge with the original diet. Relapse of signs in association with challenge followed by improvement on re-institution of the restriction diet supports a diagnosis of a cutaneous adverse food reaction.

Client compliance

It is fair to say that in a number of cases of feline pruritus it is not possible to make a specific diagnosis. In the absence of a diagnosis, client compliance should be re-evaluated to ensure exclusion diets and trial therapies have been adhered to. If clinical symptoms persist, then other disease processes should be investigated and histopathology of biopsy samples, radiography, ultrasound, virus isolation and blood tests may be indicated.

Psychogenic alopecia

When all other differentials have been evaluated, psychogenic alopecia may be considered. It is important to stress that this is not a diagnosis that should be made on clinical signs alone and there should be a history of some stressful factors, such as:

- New baby in household
- Moving house
- Boarding
- Hospitalization
- Loss of companion
- New cat in territory
- New cat in household.

The incidence of a psychogenic dermatosis as a sole cause of pruritus in the cat is considered by

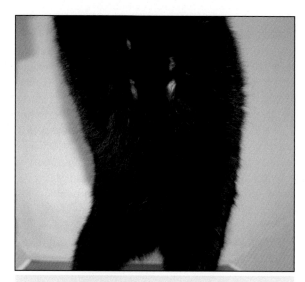

Figure 21.2 The same cat as in Fig. 21.1 after 8-week treatment with ciclosporin.

referral dermatologists to be extremely low, but in the authors' opinion, psychogenic factors may exacerbate existing pruritic skin disease. Oriental breeds of cat may be at increased risk of developing psychogenic dermatosis, and cats that are inherently nervous, hyperaesthetic, fearful or shy are at increased risk.

FOLLOW-UP

Within 8 weeks of starting treatment, there was complete regrowth of hair over the ventrum (Fig. 21.2). The frequency of administration of ciclosporin was reduced, initially to alternate-day therapy and then to twice weekly, over a 2-month period, without recurrence of self-trauma. At the time of writing, the cat is receiving monthly immunotherapy injections and twice-weekly ciclosporin at a dosage of 7 mg/kg. Over the next few months, attempts will be made to completely withdraw the ciclosporin therapy and to try and manage the pruritus on allergen-specific immunotherapy alone.

22 Hypothyroidism

INITIAL PRESENTATION

Symmetrical alopecia with hyperpigmentation and mild scaling.

INTRODUCTION

Despite being the most common endocrinopathy, hypothyroidism can be a challenging disease to diagnose. Although there are many diagnostic tests, they all have their limitations, as thyroid function can be influenced by many different intrinsic and extrinsic factors. Hypothyroidism can cause a wide variety of symptoms involving almost any organ system; however, dermatological signs are the most common. This report describes a case where the cutaneous signs were prominent.

CASE PRESENTING SIGNS

A 7-year-old, castrated male boxer dog was presented with a short history of non-pruritic symmetrical alopecia.

CASE HISTORY

The condition most commonly affects mainly middle-aged to older dogs and certain breeds are predisposed (see 'Epidemiology' section). Cutaneous signs are gradual in onset and generally non-pruritic, unless there is a concurrent secondary infection. Most clients are unaware of systemic signs such as lethargy, exercise intolerance, heat seeking and weight gain. Close questioning on changes in demeanour and general health is therefore essential during the history taking.

The relevant history in this case was:

- There was no previous history of dermatological disease.
- The non-pruritic alopecia was first noted 2 months prior to examination and was gradually becoming more extensive.
- Although, according to the owner, general health was unaffected, on closer questioning, it transpired that the dog suffered from exercise intolerance, which the owner had put down to normal ageing.
- There was no history of polyuria, polydipsia or polyphagia.
- The dog was heat seeking.
- The management had remained unchanged since the dog was acquired at the age of 3 years.
- It was fed on a proprietary commercial dry diet.
- Because of the short duration of the disease, seasonal effects were not known.

CLINICAL EXAMINATION

Physical and skin examinations may reveal a great variety of systemic and cutaneous symptoms that vary from case to case (Tables 22.1 and 22.2). The relevant findings in this case were:

- Heart rate of 58 beats per minute
- Tragic facial appearance (Fig. 22.1), due to myxoedema on the ventral neck
- Bilateral symmetrical flank alopecia with hyperpigmentation and comedone formation on the skin (Fig. 22.2)
- The hair on the dorsum was sparse and the hair was easily epilated (Fig. 22.3).

Table 22.1 Systemic signs associated with hypothyroidism

Common signs	Uncommon or rare signs
Lethargy	Bradycardia
Weight gain	Weakness
Obesity	Exercise intolerance
	Corneal lipidosis
	Neurological symptoms
	Cardiovascular disease

Table 22.2 Dermatological abnormalities in canine hypothyroidism

Common	Uncommon or rare
Thin, easily epilated hair coat	Pyoderma
Symmetrical alopecia	Ceruminous otitis externa
Failure of hair growth after clipping	Demodicosis
Scaling	Myxoedema
Hyperpigmentation	Lightening of the hair coat colour
Comedone formation	

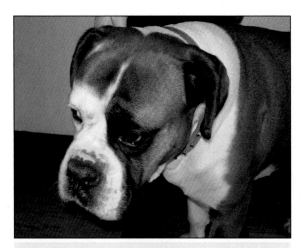

Figure 22.1 Tragic facial appearance.

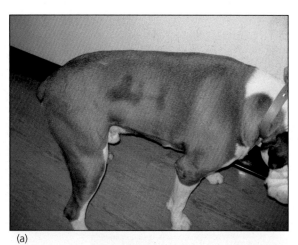

(a)

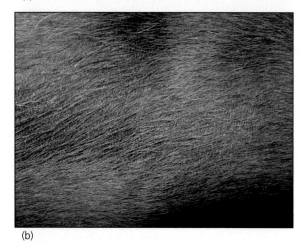

(b)

Figure 22.2
(a) Alopecia and hyperpigmentation on the lateral aspects.
(b) Close-up view.

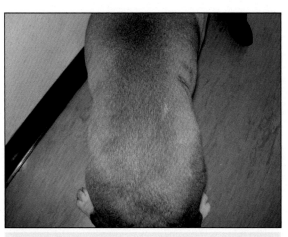

Figure 22.3 Hypotrichosis on the dorsum.

In this particular case the differential diagnoses included conditions where alopecia is the predominant sign:
- Hypothyroidism
- Cyclical flank alopecia
- Hyperadrenocorticism
- Demodicosis
- Bacterial folliculitis.

CASE WORK-UP

The following diagnostic tests were performed:
- There was no evidence of demodicosis on microscopic examination of multiple deep skin scrapes.
- Tape-strip preparations failed to reveal any coccoid bacteria on the skin surface.
- Trichography revealed mainly telogen hairs (Fig. 22.4).

At this stage, given the short duration of the disease, cyclical flank alopecia could not be ruled out, but in such cases thyroid function is unaffected. Because there was no history of polyuria, polydipsia or polyphagia, hyperadrenocorticism was unlikely.

Blood tests for hypothyroidism

Making a definitive diagnosis of hypothyroidism can prove challenging in some cases. The diagnosis is based on history, clinical signs and the demonstration of suppressed thyroid function. Because there are so many factors affecting thyroid hormone concentrations including age, breed, concurrent disease and drug therapy (see 'Anatomy and Physiology Refresher'), the diagnosis is not always easy to confirm. At the time of writing, there are no completely reliable tests that can distinguish euthyroid from hypothyroid dogs. A single thyroid assay is almost invariably misleading and multiple tests are recommended to try and confirm the diagnosis.

Haematology and biochemistry: If the history or clinical examination suggests hypothyroidism, routine haematological and biochemical examinations should be performed. This helps to exclude intercurrent disease leading to the euthyroid sick syndrome (see below). A mild, normochromic normocytic anaemia may be present in up to half of all cases of hypothyroidism. Hypercholesterolaemia is another frequent, but non-specific, finding in up to 70% of cases.

Thyroid function tests: Thyroid function tests should be performed where there are clinical signs suggestive of hypothyroidism. The clinician should rule out or treat concurrent diseases before evaluating thyroid function and, wherever possible, stop any drug treatment at least 4 weeks prior to testing. Where this is not possible, any results should be interpreted in the knowledge that drugs which could affect thyroid function have been administered. The following is a summary of the thyroid function tests currently available and their application in the diagnosis of hypothyroidism. Always use a combination of thyroid function tests to support the diagnosis.

TT4: Basal serum total thyroxine (TT4) measures protein- and non-protein-bound 'free' serum thyroxine. The concentration decreases in hypothyroidism, but also decreases with euthyroid sick syndrome and drug administration. There is a large overlap between euthyroid and hypothyroid dogs, and up to 25% of euthyroid dogs will have suppressed TT4 values; however, as a general rule, 99% of dogs with TT4 > 15 nmol/l will be euthyroid and >95% of dogs with TT4 < 5 nmol/l will be hypothyroid. Concentrations will be artificially (markedly) elevated in the presence of anti-T4 autoantibodies (AT4A), although this is an uncommon situation.

fT4ED: Basal free T4 by equilibrium dialysis (fT4ED) measures non-protein-bound circulating T4. Concentrations of fT4 will decrease in hypothyroidism, but may be maintained in early hypothyroidism, reducing the sensitivity

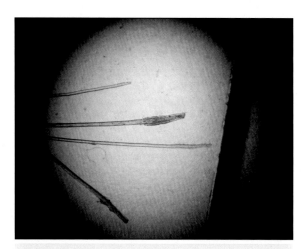

Figure 22.4 Telogen hairs on trichography.

of this test. It is expensive in comparison to TT4, but fT4 should be less affected by non-thyroidal illness than TT4 and is unaffected by the presence of AT4A. Note: some laboratories may measure free T4 using 'analogue' assay techniques, which is no more use than measuring TT4 alone.

cTSH: Canine thyroid-stimulating hormone (cTSH) measures circulating TSH. It is often used in conjunction with TT4 or fT4 as a screening test for hypothyroidism. Concentrations of cTSH increase in hypothyroidism, due to the decreased negative feedback effect of T4 and T3 on the anterior pituitary gland. This test may be affected by drug administration and by non-thyroidal illness. Between 13% and 38% of hypothyroid dogs have cTSH in the normal range (usually 0.02–0.68 ng/ml) and 7–18% of euthyroid dogs have cTSH in the hypothyroid range.

TT3 and fT3: Total and free triiodothyronine (TT3 and fT3) measurements are of little value in the diagnosis of most cases of hypothyroidism. TT3 concentrations tend to be preferentially maintained during early hypothyroidism.

TSH stim: Thyroid-stimulating hormone stimulation test (TSH stim) is considered the gold standard test in the diagnosis of canine hypothyroidism. Serum TT4 is measured before and 6 hours after intravenous injection of 0.1 IU/kg of thyrotropin (TSH). Thyroxine response to TSH is small to non-existent in hypothyroid dogs; however, a normal response may be seen in very early cases of hypothyroidism. Some drug treatments and severe non-thyroidal illness can also interfere with this test. As bovine TSH is no longer available, the use of recombinant human TSH (rhTSH) has been validated for this test.

TRH stim: In the thyrotropin-releasing hormone stimulation test (TRH stim), TT4 is measured before and 4 hours after intravenous injection of TRH. At least one study has concluded that this is not a useful test in the diagnosis of hypothyroidism, although the debate continues. Up to 25% of euthyroid dogs will fail to stimulate at all.

Thyroglobulin autoantibodies (TGAA): Thyroglobulin is a protein involved in the production and storage of thyroid hormones within the thyroid gland. The presence of TGAA is an indicator of lymphocytic thyroiditis, but does not diagnose clinical hypothyroidism.

Anti-thyroid hormone antibodies AT3A/AT4A: These antibodies are occasionally found in canine sera and can interfere with the assays for TT4, fT4, TT3 and fT3, producing spuriously increased concentrations. They are not used as a diagnostic test for hypothyroidism.

In this case, the following tests were performed:
- Routine haematology was within laboratory reference ranges. Biochemical abnormalities included hypercholesterolaemia (8.4 mmol/l; normal reference range 2.5–7.5 mmol/l) and raised creatinine (133 μmol/l; normal reference range <120 μmol/l).
- A panel of tests for thyroid function revealed low total T4 (11.1 nmol/l; normal reference range 13–52) and low free T4 by equilibrium dialysis (<2.0 pmol/l; normal reference range 7.0–40). There was an increase in thyroid stimulating hormone (1.8 ng/ml; normal reference range <0.41) and thyroglobulin autoantibodies (586%; normal reference range <200%).

Skin biopsy for histopathology was not considered necessary in this case.

DIAGNOSIS

The diagnosis of primary hypothyroidism in this case was made on a combination of history, clinical signs and laboratory tests. The increase in thyroglobulin autoantibodies supported lymphocytic thyroiditis as the cause of hypothyroidism.

PROGNOSIS

The prognosis is generally good for most hypothyroid dogs with resolution of clinical signs on thyroid hormone supplementation. Lifelong treatment is required. There is usually improved demeanour and activity levels within a few weeks of initiation of therapy but hair regrowth may take many months.

ANATOMY AND PHYSIOLOGY REFRESHER

The thyroid gland in the dog consists of two lobes, each of which lies laterally to the fifth to eighth tracheal rings. A fibrous capsule covers the external surface and intersperses into the parenchyma, dividing it into lobules. Microscopically, the parenchyma is composed of lobules, which in turn are made up of a number of hollow, spherical epithelium-lined follicles. The follicle is the basic functional unit of the thyroid gland. The centre of each follicle is composed of a viscous homogeneous substance, the colloid, that is rich in thyroglobulin.

The process of formation and secretion of thyroid hormones is complex. Iodide, the main building block of the thyroid hormones, is actively transported from the extracellular fluid (capillaries) into the thyroid follicular cells. Within the cell, inorganic iodide is oxidized by thyroid peroxidase in the presence of H_2O_2 into a reactive intermediate that is incorporated into tyrosine residues of thyroglobulin to make monoiodotyrosine (MIT) or diiodotyrosine (DIT). This iodination of thyroglobulin takes place in the follicular (apical) border of the cell, and MIT and DIT are transported into the colloid by exocytosis.

The process of excretion of thyroid hormone involves MIT- and DIT-bound thyroglobulin being taken up by the epithelial cells by endocytosis of colloid droplets, which are processed and degraded by proteolytic enzymes into the thyroid hormones thyroxine (T4) and triiodothyronine (T3). T4 is formed by coupling two DIT molecules, T3 by coupling one DIT with one MIT molecule. The thyroid favours the production of thyroxine; however, in an iodine-deficient state, or during thyroid failure, T3 is produced in preference.

The circulatory levels of thyroxine regulate thyroid function by a negative feedback mechanism, involving the hypothalamus and the pars distalis of the pituitary gland. Thyroid-releasing hormone (TRH), produced by the hypothalamus in a tonic fashion, induces the transcription and secretion of thyroid-stimulating hormone (TSH) by the pars distalis. In addition, TSH is also secreted by a direct negative feedback, in response to reduced circulatory levels of T4. TSH stimulates the synthesis and secretion of thyroid hormone. It also promotes the growth of thyrocytes and deiodination of T4 to T3. T3 has three to four times the metabolic potency of T4 and 80% of secreted T4 is deiodinated to form T3 and rT3 (metabolically inactive form) in the peripheral tissues.

Maintaining circulatory levels of thyroid hormone involves complex interactions between the production, secretion, distribution, metabolism and excretion of the hormone. Thus, any factors influencing any of these processes will eventually affect the serum concentration of thyroxine. Ninety-nine per cent of thyroid hormone (both T4 and T3) in serum is protein bound to thyroxine-binding globulin (TBG) and other proteins. The factors that influence the concentration of TBG will also influence the total serum concentration of thyroid hormone.

These factors include a variety of diseases and pharmacological agents. Only unbound thyroid hormone is able to enter the cells and undergo excretion; therefore, for assessment of thyroid function, measurement of unbound thyroid hormones may provide a more accurate indication of thyroid status (see above section on thyroid tests).

Factors affecting thyroid function

As previously stated, age, breed, diurnal variation, drug administration and concurrent illness all affect serum thyroid hormone concentrations.

Age: Puppies in the first 3–4 months of life have serum total T4 concentrations two to five times higher than those of healthy adults, and healthy sighthounds have lower resting serum T4 concentrations than do mixed breed dogs.

Drugs: Drugs known to affect serum thyroid hormone concentrations include phenobarbitol, phenytoin, diazepam, glucocorticoids, sulphonamides, amitriptyline, clomipramine and some (although not all) non-steroidal anti-inflammatory drugs.

Illness: Illness of any type can alter hormone secretion, serum protein binding, distribution, metabolism and excretion, and the effect varies depending on the disease involved.

Euthyroid sick syndrome: Euthyroid sick syndrome is thought to be a protective mechanism in sick animals to prevent the catabolic effects of the metabolically active thyroid hormones T4 and, in particular, T3. The patients with this syndrome are euthyroid and will not benefit from thyroid hormone supplementation. In this syndrome total thyroid hormone concentrations tend to be decreased, but the free hormone fraction remains within reference ranges, thus the diagnosis of hypothyroidism based on basal total T4 serum concentrations is inherently unreliable because of the large overlap between concentrations in healthy, euthyroid sick and hypothyroid dogs.

AETIOPATHOGENESIS OF HYPOTHYROIDISM

Hypothyroidism results from decreased concentrations of circulating and tissue triiodothyronine (T3) and thyroxine (T4). More than 95% of cases of hypothyroidism in adult dogs are due to the destruction of the thyroid gland, as a result of a lymphocytic thyroiditis or idiopathic thyroid atrophy (thought to be the end stage of lymphocytic thyroiditis). Very rarely, a failure in the production of thyroid-stimulating hormone (TSH) from the anterior pituitary or thyrotropin-releasing hormone (TRH) from the hypothalamus can result in secondary or tertiary hypothyroidism respectively.

There are thyroid hormone receptors in cells of all organ systems, and therefore hypothyroidism causes a wide variety of systemic (Table 22.1) and dermatological (Table 22.2) signs. Dermatological signs are seen in around 80% of cases of canine hypothyroidism. Lack of thyroid hormone results in the inhibition of hair growth (anagen) and the majority of hair follicles remain in the resting phase (telogen). Hairs are either retained for long periods, leading to bleaching, or shed and not replaced, leading to alopecia. Alopecia over the tail, pinnae and bridge of the nose, as well as the flanks, are commonly seen in hypothyroidism. Hypothyroidism causes alterations in epidermal fatty acid composition, which in turn results in defective barrier function, as well as defects in humoral and cellular immune responses, both of which predispose to pyoderma. Scaling and pigmentary changes are also quite frequent findings in hypothyroidism.

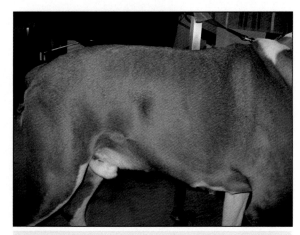

Figure 22.5 Complete hair regrowth 3 months after the start of treatment.

EPIDEMIOLOGY

Hypothyroidism is the commonest of the endocrine diseases. Breed predispositions are reported in Airedales, boxers, dachshunds, Dobermanns, golden retrievers, miniature schnauzers, Irish setters and Great Danes. In general, hypothyroidism is seen in middle-aged and older dogs, but can occur at a younger age, particularly in the predisposed giant breeds. However, it is very rare to see hypothyroidism in a dog less than 2 years old.

TREATMENT

Lifelong treatment is required and therefore a firm diagnosis should be made prior to starting thyroid supplementation. The use of therapeutic trials is not recommended. Treatment in this case was an oral supplementation of levothyroxine administered at 0.02 mg/kg twice daily. The majority of cases of canine hypothyroidism, however, are reported to respond satisfactorily to once-daily dosage. When treating dogs suffering from congestive cardiac failure, renal failure, hepatic disease or diabetes mellitus, the starting dose should

be 0.005 mg/kg and increased gradually over 3–4 weeks. Lethargy and mental demeanour will be the first symptoms to improve, generally within 2 weeks, but hair coat changes frequently take months to resolve. In this case the demeanour improved within 3 weeks and complete hair regrowth was seen within 3 months (Fig. 22.5).

THERAPEUTIC MONITORING

Post-pill monitoring of serum thyroxine concentrations is advisable, to ensure adequate supplementation and avoid the potentially harmful effects of thyrotoxicosis. Two to four weeks after commencement of therapy, serum TT4 concentration should be measured 4–6 hours after levothyroxine administration. Post-pill serum TT4 levels of between 30 and 65 nmol/l indicate that there is good absorption of T4. However, if the individual shows signs of thyrotoxicosis (weight loss, tachycardia, panting, anxiousness, polydipsia, polyphagia, polyuria, gastrointestinal signs) at the higher level, consider reducing the dosage slightly. Dogs with post-pill TT4 of less than 35 nmol/l usually require an increase in levothyroxine dosage to achieve clinical improvement. Post-pill TT4 measured at 6 hours in this case was 64 mmol/l. Post-pill cTSH was not measured in this case, but it may be of value to identify dogs which have been undertreated but will not distinguish between those that are adequately or oversupplemented.

Most nurses will be involved in sample collection, storage and transportation, and therefore should be aware of the factors that may influence the assay:

- Lipaemia can interfere with assays; therefore, make sure that the animal has been starved appropriately prior to sampling.
- Samples should be centrifuged within 30 minutes of sampling, shortly after the blood has clotted.
- Haemolysed samples should be discarded.
- The serum should be separated into a plain tube (it has been suggested that the separator serum gel may influence the results of the assay).
- The samples should be kept cool to reduce deterioration.
- The samples should be packaged and transported to the laboratory as soon as possible.

- Always measure both TT4 and cTSH, and perform haematology and biochemistry where indicated.
- Measure fT4 in addition to TT4 if non-thyroidal illness is suspected or if the animal is on drugs that cannot be withdrawn prior to testing.
- If the results are non-diagnostic, either repeat the tests after 4–6 months or, if a more rapid result is required, perform an rhTSH stimulation test (see above section on tests for hypothyroidism).
- A thyroid function panel, including TT4, cTSH, fT4, TGAA AT3A and AT4A, may be useful.
- Avoid therapeutic trials based on single assays, as this will tend to jeopardize future assays.

FOLLOW-UP

In this case the dog had a good response to therapy and the owner reported that, within 2 weeks, the dog was obviously more energetic. Full hair regrowth took several months. Over a 2-year period, the dog has been maintained on twice-daily levothyroxine treatment at the same dosage and is having 6-monthly post-pill monitoring of TT4.

23 Colour dilution alopecia

INITIAL PRESENTATION

Progressive alopecia.

INTRODUCTION

Colour dilution alopecia is a developmental disorder resulting in the weakening of hair shafts and progressive alopecia due to abnormal melanin pigment distribution within hair shafts, and within epidermal and follicular keratinocytes. It is a common condition in dogs with blue or fawn dilute colour hair coats. This case report describes a case of colour dilution alopecia in a collie with a blue hair coat.

CASE PRESENTING SIGNS

A 13-month-old, entire male Border collie was presented with a history of progressive alopecia.

CASE HISTORY

The onset of symptoms in colour dilution alopecia is usually between 6 months and 3 years of age and may present initially as gradual onset dorsal alopecia or as dorsal folliculitis. Only hairs in the dilute coat colour area are involved. When dogs present with folliculitis, there is a gradual progression of alopecia following each episode of folliculitis. Unless there is pyoderma, this is a non-pruritic disease and there is no systemic involvement. The history in this case was as follows:

- The dog had always had a dilute, blue-coloured hair coat.
- Over the past 6 weeks, there had been a progressive alopecia affecting predominantly the trunk and pinnae. White areas of hair coat were unaffected.
- There had been no evidence of pruritus and no other skin lesions.
- There were no signs suggestive of systemic involvement.
- There were no other in-contact animals.
- There was no evidence of zoonosis.
- Diet consisted of a relatively poor quality complete dried food with occasional scraps, dog chews and dog biscuits.
- The dog was regularly wormed and received routine vaccinations as a puppy.
- Flea control consisted of applications of a fipronil spot-on every 2 months.
- There had been no evidence of hair regrowth in response to 3 weeks of systemic antibacterial therapy using clindamycin at a dosage of 10 mg/kg q24 h.

CLINICAL EXAMINATION

General physical examination was unremarkable.

Examination of the skin revealed generalized, partial to complete alopecia over the pinnae and trunk (Figs 23.1 and 23.2). White areas were unaffected.

There was loss of primary hair shafts over the pigmented areas, revealing a blue to brown, dilute coloured undercoat.

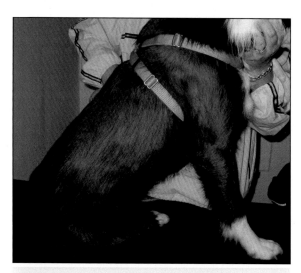

Figure 23.1 Initial presentation. Generalized partial alopecia over the trunk.

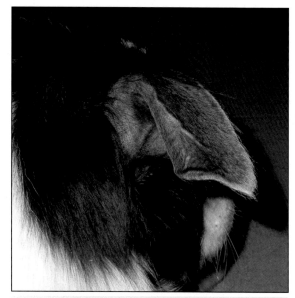

Figure 23.2 Initial presentation. Pinnal alopecia.

DIFFERENTIAL DIAGNOSES

In this case, the history and clinical signs were strongly suggestive of colour dilution alopecia, although other causes of non-pruritic alopecia were potential rule-outs. The involvement of a staphylococcal folliculitis could be ruled out on the basis of no response to the previous antibacterial therapy. In tardive onset cases, causes of hair follicle arrest, such as hypothyroidism and hyperadrenocorticism, should also be considered as differentials.

Therefore, the differential diagnosis list was:

- Colour dilution alopecia
- Other causes of follicular dysplasia
- Pattern alopecia
- Demodicosis
- Dermatophytosis.

CASE WORK-UP

Skin scraping examination and fungal cultures are indicated where a folliculitis is on the list of differential diagnoses. Trichographic examination of plucked hair shafts should show evidence of macromelanosome formation, resulting in distorted, or fractured, hair shafts, and the hair shafts should appear dysplastic ('deformed'). Histopathological examination helps support the clinical and trichographic diagnosis of colour dilution alopecia. Trial antibacterial therapy would also have been indicated if a staphylococcal infection had still been suspected.

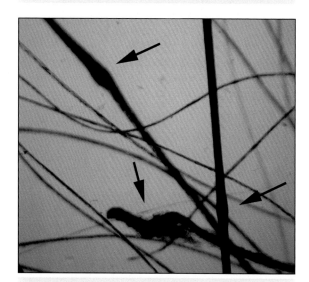

Figure 23.3 Photomicrograph of hair shafts from the dog in Fig. 23.1 showing melanin clumping and dysplasia (arrows).

The following diagnostic tests were performed:
- Multiple deep skin scrapings from affected areas, which showed no evidence of ectoparasitism.
- Trichographic examination of plucked hair shafts showed deformed dysplastic appearing hairs, with numerous large macromelanosomes resulting in distortion of hair shafts (Figs 23.3 and 23.4).
- Three samples of skin were harvested using a 6-mm biopsy punch and submitted for histopathological

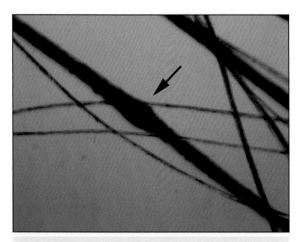

Figure 23.4 Photomicrograph of hair shafts from the dog in Fig. 23.1 showing melanin clumping and dysplasia (arrow).

examination, which revealed dysplastic hair shafts and clumped melanin pigment, both within hair follicles and hair shafts, and within the basal layer of the epidermis. These changes were consistent with a diagnosis of colour dilution/colour mutant alopecia.

DIAGNOSIS

The history, clinical signs, trichography and histopathology were consistent with a diagnosis of colour dilution alopecia.

PROGNOSIS

The prognosis for colour dilution alopecia is guarded. Although a purely cosmetic condition, the hair loss is gradually progressive, with complete alopecia developing after a few years. Episodes of secondary bacterial folliculitis are common. Because of the lack of sun protection there may be increased risk of ultraviolet light-induced skin disease and there may be an increased risk of cutaneous neoplasia.

AETIOLOGICAL AND PATHOPHYSIOLOGICAL ASPECTS OF COLOUR DILUTION ALOPECIA

Colour dilution alopecia is a form of hair follicle dysplasia. Dysplastic hair follicle diseases are characterized by abnormal growth and development of the hair follicle or associated glands. Hair follicle dysplasia may result in distortion, abnormal deposits, attenuation, absence, proliferation or degeneration. Colour dilution alopecia is a relatively common condition seen in dogs with a blue

or fawn 'dilute' hair coat colour. In general, the lighter the hair coat colour, the more severe the disease.

Colour dilution alopecia is a genodermatosis and an autosomal mode of inheritance has been suggested. A colour dilution gene has been linked to the d-locus. It is not known whether this gene is directly responsible for initiating the disease or whether this is a polygenic condition with other genes involved. In colour dilute breeds, there are abnormalities of melanosome storage and transfer from the melanocyte to surrounding keratinocytes. A recent study of black-haired follicular dysplasia (a condition similar to colour dilution alopecia but affecting dogs with black, rather than dilute, hair coat colour) concluded that the condition was analogous to Griscelli syndrome in man. This condition is caused by a defect of melanocytic intracellular transport proteins, resulting in a similar phenotypic appearance.

It should be remembered that all dilute colour hairs contain larger than normal accumulations of melanin, regardless of whether there is evidence of colour dilution alopecia. In dogs with colour dilution alopecia, there is evidence of hair shaft distortion due to the presence of large clumps of pigment (Figs 23.3 and 23.4) that probably weakens the hair shaft, leading to fracture. This is likely to be the main cause of alopecia early in the course of the disease. Folliculitis is also common in these dogs and will lead to further alopecia; however, these factors alone would not usually explain the extent of hair loss. Signals from melanocytes are important in the initiation of anagen, the growth phase of the hair follicle, and it is possible that the abnormal transfer of melanosomes in colour dilution alopecia could result in a lack of stimulation of the hair bulb keratinocytes, leading to resting, non-cycling follicles.

EPIDEMIOLOGY

Colour dilution alopecia is most frequently seen in the blue Dobermann pinscher, but many other dilute coat colour breeds including the Great Dane, whippet, Italian greyhound, Yorkshire terrier, chihuahua, miniature pinscher, chow-chow, silky terriers and mongrels with dilute coat colours are affected. Dogs with light blue coats usually first develop symptoms at around 6 months of age, whereas those with less marked coat colour dilution may have a more tardive onset between 2 and 3 years of age.

TREATMENT OPTIONS

As colour dilution alopecia is a progressive incurable genodermatosis, there is no effective treatment;

however, there are some palliative measures that can be taken. Early in the course of the condition the hair coat becomes dry and brittle, and scaling may become evident. The hair loss is due to hair shaft fracture and so excessive brushing and vigorous shampooing should be avoided, but moisturizers may improve the appearance of the hair coat and perhaps make it less brittle and liable to fracture. Episodes of folliculitis should be treated with systemic and gentle topical antibacterial therapy. Some cases develop quite severe scaling and oral vitamin A or synthetic retinoids (see Chapter 13) have been advocated to control the scale, and perhaps help to reduce the frequency and severity of bacterial folliculitis. Anecdotally, melatonin (see Chapter 24), given as a non-specific hair cycling inducer may be effective in promoting hair growth in colour dilution alopecia.

In this case, the following treatments were administered:

- Daily administration of an omega-6- and omega-3-containing fatty acid supplement at a dosage of 15 mg/kg γ-linolenic acid p.o., s.i.d.
- Daily or alternate-day applications of propylene glycol diluted 50:50 with water and applied using a plant hand sprayer.
- Treatment was started with melatonin at a dosage of 3 mg p.o., t.i.d. Melatonin is unlicensed for veterinary use but can be obtained with a special import certificate.

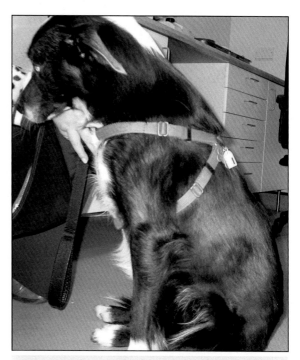

Figure 23.5 Same dog as in Fig. 23.1 after 3 months of treatment. There is some hair regrowth over the trunk.

CLINICAL TIPS

Examination of hair shafts is a useful diagnostic technique in colour dilution alopecia. However, large accumulations of pigment will be evident in the hair shafts of all dogs with a dilute coat colour, regardless of whether they have colour dilution alopecia. There should be evidence of dysplastic and distorted hair shafts, as in this case, to make the diagnosis of colour dilution alopecia.

The best sites from which to take samples for histopathological examination are those with complete alopecia. As usual, three to five areas should be sampled.

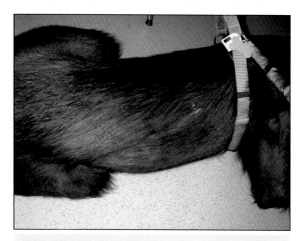

Figure 23.6 After 5 months of treatment. Further hair loss is evident over the flanks.

FOLLOW-UP

Re-examination after 3 months of treatment revealed no progression of the alopecia, with minimal scaling (Fig. 23.5), and so treatment was continued. After a further 2 months, there had been further progression of the alopecia (Fig. 23.6) and the owner elected to stop melatonin therapy on the grounds of lack of efficacy. The topical therapy and essential fatty acid supplement were continued. In a follow-up telephone call a year later, the owner reported that there had been no further progression and there had in fact been an apparent waxing and waning of the degree of alopecia. There had been no evidence of pruritus or folliculitis.

24 Alopecia X in a Pomeranian

INITIAL PRESENTATION

Symmetrical, truncal, non-inflammatory alopecia in a Pomeranian.

INTRODUCTION

Symmetrical, truncal, non-inflammatory alopecia can occur for a number of different reasons, including follicular dysplasias and endocrinopathies. The most common endocrinopathies resulting in these symptoms are hypothyroidism and hyperadrenocorticism. There is a form of alopecia that occurs in plush-coated Nordic breeds characterized by bilaterally symmetrical, non-inflammatory alopecia with hyperpigmentation. The exact aetiology is not known and the condition has been designated 'alopecia X'. This case report describes a case of alopecia X in a Pomeranian.

CASE PRESENTING SIGNS

A 4-year-old, spayed female Pomeranian was presented because of non-pruritic alopecia.

CASE HISTORY

The history in cases of alopecia X is of gradual, progressive onset of alopecia without systemic signs. There may be a history of hair regrowth over skin scrape, biopsy or other surgical sites.

The history in this case was as follows:

- There was a 12-month history of, initially, thinning of the hair coat over the dorsal neck, with later complete alopecia over the trunk but sparing the head and limbs.
- There had been no evidence of pruritus nor any evidence of inflammation.

- The areas of alopecia had become markedly pigmented.
- No polyuria, polydipsia or polyphagia, no weight change, no lethargy and no other signs suggestive of systemic involvement were seen.
- There was no regrowth of hair following 1 month of treatment with levothyroxine at a dosage of 10 µg/kg b.i.d.
- There was no regrowth of hair following 2 months of treatment with melatonin at a dosage of 2 mg t.i.d.
- A routine ovariohysterctomy had been performed after the onset of hair loss, and there had been hair regrowth over the spay wound site.
- There were six other related dogs within the household, none of whom had been affected, although the sire of the affected dog had developed similar symptoms that had remained undiagnosed.
- There was no zoonosis.
- The dog was fed a standard tinned dog food and biscuit mixer along with biscuits and dog chews.

CLINICAL EXAMINATION

There were no abnormalities on full physical examination.

The significant findings on examination of the skin were:

- Well-demarcated areas of partial to complete alopecia and hyperpigmentation over the trunk.
- The head and limbs were spared (Figs 24.1, 24.2 and 24.3).

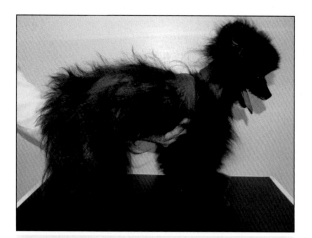

Figure 24.1 Hair loss on flank at presentation.

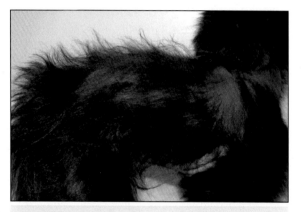

Figure 24.2 Hair loss on flank at presentation (close-up).

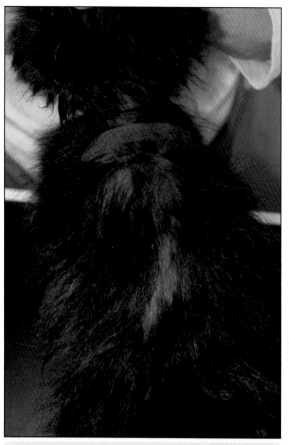

Figure 24.3 Hair loss on dorsum at presentation.

DIFFERENTIAL DIAGNOSES

The symptoms of symmetrical, non-inflammatory, truncal alopecia were supportive of a hair growth cycle disorder due to an endocrinopathy, although the differential diagnosis would include other causes of non-pruritic hair loss, including:

- Alopecia X
- Hypothyroidism
- Hyperadrenocorticism
- Seasonal or cyclical flank alopecia
- Telogen defluxion
- Sebaceous adenitis
- Alopecia areata
- Pseudopelade
- Demodicosis.

CASE WORK-UP

As with any case of alopecia, skin scrapes should be performed to rule out demodicosis. Routine haematological and biochemical examinations and further tests for hyperadrenocorticism and hypothyroidism were also indicated. In addition to a standard ACTH stimulation test measuring pre- and post-ACTH cortisol concentrations, the same test, measuring pre- and post-17-hydroxy-progesterone concentrations, has been used as an indicator of adrenal dysfunction. Post-ACTH 17-hydroxy-progesterone concentrations are frequently elevated in cases of alopecia X. Histopathological examination is unlikely to give a definitive diagnosis in a case of alopecia due to an endocrinopathy but would be helpful in ruling out other causes of hair loss.

The following diagnostic tests were performed:

- Microscopic examination of multiple deep skin scrapes showed no evidence of ectoparasitism.
- Histopathological examination revealed an atrophic dermatosis with epidermal atrophy, mild orthokeratotic hyperkeratosis, mild hypermelanosis and mild to moderate follicular keratosis. There was miniaturization of some hair follicles and fewer than expected anagen hair bulbs in the sections. Most hair follicles were in telogen.
- Apart from eosinopaenia, there were no other significant abnormalities on haematological and biochemical examination.
- ACTH stimulation provoked a markedly exaggerated response of 17-hydroxy-progesterone:
  Cortisol concentrations:
  - Basal, 184.0 nmol/l (50.0–250.0)
  - Post-ACTH, 462.0 nmol/l (150.0–550.0).
  17-Hydroxy-progesterone concentrations:
  - Basal, 1.6 nmol/l (<3)
  - Post-ACTH, 15.2 nmol/l (<4).

DIAGNOSIS

The history, clinical signs and results of laboratory tests were consistent with a diagnosis of alopecia X.

PROGNOSIS

Alopecia X is a benign, essentially cosmetic, condition. There are no reported cases with severe systemic involvement. If left untreated, the hair loss can progress to involve the entire trunk but will spare the head and legs. There are treatment options that seem to be effective in inducing hair regrowth, although hair loss may recur after apparently successful therapy.

AETIOLOGICAL AND PATHOPHYSIOLOGICAL ASPECTS OF ALOPECIA X

The control of hair growth is complex and poorly understood but is influenced by many extrinsic and intrinsic growth factors. Extrinsic factors include hormones, neuropeptides and signals from immunologically active cells. Intrinsic factors include hormones working in a paracrine or autocrine fashion, cytokines and growth factors, neuropeptides, adhesion molecules and enzymes.

The aetiopathogenesis of alopecia X remains obscure. The controversial name was coined 10 years ago to encompass a number of clinical entities, affecting mainly the plush-coated breeds, with a similar clinical picture and named according to endocrinological abnormalities and/or response to various treatment regimes. These conditions include congenital adrenal hyperplasia-like syndrome, pseudo-Cushing's syndrome, growth hormone-responsive alopecia, castration-responsive dermatosis and black skin disease of Pomeranians, amongst many others.

There have been various hypotheses put forward as to the cause of the hair loss in alopecia X, including a genetic predisposition to a hormone imbalance and/or a defect in hair follicle receptors, that seem to vary according to the breed involved. A deficiency of the steroidogenesis hormone, 21-hydroxylase, leading to an increase in the concentration of progesterone (Fig. 24.4), has been postulated to be a factor in the pathogenesis of alopecia X. This abnormality has been demonstrated in poodles, Pomeranians and Alaskan malamutes. There is also evidence that dogs with alopecia X have some increase in cortisol production. These factors are behind the rationale of treating alopecia X with trilostane. However, the significance of these apparent abnormalities in corticosteroid and sex hormone concentrations in relation to the alopecia is still in some doubt, as sex hormone concentrations did not return to the expected reference range concentrations in dogs with alopecia X successfully treated with either melatonin or mitotane. To date, although breed-specific hormonal abnormalities have been demonstrated (i.e. Pomeranians and Alaskan malamutes), these abnormalities do not consistently affect other plush-coated breeds affected by alopecia X, and no consistent hormonal abnormalities have been demonstrated in breeds such as the chow-chow and samoyed. Based on the results of one study, there is no single hormonal abnormality associated with the hair loss in alopecia X and it might be better to consider this condition to be one of hair follicle arrest rather than equating it with an adrenal hormone imbalance. Thus, at the time of writing, work still needs to be done to establish the aetiology of this condition.

EPIDEMIOLOGY

Alopecia X has been recognized most frequently in the plush-coated breeds, including Pomeranians, samoyeds, malamutes, huskies, chow-chows and keeshonds. Miniature poodles are also predisposed. Any age of dog can be affected, from early adulthood to 11 years of age. It is seen more frequently in neutered dogs.

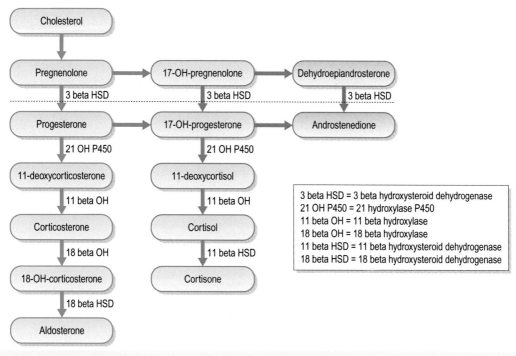

Figure 24.4 Simplified outline of steroidogenesis pathways in the adrenal cortex.

TREATMENT OPTIONS

As this is a cosmetic condition with no serious systemic effects, some owners may decline treatment after counselling; however, there are numerous treatment options which may result in some hair regrowth.

Neutering: Neutering results in hair regrowth in some intact male and female animals, and should be considered as a first-line treatment.

Melatonin: In neutered animals, for reasons of cost and safety, melatonin is now considered the treatment of choice by most veterinary dermatologists. At the time of writing, in the USA, melatonin is considered to be a food supplement and is available over the counter. However, in the UK it is considered a drug; it is therefore an unlicensed product and its import is subject to restrictions. Work still needs to be done to optimize dosage and duration of treatment, but oral melatonin, at the rate of 3 mg/dog (b.i.d. or t.i.d.) for up to 3 months, is commonly used to treat alopecia X. Around one-third of cases can be expected to exhibit hair regrowth with this treatment.

Mitotane: Mitotane causes necrosis and atrophy of the adrenal cortex and, prior to licensing of trilostane, was routinely used for the treatment of hyperadrenocorticism. Mitotane has also been used successfully for the treatment of alopecia X, although this is a potent and unlicensed therapy.

Trilostane: More recently, there have been reports that trilostane, a competitive inhibitor of 3β-hydroxysteroid dehydrogenase which interferes with adrenal steroidogenesis, has resulted in hair regrowth in affected Pomeranians, miniature poodles and Alaskan malamutes. This is a treatment that has been shown to be effective in cases of spontaneous hyperadrenocorticism.

Treatment in this case: The owner was particularly keen to try further treatment and, as there had been no response to melatonin, the decision was made to start treatment with trilostane.

The initial dosage of trilostane administered was 3.5 mg/kg s.i.d. with food.

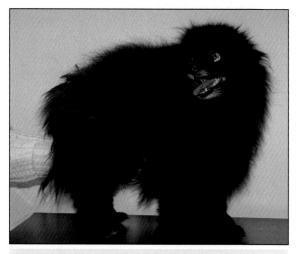

Figure 24.5 Hair regrowth after 7 months of continuous trilostane treatment, right flank.

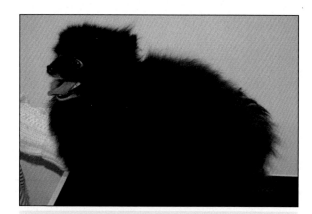

Figure 24.6 Hair regrowth after 7 months of continuous trilostane treatment, left flank.

FOLLOW-UP

Routine monitoring of this case involved re-examination at 10 days, 4 weeks, 3 months and every 3 months thereafter for routine biochemistry and repeat ACTH stimulation tests.

There were no abnormalities on any of the serum biochemical examinations.

After 10 days' treatment with trilostane, pre- and post-ACTH cortisol concentrations were 134 and 375 nmol/l respectively, and the dosage of trilostane was increased to 7 mg/kg s.i.d.

Within 4 weeks of increasing the dosage of trilostane, there was some evidence of hair regrowth.

After 4 months of therapy, there was almost complete regrowth of hair, although some thinning of secondary hairs remained.

After 7 months of continuous trilostane treatment, hair regrowth was considered acceptable by the owner (Figs 24.5, 24.6 and 24.7) and the trilostane dosage was reduced to 7 mg/kg given on alternate days.

On re-inspection 6 weeks later, patches of alopecia had developed over the neck and caudal dorsum, and the trilostane dosage was once again increased to 7 mg/kg s.i.d. At the time of writing, the response to the increased trilostane dosage is not known.

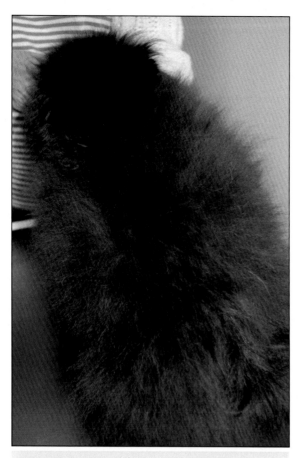

Figure 24.7 Hair regrowth after 7 months of continuous trilostane treatment, dorsum.

INITIAL PRESENTATION

Symmetrical alopecia with mild scaling and hyperpigmentation.

INTRODUCTION

Canine recurrent flank alopecia is characterized by symmetrical seasonal hair loss affecting the thorax and flanks. In the past, it has been referred to as seasonal flank alopecia, canine idiopathic cyclic flank alopecia and cyclic follicular dysplasia. The condition mimics other endocrine disorders but the aetiology of canine recurrent flank alopecia is not known. There is seasonal hair regrowth in most dogs affected by this condition; however, in a small number of cases it may only be partial, or even non-existent. Clinically, canine recurrent flank alopecia is most often confused with hypothyroidism and, being only an aesthetic problem, it is important to distinguish between the two at the first instance to avoid unnecessary lifelong therapy. This report describes such a case.

CASE PRESENTING SIGNS

A 4-year-old spayed, female Rhodesian ridgeback was presented, in spring 2006, with symmetrical truncal alopecia and excessive hyperpigmentation of the skin.

CASE HISTORY

Most cases are presented for the alopecia, which appears to be visually more marked because of the hyperpigmentation. Most dogs do not exhibit signs of pruritus unless there is secondary pyoderma. The affected dogs are healthy and usually the onset of the condition is of short duration.

The history in this case was:
- The dog's general health was unaffected.
- The familial history was unknown.
- The dog's routine management had not been changed.
- The hair loss was first noticed in late December/early January.
- It had started on the flanks and progressed anteriorly to involve the lateral thorax.
- There was poor hair regrowth at the site of clipping for skin scrapes.
- The condition was non-pruritic.

CLINICAL EXAMINATION

Generally the alopecia is bilaterally symmetrical, mostly involving the lateral thorax and flanks, but in some dogs it may also affect the dorsal aspects. In a minority of cases, it may also involve the bridge of the nose, convex aspects of the ears, the tail base and the perineum. The alopecia is usually irregular but well demarcated, and both primary and secondary hairs are lost. On regrowth, a change in hair colour – lighter (aurotrichia) or darker (melanotrichia) – may be evident and, in some dogs, the new hair is dry, coarse and brittle. General physical examination in all cases is unremarkable, unless there is a concurrent disease.

The key findings in this case were:
- No abnormalities were detected on physical examination. The heart rate was 90 beats per minute.
- A symmetrical alopecia affected the lateral aspects of the thorax and the flanks (Fig. 25.1).
- The skin was grossly hyperpigmented (Fig. 25.2).
- The hair was easily epilated during examination.

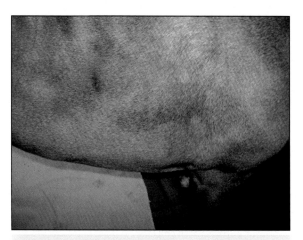

Figure 25.1 Alopecia and hyperpigmentation on the lateral thorax and abdomen (note the biopsy site).

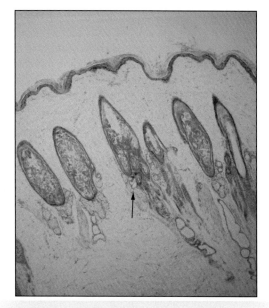

Figure 25.3 Histological section showing marked hyperkeratosis of the follicular infundibula, giving the appearance of 'witches' feet'.

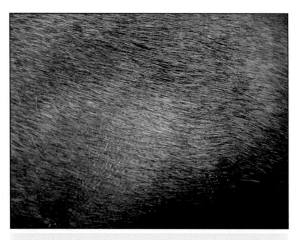

Figure 25.2 Marked hyperpigmentation and hypotrichosis on the lateral thorax.

DIFFERENTIAL DIAGNOSES

These include all the potential causes of symmetrical alopecia of dogs, which are:
- Canine recurrent flank alopecia
- Hypothyroidism
- Hyperadrenocorticism
- Sex hormone imbalance (oestrogen-responsive dermatosis)
- Alopecia X
- Demodicosis.

CASE WORK-UP

Although the main differential diagnoses for canine recurrent flank alopecia are endocrinopathies, demodicosis should always be ruled out with skin scrapings. A trichogram is useful in showing that the hair loss is not self-induced and will provide information on the stage of hair cycle.

The following tests were performed:
- No evidence of demodicosis was found on examination of deep skin scrapings.
- Trichographic examination revealed almost entirely telogen hair roots.
- There were no abnormalities on haematological and biochemical examination.
- Basal thyroxine and endogenous TSH were within laboratory reference ranges.

Four skin samples were taken by punch biopsy from both flanks, one from each of the areas of maximum hair loss and also from the lesion margins.

The histology revealed an epidermis of normal thickness, which was hypermelanotic. Marked orthokeratotic hyperkeratosis of the follicular infundibulum, giving the appearance of witches' feet (Fig. 25.3), was evident.

These changes are typically seen during the active phase of the hair loss in dogs affected with canine recurrent flank alopecia. In later stages, when only atrophic follicles are present, it can be difficult to distinguish canine recurrent flank alopecia from hypothyroidism. Indeed, histology alone does not rule out the other differential diagnoses but hypothyroidism could be ruled out on history, physical examination and thyroid function tests. Dogs with hyperadrenocorticism have a history of polyuria, polydipsia and polyphagia and clinical examination usually reveals systemic signs such as hepatomegaly, abdominal enlargement, and muscle weakness and wasting. The skin lesions include comedones, recurrent pyoderma and thin hypotonic skin with prominent vasculature. In this case, the history and clinical signs were not suggestive of hyperadrenocorticism, nor was it supported by the haematology and biochemistry as raised serum alkaline phosphatase is a fairly consistent finding in dogs with hyperadrenocorticism.

DIAGNOSIS

In this case, the history, examination and results of the laboratory tests were consistent with a diagnosis of canine recurrent flank alopecia.

PROGNOSIS

The prognosis for canine recurrent flank alopecia is variable. Most cases show ongoing seasonal hair loss followed by hair regrowth. Approximately 20% of cases may have only one isolated episode of flank alopecia during their life but in others, there may be a progression to complete failure of hair regrowth. The area of alopecia is variable: some dogs develop virtually the same hair loss (size and duration) year after year whilst others develop progressive larger areas and/or longer episodes of hair loss as years go by. There is no systemic involvement.

ANATOMY AND PHYSIOLOGY REFRESHER

Hair growth occurs in cycles, and is influenced by local and systemic, intrinsic and extrinsic factors and external factors, such as seasons and the photoperiod (see Chapter 20). The aetiology of canine recurrent flank alopecia is not known but, because it is seasonal and occurs annually, photoperiodicity has been implicated, but not proven. Moulting is associated with external stimuli such as the photoperiod, via its action on the pineal gland. Melatonin is produced by the pineal body during the hours of darkness and initiates hair growth, which provides the link between external factors and systemic hormonal influences on hair growth and the hair cycle. Circulating levels of prolactin have the opposite effect to that of melatonin.

EPIDEMIOLOGY

The condition may occur in any breed but is most frequently seen in the boxer. Other predisposed breeds include Airedale terriers, English bulldogs, miniature schnauzers and bearded collies, suggesting a genetic predisposition. Increased risk is also reported in Rhodesian ridgebacks, Dobermann pinschers, Scottish terriers, and German short-haired and wire-haired pointers. Geographically, the incidence is greater where the changes in seasons are well defined. In most cases, the hair loss occurs between November and March. In a small percentage of cases the reverse occurs. There is no known sex predisposition and it can occur at any age in adult dogs, with a mean age of onset of the first episode of approximately 4 years.

TREATMENT

Canine recurrent flank alopecia is an aesthetic condition and although most dogs will have spontaneous hair regrowth without treatment, the clinical course is variable and some dogs fail to regrow their coat.

Melatonin: Melatonin is used by some dermatologists and is helpful in some cases in either preventing recurrence of alopecia or reducing the duration of the alopecic episode. This is an unlicensed treatment and currently requires a Special Treatment Authorization in the UK. Melatonin is administered at the dose of 3–6 mg/dog every 8–12 hours for up to 2 months. The use of melatonin is at present experimental and, in the short term, its use appears to be safe, but the effects of its long-term use are not known.

Treatment in this case

In this case, the dog had completely regrown all its lost hair by the end of August (Fig. 25.4), and treatment was not required.

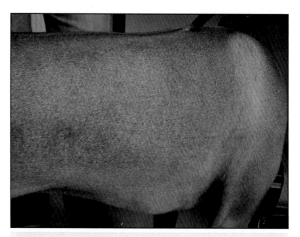

Figure 25.4 Spontaneous regrowth of hair at the end of summer.

Canine recurrent flank alopecia is easily confused with hypothyroidism, so always rule out thyroid dysfunction before making a definitive diagnosis.

Remember that the two conditions can occur concurrently in older animals, so re-evaluate the case if there are systemic signs or a failure of hair regrowth as the dog gets older.

FOLLOW-UP

There was no recurrence of the alopecia in the subsequent year up to the time of writing.

Demodicosis

Multifocal alopecia, crusting and scaling in a West Highland terrier.

INTRODUCTION

Canine demodicosis is a common skin disease resulting from a proliferation of *Demodex* spp. mites within hair follicles or, depending on the species of mite involved, in the stratum corneum. The disease usually presents as focal or multifocal patches of alopecia, with or without secondary pyoderma. This case report describes a case of demodicosis in an adult West Highland terrier that had a long history of glucocorticoid-responsive pruritus and concurrent respiratory disease.

CASE PRESENTING SIGNS

A 6-year-old, spayed female West Highland white terrier was presented with multifocal alopecia, crusting and scaling.

CASE HISTORY

The disease is most commonly seen in puppies and young dogs, with no history suggestive of systemic involvement. In around 50% of adult-onset cases there is some underlying immunosuppressive disorder and the history may reflect this. There may be a history of long-standing pruritic skin disease that has been reasonably well controlled by the use of glucocorticoids, but therapy has recently been ineffective and the skin lesions have become more severe. Demodicosis is not zoonotic and only very rarely contagious.

The history in this case was as follows:

- Non-seasonal dorsal, ventral, pedal and limb pruritus developed from around 6 months of age.

- The pruritus had been controlled effectively with methylprednisolone at dosages of between 0.25 and 0.5 mg/kg on alternate days.
- Eight months prior to presentation, patchy alopecia with later crusting and scaling had developed over the trunk and limbs. There had been no increase in pruritus associated with the lesions.
- Increasing the methylprednisolone dosage to 0.5 mg/kg s.i.d. had resulted in no clinical improvement.
- An 8-week course of enrofloxacin at a dosage of 5 mg/kg s.i.d. resulted in reduction in crusting and scaling, but no regrowth of hair.
- There was no evidence of zoonosis.
- There were no other pets in the household.
- Routine flea control was not used.
- The diet consisted of a commercial turkey and rice kibble, with additional dog biscuits and water.

CLINICAL EXAMINATION

Demodicosis usually presents as focal or multifocal patches of alopecia with variable crusting, scaling and pruritus. Canine localized demodicosis (CLD) is usually defined as involving up to five individual patches of alopecia, while generalized disease (CGD) involves six or more patches, an entire body region, or presents as pododemodicosis. Squamous demodicosis is characterized by patches of alopecia, scaling, erythema, folliculitis and comedone formation. Pustular demodicosis is diagnosed when secondary bacterial infection is present, and is characterized by lesions of deep pyoderma and cellulitis. Most cases of CLD are squamous, whereas CGD may initially present as squamous, but frequently

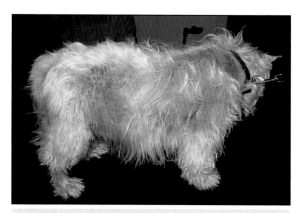

Figure 26.1 Adult-onset generalized demodicosis. Extensive truncal alopecia, erythema and hyperpigmentation.

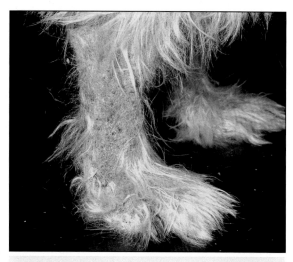

Figure 26.2 Close-up of the hind leg of the dog in Fig. 26.1, showing alopecia, scaling, crusting and erythema.

progresses to the pustular form of the disease. Extensive pustular demodicosis is a severe, potentially life-threatening systemic disease. Secondary infection with *Staphylococcus intermedius* is common and more rarely *Pseudomonas aeruginosa* or *Proteus mirabilis* may be involved. Peripheral lymphadenopathy is usually present in pustular demodicosis.

Examination in this case revealed:
- The patient had a slightly pot-bellied appearance and was hyperpnoeic at rest.
- Rectal temperature was 102°F; mucous membranes were pale. There was marked prescapular and popliteal lymphadenopathy.
- Auscultation of the chest revealed a grade 3/6 systolic cardiac murmur and severe generalized crackles over lung fields.
- Examination of the skin revealed generalized hypotrichosis. Additionally, there were multifocal, partial to complete, poorly demarcated patches of alopecia, with variable erythema, crusting, scaling and hyperpigmentation over the trunk and limbs (Figs 26.1 and 26.2).

DIFFERENTIAL DIAGNOSES

There was a long history of glucocorticoid-responsive pruritus that was very suggestive of a hypersensitivity disorder. The recent exacerbation of skin disease associated with multifocal alopecia, crusting and scaling was consistent with the development of an additional disease such as

pyoderma or demodicosis. Additionally, there were signs of systemic disease, probably related to hypercortisolaemia and also respiratory involvement.

Therefore, the differential diagnosis list included:
- Demodicosis
- Pyoderma
- Dermatophytosis
- Atopic dermatitis
- Cutaneous adverse food reaction
- Iatrogenic hyperadrenocorticism
- Congestive cardiac failure
- Pulmonary interstitial fibrosis.

CASE WORK-UP

The diagnosis of demodicosis is generally made on the microscopic demonstration of mites or eggs. Skin scrapes are the most sensitive method of finding mites, although they may also be found on examination of exudate or on trichography (see Chapter 2). Skin scrapes and cytology should always be the first diagnostic tests performed where there is evidence of alopecia, crusting and scaling.
- Numerous adult and immature *Demodex canis* and eggs were found on hair plucks and multiple skin scrapes from the trunk (Fig. 26.3).

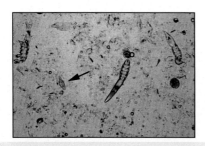

Figure 26.3 *Demodex canis* mites and egg (arrowed) in a skin scrape taken from the dog in Fig. 26.1.

- Cocci were seen on an impression smear from a crusted area.

Further investigation of the respiratory disease was indicated because not only was the disease affecting the patient's quality of life, but also because any treatment required to control the respiratory symptoms could have a bearing on the management of the demodicosis. The dog was thus referred to a cardiologist.
- Thoracic radiography revealed an enlarged cardiac silhouette and marked generalized increase in bronchointerstitial markings over the lung fields. There was marked hepatomegaly.

DIAGNOSIS

The cause of the recent severe skin disease was generalized, adult-onset, demodicosis.

Adult-onset demodicosis is usually associated with underlying immunosuppression and, in this case, the long-term use of glucocorticoids to control pruritus was very likely to be the cause. Additionally, the chronic respiratory disease and secondary pyoderma would have lead to further immunosuppression. The long-term pruritus was suggestive of a hypersensitivity disorder. There was evidence of cardiac enlargement and a heart murmur but no clinical signs suggestive of congestive cardiac failure. The provisional diagnosis for the thoracic disease was pulmonary interstitial fibrosis.

PROGNOSIS

The prognosis for adult-onset canine generalized demodicosis is guarded because, despite apparent elimination of mites, around 10–15% of cases of CGD relapse within several months of treatment withdrawal, unless the cause of the underlying immunosuppression can be identified and resolved.

In this case, the situation was made more complex by the presence of the respiratory disease. Pulmonary interstitial fibrosis is an irreversible condition and ongoing glucocorticoid treatment was likely to be required to control the respiratory symptoms. This medication would complicate management of the demodicosis and probably necessitate the use of ongoing miticidal therapy to prevent recurrence of demodicosis in the face of glucocorticoid treatment.

AETIOPATHOGENESIS OF DEMODICOSIS

Demodex mites are normal residents of mammalian skin and are acquired from the dam when young suckle. Three different species of mite with different morphologies have been identified in the dog. *Demodex canis* and a long-tailed mite recently named *Demodex injai* are the species that inhabit canine hair follicles and sebaceous glands. A short, unnamed form is considered to inhabit the surface layers of the epidermis and may be detected on tape-strip preparations. Clinical disease comes with the accumulation of large numbers of mites within hair follicles, resulting in first folliculitis and loss of hair, and subsequently furunculosis and deep pyoderma.

Evidence has been accumulated that supports the likelihood that dogs susceptible to demodicosis have a *Demodex*-specific T-cell immunodeficiency of varying severity that allows the proliferation of mite numbers. This immunodeficiency may be exacerbated by stress in young puppies and, in older dogs, by underlying immunosuppressive diseases such as hypothyroidism, hyperadrenocorticism, diabetes mellitus and leishmaniosis, or immunosuppressive treatment with immunosuppressive or cytotoxic therapies. However, in 30–50% of cases of adult-onset demodicosis, an underlying disease is not found. Once the disease has established, further immunosuppressive humoral factors are thought to be produced by the large numbers of mites and secondary pyoderma, resulting in greater proliferation of mite numbers.

EPIDEMIOLOGY

Demodicosis is seen most commonly in puppies and young dogs; the majority of cases start between 3 and 18 months of age. Many of these juvenile cases spontaneously resolve but the disease may persist into adulthood.

Adult-onset demodicosis is used to describe cases where the disease first appeared when the dog was 4 years or older.

Differing breed predispositions for juvenile- and adult-onset demodicosis have been recognized. Demodicosis is more common in pure bred dogs and predisposed breeds include the Shar Pei, West Highland white terrier, Scottish terrier, English bulldog, Staffordshire bull terrier, boxer and Great Dane.

Sex predilections are not noted with canine demodicosis.

TREATMENT OPTIONS FOR THE RESPIRATORY DISEASE

Interstitial pulmonary fibrosis results in loss of lung tissue elasticity with increased airway resistance and airway collapse during expiration. Despite fairly severe radiographic changes, the patient was relatively asymptomatic and it was considered that the previous glucocorticoid administration had been controlling the symptoms. On the advice of the cardiologist, it was decided that glucocorticoid therapy should be continued, albeit at the lowest possible dosage, with the option of introducing bronchodilating drugs such as theophylline or terbutaline if required. It was also likely that the glucocorticoid therapy would additionally control the symptoms due to the putative hypersensitivity disorder.

TREATMENT OPTIONS FOR DEMODICOSIS

Basic principles: Concurrent pyoderma has been shown to contribute to the immunosuppression in demodicosis and should be thoroughly treated. Failure to treat pyoderma is one reason for the recurrence, or persistence, of demodicosis. A bactericidal antibacterial should be used, and treatment should be continued for at least 2 weeks past resolution of pyoderma. In the case of adult-onset disease, every attempt should be made to identify and resolve any underlying immunosuppressive disorder. In general, concurrent glucocorticoid administration of any kind is contraindicated although there were exceptional circumstances in this case.

Miticidal treatment is indicated in cases of canine generalized demodicosis. An effective miticide should be used and treatment should be continued until complete elimination of mites. As a clinical cure will occur before all mites are eliminated, it is essential to determine the end point of treatment by taking repeat skin scrapings. Note that miticidal therapy is frequently not required in cases of localized, juvenile-onset demodicosis, where the disease frequently resolves spontaneously.

Many treatments and differing protocols have been described and published for the treatment of canine demodicosis. These studies should be carefully appraised bearing in mind that spontaneous resolution of the disease is common. Furthermore, a treatment should only be considered as effective if the dog is still free of disease after a year.

In view of the apparent inheritability of the disease, it is recommended that all dogs that have developed generalized demodicosis should be neutered.

Amitraz: Amitraz is an acaricide/insecticide of the formamidine family. The undiluted product consists of a 5% w/v concentrated liquid. It is thought to act at octopamine receptor sites in ectoparasites, resulting in neuronal hyperexcitability and death. In addition to its effects on arthropods, amitraz is also a monoamine oxidase inhibitor, a potent α2-adrenergic agonist and inhibits prostaglandin synthesis.

Amitraz is licensed in the UK to treat canine demodicosis at a concentration of 500 ppm (a 0.05% w/v solution). The concentrate is diluted with water just prior to use and sponged over the entire integument of the dog. Clipping of long-haired dogs and prior shampoo treatment in dogs with pustular demodicosis with a follicular flushing agent such as benzoyl peroxide improve skin contact. Treatment is repeated weekly until complete resolution of disease. Treatment is messy and protective clothing should be worn. Owners suffering from diabetes mellitus or circulatory disorders should not do the treatments themselves. Many other amitraz treatment protocols have been described and for more in-depth information the reader is referred to an excellent, recently published, meta-analysis of treatment options for canine generalized demodicosis (Mueller, 2004).

Adverse effects to amitraz are commonly seen and can mainly be attributed to α-adrenergic effects. These include elevation of plasma glucose concentrations by suppression of insulin secretion, bradycardia, hypotension, hypothermia, depression, sleepiness, ataxia, polyphagia and polydipsia, vomiting and diarrhoea. Side-effects tend to be more severe in small dogs. Post-treatment generalized erythema and pruritus is frequently seen, particularly following the first treatment. This is presumably associated with the presence of large numbers of dead mites in the skin and can be a reason for owners requesting alternative treatment.

Macrocyclic lactones

Avermectins and milbemycins are macrocyclic fermentation products of various *Streptomyces* spp. Available avermectins include doramectin, ivermectin and selamectin, and the milbemycins, moxidectin and milbemycin. These drugs are active against a wide range of nematodes and arthropods, and may be administered orally or by injection, or as spot-on or pour-on products.

Avermectins and milbemycins induce a tonic paralysis of musculature of susceptible organisms via potentiation, direct activation, or both, of glutamate-gated chloride channels, to which macrocyclic lactones bind selectively and with high affinity.

Moxidectin: Moxidectin is available in the UK as a spot-on preparation that is licensed for the treatment of canine demodicosis. It is also available as a 1% injectable solution for sheep and cattle. Given orally, moxidectin has been shown to be effective in the treatment of canine generalized demodicosis at a dose rate of 0.2–0.4 mg/kg s.i.d.

In the UK, clinical experience with the spot-on product has not supported the original claims that this is a consistently effective treatment for canine generalized demodicosis.

Ivermectin: Orally administered ivermectin has been effective in the treatment of CGD at dosages between 0.3 and 0.6 mg/kg s.i.d. Treatment may be required for several months. In general, relapse rates were around 15–20% but were lower when higher dosages were used.

There are many concerns regarding the safety of ivermectin (see below), and its use should only be considered when licensed treatments have failed and where other, less toxic therapies such as milbemycin may be unaffordable.

It is recommended to increase the dosage gradually from 0.05 mg/kg s.i.d. to the full therapeutic dosage over the course of the first week of treatment, but adverse effects can become apparent up to 10 weeks into treatment. It has been estimated that up to 10% of *all* dogs (excluding the known ivermectin-sensitive breeds) treated with daily oral ivermectin at dosages between 0.3 and 0.6 mg/kg s.i.d. will develop mydriasis and possibly ataxia within 3 weeks of starting treatment. Decreasing the dosage or ceasing treatment usually results in resolution of these symptoms within a few days.

Milbemycin oxime: Milbemycin oxime is licensed in Europe for the prevention of heartworm at a dosage of 0.5 mg/kg once a month and as an anthelmintic in the UK. Several studies have investigated the efficacy of daily oral milbemycin oxime in the treatment of canine generalized demodicosis, and it has been shown to be an effective treatment when used at dosages of between 0.5 and 1.6 mg/kg s.i.d. One current recommendation for treatment is to start therapy at 1 mg/kg s.i.d. and, if mite numbers apparent on skin scraping have not decreased after 30 days, then the dosage should be increased to 2 mg/kg s.i.d. It has been stated that milbemycin has a higher safety margin than ivermectin and is less likely to result in side-effects in ivermectin-sensitive breeds. However, at the high dosage of 10 mg/kg it did induce toxic reactions in ivermectin-sensitive collies and great care should be taken when treating these breeds. The major drawback of the use of milbemycin is its cost.

Adverse effects: Adverse effects to high dosages of macrocyclic lactones, and in particular ivermectin, are common and are primarily neurological. Both acute and chronic toxicity may be seen. Accidental overdosage has the potential to result in acute toxicity in any breed; however, acute toxicity following administration of standard therapeutic doses (0.2–0.6 mg/kg s.i.d.) may be seen in ivermectin-sensitive breeds such as Shetland collies, Australian shepherds, Old English sheepdogs and Border collies. These reactions are manifested by hypersalivation, ataxia and lethargy, sometimes followed by coma and rarely death. These reactions are most likely to be due to a defect of the Mdr1a gene encoding P-glycoprotein, a protein responsible for pumping ivermectin out of the endothelial cells of blood–brain barrier vessels.

Chronic toxicity consisting of mild to moderate, non-lethal, progressive neurological signs including lethargy, anorexia, ataxia, mydriasis, blindness and tremors may occur after days, weeks or months of administration of ivermectin (0.2–0.6 mg/kg s.i.d.), milbemycin (1–2 mg/kg s.i.d.) or moxidectin (0.3 mg/kg s.i.d.).

Monitoring response to treatment

As already stated, clinical cure will occur before elimination of parasites and there is an increased likelihood of recurrence of disease if clinical signs alone are used to determine the end point of treatment. For this reason, most dermatologists assess the end point of treatment to be when two negative sets of skin scrapes have been obtained with an interval of 4 weeks between each set of scrapings. One 'set' of scrapes would consist of three to five individually scraped sites on the dog.

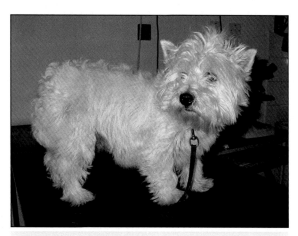

Figure 26.4 The same dog as in Fig. 26.1 after 14 weeks of amitraz therapy.

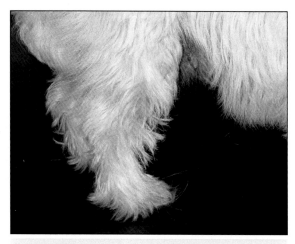

Figure 26.5 Close-up of the hind leg of the dog in Fig. 26.1 after 14 weeks of amitraz therapy.

Treatment selected in this case was as follows:

- Methylprednisolone was given at a total dosage of 2 mg s.i.d.
- Pyoderma was treated with cefalexin at a dosage of 25 mg/kg b.i.d. for 8 weeks.
- Initial miticidal therapy consisted of weekly amitraz dips at a concentration of 500 ppm. The dog was bathed in benzoyl peroxide immediately prior to each amitraz dip. The dog was thoroughly rinsed and then patted dry before the dip so the concentration of the amitraz was not diluted.

After 8 weeks of therapy, the patient was brighter and more active, and her hyperpnoea and pruritus had improved. Examination revealed resolution of crusting and hair regrowth over the affected areas; however, some scaling persisted. Examination of five deep skin scrapings from previously affected areas revealed only one dead *Demodex* mite.

- Antibacterial therapy was withdrawn but weekly amitraz dips continued. The methylprednisolone dosage was reduced to 2 mg s.i.d. on alternate days.

No *Demodex* mites were found on examination of skin scrapings repeated after 14 and 18 weeks of treatment, and by the 14 week examination, the skin lesions and pruritus had resolved (Figs 26.4 and 26.5). The dog remained mildly hyperpnoeic with some crackles over lung fields although, overall, the respiratory signs were

much improved. On the advice of the cardiologist, it was decided that glucocorticoid therapy should be continued at the same dosage. Long-term miticidal therapy was indicated because of the possibility of recurrence of demodicosis associated with the ongoing glucocorticoid therapy. Due to the owner's poor health and difficulty with the amitraz dips, treatment was switched to oral ivermectin. Starting daily therapy was not necessary as the demodicosis was in remission.

- The dog was started on a dosage of 0.2 mg/kg twice weekly, increasing by 0.1 mg/kg fortnightly to 0.4 mg/kg twice weekly.

> ### NURSING ASPECTS
>
> - Amitraz is a potent drug and contact with human skin should be avoided when using the product. It should be used in a well-ventilated area and protective clothing should be worn.
> - Once a bottle of amitraz has been opened, it quickly oxidizes and loses its potency. Opened and partly used bottles should therefore be discarded.
> - Many veterinary practices prefer to apply amitraz to the animal themselves, but if owners are to use the product they should be instructed carefully on correct usage.

CLINICAL TIPS

It is good practice, and helpful when it comes to reassessing cases, if careful clinical notes are kept of which skin sites were scraped, approximately how many mites and eggs were found on the slide, and whether the mites were alive or dead. At subsequent examinations, the same sites should be sampled and a comparison may be made which will give an indication of whether treatment is effective. Many owners (and sometimes vets) tend to be impatient when treating demodicosis and if mites are still present after 1–2 months of therapy, treatment is deemed to have failed. However, provided the clinical signs are not deteriorating, treatment should be continued for at least 3 months before making any sort of decision on efficacy and in severely affected cases it can take many months of therapy to obtain remission.

FOLLOW-UP

Follow-up 1 year later revealed that the dog was still receiving methylprednisolone (2 mg on alternate days). The ivermectin dosage had been reduced to 0.4 mg/kg once weekly. There had been no recurrence of pruritus or alopecia and, although the dog was still mildly dyspnoeic, there had been no progression of the respiratory symptoms.

27 Staphylococcal pyoderma

INITIAL PRESENTATION

Non-pruritic, multifocal patches of alopecia and hyperpigmentation in a dog with idiopathic superficial folliculitis.

INTRODUCTION

Pyoderma is one of the most common causes of skin disease in dogs and yet one of the most underdiagnosed, perhaps in part because the clinical signs are so variable between individuals, and because pyoderma can mimic almost any dermatosis. It is defined as a pyogenic infection of the skin but to some extent the definition is a misrepresentation, because in many cases there are no pustules and/or pus. The clinical signs include papules, pustules, follicular papules, crusting, comedones, epidermal collarettes, scaling, follicular casting, alopecia, erythema, excoriations, ulceration, hyperpigmentation and lichenification. The lesions seen depend on the depth of the infection and also on the duration of disease.

The majority of cases of canine pyoderma involve infection with resident bacteria, in particular, *Staphylococcus intermedius*, and arise because of an underlying systemic or cutaneous disease that renders the cutaneous microenvironment more favourable for bacterial proliferation and infection. Ectoparasitic disease, hypersensitivity disorders, endocrinopathies and primary scaling disorders are amongst the recognized underlying diseases. Some cases of canine pyoderma, however, are idiopathic. Pyoderma is classified as either surface, superficial or deep depending on the depth of infection. Surface infection is limited to the surface of the stratum corneum (Fig. 27.1), and includes intertrigo (skin fold dermatitis), pyotraumatic dermatitis (acute moist dermatitis) and some mucocutaneous pyodermas. Superficial infection involves the epidermis and/or the follicular infundibulum (Fig. 27.2), and includes impetigo, superficial folliculitis, superficial spreading pyoderma and some mucocutaneous pyoderma. Deep

pyoderma involves all the portions of the hair follicle and the dermis (Fig. 27.3). This group includes deep folliculitis, furunculosis and cellulitis, German shepherd pyoderma and pyotraumatic folliculitis and furunculosis. In addition, localized deep infections are classified as: pedal pyogranulomas, or as nasal, muzzle, chin, callus and pedal folliculitis, or furunculosis. This case describes a case of superficial folliculitis, which is a common presentation in short-coated dogs and results in a characteristic moth-eaten appearance.

CASE PRESENTING SIGNS

An 11-month-old, entire male Rhodesian ridgeback was presented with patchy truncal alopecia appearance.

CASE HISTORY

As already stated, because pyoderma is usually a secondary problem, a detailed history is an essential step in establishing the nature of the primary disease process.

The level of pruritus in dogs with pyoderma varies from none to severe but dogs with an underlying allergic skin disease are usually pruritic. However, a ventral pyoderma in a young dog without a previous history of pruritus may be the first harbinger of the onset of atopic dermatitis. A history of a generalized scaling skin disease and possibly alopecia prior to the onset of more typical pyoderma lesions might suggest a primary seborrhoea or a genodermatosis such as colour dilution alopecia. The owner should be questioned regarding symptoms

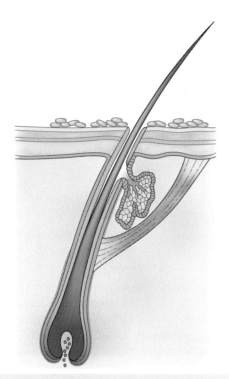

Figure 27.1 Diagrammatic representation of surface bacterial infection.

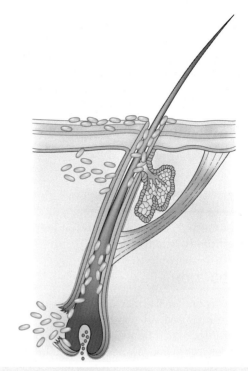

Figure 27.3 Diagrammatic representation of deep infections which can result in rupture of hair follicles.

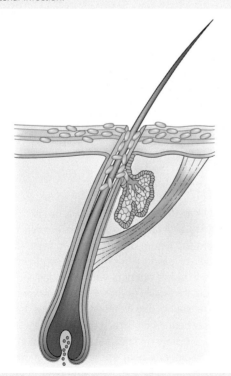

Figure 27.2 Diagrammatic representation of superficial infection.

suggestive of systemic involvement. For example, lethargy and weight gain might suggest hypothyroidism, and polyuria, polydipsia and polyphagia should alert the clinician to the possibility of hyperadrenocorticism or diabetes mellitus. Owners may report that the dog's skin is greasy and malodorous, especially when deep pyoderma is present.

In this case the relevant history was:

- Skin lesions had first started 8 weeks previously on the head with later involvement of the dorsal neck and thorax.
- A 2-week course of clindamycin (5 mg/kg b.i.d.) had resulted in resolution of lesions but they had recurred again within 2 weeks of antibiotic withdrawal.
- There had been no evidence of pruritus.
- There was no evidence of zoonosis or spread to a recently acquired, in-contact 4-month-old puppy.
- The affected dog was being treated with fipronil spot-on every 8 weeks, regularly wormed and vaccinated. The puppy had been treated once with fipronil spot-on.
- The dog's diet included raw chicken wings, raw tripe, dairy products (cheese, cottage cheese and yogurt), fruit (berries and apples) and a kibbled food.

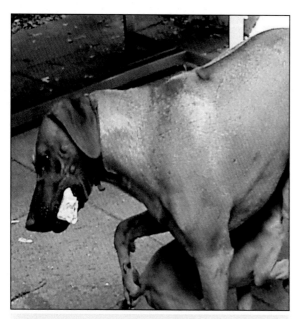

Figure 27.4 Multifocal areas of hypotrichosis and raised tufts of hair on the neck and thorax.

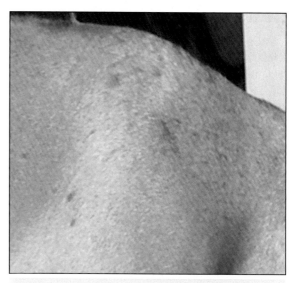

Figure 27.5 Close-up view of the opposite side.

- There had been frequent episodes of diarrhoea and vomiting since puppyhood but no other symptoms of systemic disease.
- The dog had not travelled abroad.

CLINICAL EXAMINATION

Pyoderma commonly involves the ventral abdomen and groin, but a wide variety of cutaneous signs may be evident and it is important to thoroughly examine the entire integument. Similarly, a full physical examination is required in order to carefully evaluate the patient for evidence of underlying systemic disease. Deep pyoderma may result in localized lymphadenopathy of the draining lymph node – for example, prescapular or popliteal lymph node enlargement is usually evident when the feet are affected.

The relevant findings in this case were:
- The cutaneous lesions were symmetrically distributed over the dorsal aspects of the neck and thorax.
- Raised tufts of hair and patchy alopecia were evident, giving the dog a moth-eaten appearance (Figs 27.4 and 27.5). There was hyperpigmentation of affected areas but there were no comedones.
- The hair surrounding these areas was easily epilated.
- There was minimal scaling of the skin.
- Physical examination was unremarkable.

DIFFERENTIAL DIAGNOSES

Although the clinical signs and previous response to antibiotic treatment supported a pyoderma, there were other possible differential diagnoses. The presence of multifocal, patchy alopecia is suggestive of a folliculitis which is most commonly the result of staphylococcal pyoderma, demodicosis or dermatophytosis. The age of the dog and the lack of pruritus were important factors to consider.

Based on the history and examination, the differential diagnoses included:
- Idiopathic or secondary superficial pyoderma
- Demodicosis
- Dermatophytosis
- Urticaria
- Pemphigus foliaceus.

If this was a pyoderma, possible underlying causes included an adverse food reaction, particularly given the history of predisposition to gastrointestinal disease, and despite the lack of pruritus, atopic dermatitis. In addition, underlying immunosuppressive disorders should also be considered.

CASE WORK-UP

The history and clinical signs were suggestive of a pyoderma and, in general, the most convenient way to confirm bacterial involvement is on cytological examination (see Chapter 2).

The following diagnostic tests were performed:

- Tape-strip preparations from affected areas, rather than direct impression smears, were taken for cytological examination. These failed to reveal any valuable diagnostic information. However, in some cases, coccoid bacteria and smaller numbers of degenerating and disintegrating neutrophils, some with phagocytosed cocci, may be evident.
- Microscopic examination of multiple deep skin scrapings and hair plucks was negative for demodicosis and dermatophytosis.
- Hair plucks and scrapings from several lesions were submitted for fungal culture, which was negative.
- In view of the previous antibacterial therapy, a bacteriological swab, moistened with sterile saline, was rubbed on the lesional skin and submitted for culture and sensitivity (*S. intermedius* sensitive to amoxicillin/clavulanate, enrofloxacin, trimethoprim/sulphonamide and cefalexin was isolated).

These findings supported the diagnosis of a bacterial folliculitis.

Trial therapy

Trial antibacterial therapy was started using cefalexin (20 mg/kg b.i.d. for 3 weeks) along with twice weekly bathing using a 10% ethyl lactate shampoo. In addition, the owner was advised to increase the frequency of application of the fipronil spot-on to monthly to both dogs. This resulted in complete resolution of all skin lesions after 2 weeks and treatment was continued for a further week (Fig. 27.6). Histopathological examination would have been indicated if there had been no response to antibacterial therapy, particularly to rule out pemphigus foliaceus.

FURTHER INVESTIGATION

As most cases of pyoderma are secondary problems, identification and correction of the underlying cause is paramount in preventing recurrence. As already discussed, there may be clues to the underlying cause from the history and examination. Since the pyoderma itself can contribute to the pruritus, it is important to treat the infection before assessing any further conditions.

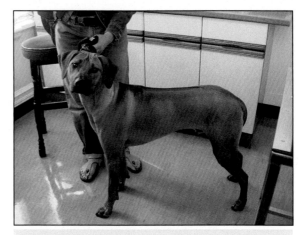

Figure 27.6 Complete resolution after 3 weeks of antibiotic therapy.

As there had been a complete response to antibacterial therapy, the owner was reluctant to pursue further investigation at this stage. However, 4 weeks after antibiotic withdrawal, the pyoderma recurred again despite continuation of the weekly antibacterial shampoos. Antibiotic treatment was restarted using cefalexin at a dosage of 20 mg/kg. At the same time, the dog was started on a restricted diet trial by feeding a chicken hydrolysate. After 2 weeks of treatment, the pyoderma had completely resolved again and antibiotic therapy was withdrawn after a total of 4 weeks therapy. However, the diet trial, shampoo treatment and flea control were continued following treatment withdrawal. After the dog had been on the diet for 6 weeks, the owner reported that the dog was no longer flatulent and there had been no further episodes of diarrhoea in the 6 weeks of the trial. Despite this, 5 weeks after the withdrawal of cefalexin, the pyoderma once again recurred.

The recurrence of the pyoderma despite the ongoing diet trial supported the likelihood that an underlying adverse food reaction was not the cause of the pyoderma. Further options for investigation into underlying causes of the pyoderma at this stage included haematological and biochemical examinations, including basal thyroxine and thyroid-stimulating hormone concentrations. In addition, as some dermatologists believe that recurrent pyoderma in the absence of pruritus can be the only presenting symptom of atopic dermatitis, intradermal testing with the view to starting the dog on allergen-specific immunotherapy might also have been indicated.

- Routine haematology and biochemistry were unremarkable and thyroid parameters indicated normal thyroid function at the time of the tests.

Intradermal testing was declined by the owner. As the restricted diet had helped in regard to the dog's GI symptoms, this was continued.

DIAGNOSIS

The history, clinical signs, laboratory tests and response to treatment confirmed a diagnosis of superficial folliculitis caused by *S. intermedius*. An underlying cause for the pyoderma could not be established and the pyoderma was considered to be idiopathic.

PROGNOSIS

The prognosis for resolution of the pyoderma is good, provided the infection is appropriately treated. However, unless the underlying cause is identified and corrected, the pyoderma is very likely to be recurrent.

ANATOMY AND PHYSIOLOGY REFRESHER

The skin and hair provide an individual with an effective physical, chemical and microbial barrier to a hostile external environment. At the same time, the microenvironment at the skin surface should be viewed as a modified niche that is ideal for the survival of some microorganisms. It is important to remember that the microenvironment is dynamic and therefore subject to constant change, depending on host and microbial factors. Certain host and microbial factors play an important role in both protecting individuals against infections and, in others, predisposing them to infections.

Host factors

Skin structure and function: The stratum corneum, the outermost layer of the epidermis, forms a normally impermeable barrier to the external environment. It is formed of highly keratinized cells, the corneocytes, that are permeated by an emulsion of sweat and sebum. Corneocyte desquamation aids in physical removal of colonizing microorganisms. The sweat/sebum emulsion contains immunoglobulins, complement, cytokines and antimicrobial peptides, all of which play an active role in providing the skin surface with its first line of defence against microbial invasion. Sweat is also the source of

inorganic ions such as sodium, potassium, chloride, phosphates, calcium and lactates that can also have antimicrobial effects. There are numerous cells within the skin that play a highly active role in both the innate and adaptive immune systems and defend against microbial invasion. These cells include keratinocytes, Langerhans' cells, lymphocytes, dermal dendritic cells and mast cells.

Anatomical sites: Intertriginous areas such as the interdigital skin, ventral neck, groin and perineum, and also the ear canals provide a suitable local microenvironment for microbial proliferation due, amongst other factors, to the effects of higher humidity and maceration of the outermost layers of the stratum corneum.

Coat type: The length and density of the hair coat influences both the temperature and the humidity at the skin surface, and can affect microbial colonization.

Skin pH: Canine skin is reported to have a variable pH of between 5.5 and 8.6. There are suggestions that a low pH inhibits microbial growth.

Microbial factors

There are complex interactions between microorganisms on the skin. The microorganisms themselves produce organic and inorganic substances that may enhance or prevent growth of other microorganisms in the same area. The production of antibiotics, bacteriocins, small metabolic end-products and fatty acids by microorganisms may play an important role in preventing the establishment of pathogens. This combination of the individual's innate immunity and the ability of resident bacteria to enhance this defence, while thriving on nutrients on the skin's natural lipids, demonstrates a symbiotic relationship between these resident bacteria and their hosts.

Bacteria: The bacteria found on the human skin surface and hairs have been categorized as being residents, transients and nomads. This categorization has been extended to canine skin and is used in this chapter. Resident organisms are those that are well established and able to live and multiply on the skin without any detriment to the host. Transients are those that, once deposited on the surface of the skin, are able to survive for only a limited time. Nomads are not normally resident, but are able to colonize the skin if the micro- and macroenvironmental factors are suitable at the time of seeding. Nomads can cause harm to the individual if the host's defences are disrupted. Where individual species are concerned, there may well be an overlap in the relationship between the bacteria and the host, and too rigid a classification of their status is inappropriate.

Staphylococcus intermedius is the most common staphylococcal species involved in canine pyoderma and is considered to be a resident organism on canine skin and mucous membranes. It has been found at carrier sites, such as the anterior nares, the oral cavity and the anal mucosa, from where it is seeded onto other sites during grooming. Gram-negative organisms such as *Escherichia coli*, *Proteus mirabilis* and *Pseudomonas* spp. are transients and may be involved as secondary pathogens in deep pyoderma and in dogs with demodicosis. *Staphylococcus aureus*, *S. schleiferi* subsp. *coagulans* and *Pseudomonas* spp. have also been reported as pathogens in dogs with pyoderma.

Why does pyoderma occur?

A full discussion of all the possible factors currently thought to contribute to the development of pyoderma is way beyond the scope of this chapter and could potentially be the subject of an entire textbook. However, compared to other species, the dog is uniquely predisposed to developing pyoderma and it has been speculated that, amongst other factors, this may be due to the fact that they have a thinner stratum corneum, a higher skin pH and lack a lipid follicular plug to seal the opening to the hair follicle infundibulum.

As already indicated, anything that disturbs the delicate balance between microbe and host defence can favour microbial proliferation and infection. The common primary skin diseases that can result in secondary pyoderma include ectoparasitic, allergic and scaling skin disorders but just about any skin disease can result in increased bacterial colonization and bacterial infection. Underlying atopic dermatitis is a very common cause of recurrent pyoderma and the skin of atopic dogs and humans is heavily colonized by staphylococci. On this note, one of the prerequisites for bacterial infection of the skin is adhesion of the microbe to the skin surface and increased staphylococcal adherence has been demonstrated to keratinocytes from atopic, compared to those from healthy, humans and dogs. Self-trauma resulting in degradation of the cutaneous barrier, increased moisture content from licking, alteration of lipid content of the epidermal barrier and long-term immunosuppressive therapy are other factors predisposing to pyoderma in atopic individuals. Similarly, dis-ordered desquamation, degradation of the cutaneous barrier, altered lipid content, and follicular hyperkeratosis and obstruction are factors predisposing to pyoderma in scaling skin disorders. Endocrinopathies and metabolic diseases predispose to pyoderma because of immunosuppressive effects and/or altered keratinization. Additionally, congenital or acquired immunosuppressive disorders or any anti-inflammatory or immunosuppressive treatment can predispose to pyoderma. Lastly, iatrogenic factors such as over-bathing, poor nutrition or a dirty environment may precipitate the onset of pyoderma.

Unfortunately, as in this case, it is not always possible to identify an underlying cause and it is considered to be idiopathic.

EPIDEMIOLOGY

Pyoderma can occur at any age, in either sex and in any breed, although some breeds such as bull terriers and German shepherd dogs are predisposed. Short-coated breeds such as Dobermann pinschers, Great Danes, boxers and dachshunds are predisposed to superficial folliculitis.

TREATMENT

The treatment should be tailored to the individual animal, in each case, and should include:
* Systemic antibiotic therapy
* Topical therapy and
* Management of any underlying disease.

Systemic treatment

Traditionally, culture and sensitivity testing has not been routinely performed when treating canine pyoderma because *Staphylococcus intermedius* is the organism most commonly involved and its spectrum of antibiotic sensitivity is well known. However, most dermatologists would perform culture and sensitivity testing if: unusual organisms are identified on cytology; there have been several previous courses of treatment; there has been a previous poor response to treatment; or if a long course of treatment may be required for treatment of deep pyoderma. However, because of the recent increase in antimicrobial resistance and the identification of atypical staphylococci such as *Staphylococcus schleiferi* that can have very different antibacterial sensitivity, this situation is changing and increased consideration should be given to culture and sensitivity testing prior to starting antibiotic treatment.

Table 27.1 Dosage and frequency of administration of antibiotics used in canine pyoderma

Antibiotic	Dosage (mg/kg)	Dose interval (hours)	Route
Amoxicillin/clavulanate	12.5	12	P.o.
Cefalexin	15–30	12	P.o.
Enrofloxacin	5	24	P.o.
Marbofloxacin	2	24	P.o.
Trimethoprim sulphonamide	15–30	12	P.o.
Clindamycin	11	24	P.o.
Cefovecin	8	14 days	S.c.

The antibiotic selected to treat a pyoderma:
- Has to be tolerated by the patient.
- Has to be administered at the appropriate dose, frequency and duration, and the owners should be capable of doing this, i.e. there is little point in prescribing treatment that needs to be administered three times daily if the owners are away for 12 hours at a time.
- Should ideally be narrow spectrum and effective against *Staphylococcus* spp.
- Should not favour development of resistant strains.
- Should be cost-effective.
- Should be licensed for veterinary use (Table 27.1), unless otherwise indicated by sensitivity testing (and conform to the cascade for prescribing unlicensed drugs).
- Should be bacteriocidal, especially in animals with immunosuppressed.

In general:
- Superficial pyoderma should be treated for 7–14 days beyond clinical cure, and on average this tends to vary between 3 and 6 weeks in practice.
- Deep pyoderma should be treated for 14–28 days beyond clinical cure, and on average this tends to vary between 8 and 12 weeks in practice.
- The integrity of the host immune response is crucial when using bacteriostatic drugs such as clindamycin, lincomycin and erythromycin.
- Recently, licensed injectable third-generation cephalosporin/cefovecin is promising, particularly in cases where owner and/or pet compliance is an issue.

Topical treatment

Topical treatments include shampoos, ointments, sprays, gels and creams. In most cases ointments, gels and creams are of limited value because of the hair coat, the widespread distribution of lesions and licking. In addition, most ointments, creams and gels licensed for

Table 27.2 Activity of agents in shampoo commonly used in canine pyoderma

Active ingredient	Mode of action
Chlorhexidine	Cleansing and antibacterial
Ethyl lactate	Antibacterial
Benzyl peroxide	Antibacterial, follicular flushing, degreasing and keratolytic
Hexetidine	Antibacterial and cleansing
Piroctone olamine	Antibacterial and cleansing

animal use in the UK contain glucocorticoids, which should be avoided in pyoderma. It has been suggested that treatment of carriage sites such as the nares with fusidic acid may reduce the incidence of recurrent infections.

In most cases shampoo therapy is very useful when used in conjunction with systemic antibiotics. It helps remove crust, reduces the bacterial load on the skin surface and, in some cases, has an antipruritic effect. The choice of which shampoo to use should be tailored to the clinical signs and type of infection. In this case the dog was bathed with 10% ethyl lactate shampoo. Additional antibacterial shampoos are listed in Table 27.2 and Appendix 4. The success of shampoo therapy depends on owner and pet compliance.

Management of idiopathic recurrent pyoderma

In those cases with recurrent infection without an identifiable cause, immunostimulation may prove useful. For instance, a staphylococcal autogenous bacterin has been shown to be of value in some cases with recurrent infections. Commercial immunostimulants such as Staphage lysate (Delmont Laboratories, Swarthmore, PA) are available (it requires a special licence in the UK). In other cases antibiotic pulse therapy is useful in maintaining the individual in a disease-free state. The antibiotic of choice should not show any long-term adverse effects and the risk of antimicrobial resistance with repeated administration should be minimal. One study has demonstrated the safe use of cephalosporins for this purpose, when they are administered for 2 days, at the full dose, every 7 days (weekend therapy). The interval between the doses can be tailored to individuals needs.

NURSING ASPECTS

If the practice has dog bathing facilities, the nurses can become involved with the case. Long-haired dogs should be clipped and the appropriate contact time with the shampoo must always be allowed.

CLINICAL TIPS

Common pitfalls leading to treatment failure in canine pyoderma are:
- Failure to recognize the condition because of the wide range of clinical signs.
- Failure to treat at the appropriate dosage, dose interval and duration (i.e. well beyond clinical cure).
- Failure to manage an underlying condition adequately.
- Failure to gain owner and pet compliance for the duration of the treatment.

- Failure to recognize and appropriately treat pyoderma in atopic dogs being treated with glucocorticoids or ciclosporin.

A brief explanation of the pathogenesis of the disease improves owner understanding and compliance; however, there will always be a reluctance by some owners to administer such prolonged courses of antibiotics, especially beyond apparent cure. Always check the animal over thoroughly and do not rely on owners' observations on whether the animal is cured or not. Often, closer examination will reveal mild lesions, which necessitate continued treatment.

The investigation of the involvement of an adverse food reaction as an underlying cause of recurrent pyoderma is not straightforward when pruritus is not a symptom. As in this case, it depends on demonstrating whether or not the pyoderma recurs whilst the dog is being fed a restricted diet.

FOLLOW-UP

The dog continued to have intermittent episodes of pyoderma over the next 2 years, although as they only recurred every few months, continuous therapy was not considered necessary and the pyoderma responded to further 3- to 4-week courses of antibiotics. The dog did not develop symptoms of pruritus suggestive of underlying atopic dermatitis.

28 Dermatophytosis

INITIAL PRESENTATION

Focal alopecia with mild scaling in a cat.

INTRODUCTION

Dermatophytosis is a superficial infection of the skin by pathogenic dermatophytes belonging to species *Microsporum*, *Trichophyton* and *Epidermophyton*, which are known to invade keratinized tissues in animals and humans. The dermatophytes are classified according to their natural habitats, i.e. animals, humans or soil. Zoophilic species such as *M. canis* and *T. equinum* are adapted to inhabit animals, although the spores can survive in the environment for long periods. Anthropophilic dermatophytes are adapted to man, and these species include *Epidermophyton* spp. and *M. audouinii*. Geophilic dermatophytes inhabit the soil and include *M. gypseum* and *M. nanum*. Dermatophytosis is a zoonotic condition and therefore vets require an understanding of the pathogenesis of the disease, not only as regards its treatment in animals, but also as regards limiting further infections in both people and animals. This case report describes the steps involved in the diagnosis and management of cats infected with *M. canis*.

CASE PRESENTING SIGNS

A 9-month-old, male neutered domestic short-haired cat was presented with a circumscribed patch of alopecia on the upper lip.

CASE HISTORY

Although dermatophytosis can occur at any age, younger animals are more predisposed to infection. The condition is spread between animals or from environmental contamination of the hair coat. Studies have reported a higher incidence in rescue centres, in show cats and in breeding establishments. There is reported breed predisposition in Persian cats.

In this case the relevant history was:
- The owner acquired the cat from a cat rescue centre about 4 weeks prior to presentation.
- The cat's history prior to its rescue was not known.
- It had been vaccinated, wormed and neutered while at the rescue centre.
- Recent FIV and FeLV serology had been negative.
- There was no history of zoonosis and there were no other in-contact cats in the household.
- The cat had not yet been allowed out, but it had access to all the rooms in the house.
- The condition was non-pruritic.
- It was fed on a proprietary commercial cat food.

CLINICAL EXAMINATION

Feline dermatophytosis can present not only with a variety of different lesions, but also with different reaction patterns, which are all common to other diseases seen in this species. The alopecia may be circumscribed or diffuse, with patches of scaling, hyperpigmentation, erythema and comedone formation, which may be present on the head or on the extremities. The hairs on the margin of lesions may be broken. In some feline cases clinical reaction patterns such as miliary dermatitis, eosinophilic granuloma complex and chin acne have been associated with dermatophyte infection. Dermatophyte pseudomycetoma, a form seen in long-haired cats, is characterized by subcutaneous nodules, which may ulcerate and/or discharge.

In dogs the clinical signs, although variable, are mainly associated with hair loss. The lesion distribution may be localized or diffuse. Circular patches of alopecia, scaling, hyperpigmentation, crusts and/or follicular papules may be seen on the head and the extremities (see Chapter 9). The lesions are usually well demarcated. Kerion, an inflammatory nodule seen in dogs, is a result of concurrent fungal and bacterial infection. Symmetric nasal or facial lesions that mimic autoimmune disease in rare cases may be associated with dermatophyte infections caused by *M. persicolor* or by *T. mentagrophytes*.

In this case the examination was performed wearing disposable gloves, because from the history dermatophytosis was high on the list of differential diagnoses. A dermatological examination in this case revealed a single expanding patch of alopecia with broken hairs at the periphery on the upper lip (Fig. 28.1). The lesion surface was scaly but non-inflammatory. The general physical examination was within normal limits.

CASE WORK-UP

A diagnosis is made on the history, clinical signs and laboratory tests. In-house screening tests may be carried out to demonstrate the presence of a dermatophyte but the services of a commercial laboratory are likely to be required to speciate the fungus. Knowing the species will help in formulating a strategy both for treatment

DIFFERENTIAL DIAGNOSES

Dermatophytosis can mimic almost any other dermatosis, particularly in cats. The differential diagnosis in this case included:

- Dermatophytosis
- Bacterial folliculitis
- Contact irritant dermatitis
- Contact allergic dermatitis
- Demodicosis
- Alopecia areata
- Pseudopelade.

and control of the fungus within the environment. In-house screening tests include Wood's lamp examination (Fig. 28.2), direct microscopy and culture on dermatophyte test medium (DTM), and are discussed in detail in Chapter 2. All these tests are dependent on good technique for their success and have their pitfalls.

The following tests were performed:

- Microscopic examination of skin scrapes was negative for demodicosis.
- Wood's lamp examination was negative but a negative result did not rule out dermatophytosis.
- In this case, microscopic examination of hairs mounted in liquid paraffin revealed hairs infected with arthrospores (Fig. 28.3).

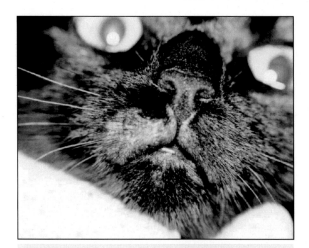

Figure 28.1 Focal alopecia with mild scaling on the skin surface.

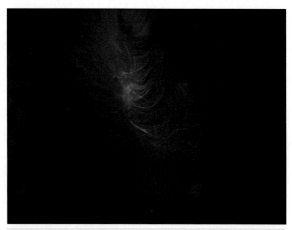

Figure 28.2 Example of apple green fluorescence of *M. canis*-infected hairs on Wood's lamp examination.

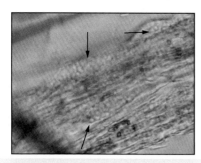

Figure 28.3 Microscopic examination of hair plucks in liquid paraffin mount showing ectothrix arthrospores (arrowed).

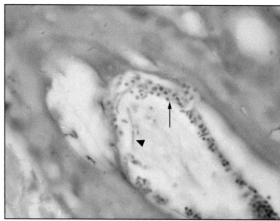

Figure 28.5 Fungal spores (arrow) and hyphae (arrowhead) in a hair follicle on a histological section.

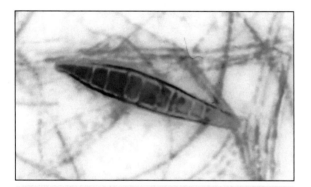

Figure 28.4 Macroconidia from *M. canis* showing thick walls, more than six cells and a knob at one end.

- Skin scrapings from the lesion surface and hairs plucked from the edge of the lesion were submitted to a laboratory for fungal culture and *Microsporum canis* was cultured from the sample.

Definitive diagnosis is made on the cultural characteristics and on the microscopic morphology of the fungal hyphae and macroconidia. *Microsporum canis* appears as cotton wool-like white colonies and the reverse side of the growth medium has a yellow–orange pigment that turns brown. The morphology of the macroconidia is determined by the flag technique. Take a small square of clear adhesive tape and place it on the surface of the colony using a pair of rat tooth forceps. Then place the tape on a microscope slide on which there is a drop of lactophenol cotton blue stain (do not forget to disinfect the instrument with heat or chemical disinfection). *Microsporum canis* macroconidia contain six or more cells and are spindle shaped with thick walls which form a knob at one end (Fig. 28.4). This technique can also be used on DTM medium to look for macroconidia.

Skin biopsies may indicate the presence of fungal elements (Fig. 28.5), but do not indicate the species involved; therefore, they are of limited value as a diagnostic aid, except where fungal infections mimic autoimmune disease, or for deep bacterial infections. Some cases may require special staining with PAS to demonstrate the presence of hyphae or spores. Histopathology is a useful tool to rule out alopecia areata and pseudopelade. In this case, given the history, clinical signs and the supporting evidence from the microscopic examination of hairs, histopathological examination was not indicated.

DIAGNOSIS

A diagnosis of focal *M. canis* infection was confirmed by culture.

AETIOPATHOGENESIS OF DERMATOPHYTOSIS

Dermatophytes invade keratinized tissue such as hair, stratum corneum and nails. Dermatophyte infections are acquired by contact with arthrospores from fomites, infected soil and infected animals. The first step in the process of infection is the adherence of the arthrospores to the stratum corneum. The second step is the germination of the spore and the production of hyphae, which secrete keratinase and invade the stratum corneum and anagen hair shafts.

Dermatophytosis is a contagious disease, and infections can spread between species by both direct and indirect contact if the predisposing conditions are favourable. These predisposing factors include both host and environmental factors.

Host predisposing factors

Young, older and immunosuppressed animals appear to be the most susceptible to infection. Cats with FIV or FeLV and animals receiving chemotherapeutic drugs may be at risk. Genetic susceptibility also may be an important predisposing factor, especially for Persian cats. Cats that have recovered from infections remain susceptible, but the time taken for recovery from a repeat infection is shorter and the disease is less severe. It is thought that the mechanical removal of spores by grooming in cats may provide a natural defence against infection. It follows that long-haired cats, including Persians, could be at higher risk, because the length of their coat may inhibit such removal. Matted fur, in older animals, may also trap spores and prevent their removal by grooming.

Innate immunity

Innate immunity, or non-specific immunity, is the body's first line of defence against infection. Transferrin, complement and neutrophils are involved in protecting against infection in its early phase. Transferrin, an iron-binding protein found in the epidermis, inhibits fungal growth by limiting the availability of iron. Complement is activated via the alternative pathway and this also inhibits fungal growth. Dermatophyte penetration into tissue will recruit neutrophils to the site within hours, where they too will inhibit fungal growth.

Cell-mediated immunity

Cell-mediated immunity provides the main mechanism for protection against, and elimination of, infection. The mechanism is not fully understood, but this is a T-cell-mediated response and involves the release of cytokines that both increase keratinocyte turnover and so aid in physical expulsion of the fungus, and also result in up-regulation of the inflammatory response directed against the fungus.

Humoral immunity

Humoral immunity, which involves production of antidermatophyte antibodies, provides little protection to the individual. In fact, some dermatologists argue that high levels of antibodies may prevent the cell-mediated response and could therefore result in chronic infections.

Behavioural factors

Whatever the level of spores in the environment, breakdown of the epidermal barrier is also a prerequisite for infection to occur. This barrier may be breached by trauma either by accident or during grooming. Microtrauma, caused by self-grooming and by ectoparasites, has been suggested as a predisposing factor in cats.

Environmental predisposing factors

Temperature and humidity are important predisposing factors, which explains the higher incidence of infection in geographical locations where the climate favours fungal growth. In some species, such as horses and cattle, excessive wetting leading to maceration is also considered a predisposing factor.

Spores in the environment can be a constant source of infection, as they may remain viable for years under natural conditions and play a substantial role in spreading infection in cat colonies.

EPIDEMIOLOGY

Reports of the incidence of the disease vary throughout the world. The variation can perhaps be explained by local breed predisposition effects, and a range of environmental factors which affect the survival of the organism. Transmission of disease is either by direct contact, with an infected or a carrier animal, or by indirect contact, via a contaminated environment.

Most of the dermatophyte infections in the UK in small animals are caused by *M. canis*. A survey based on a study of hair samples collected over 35 years from cats suspected of having dermatophytosis found that dermatophytes were isolated from 26% of samples, of which 92% were *M. canis*. Studies on the isolation of *M. canis* from asymptomatic cats have been reported to range from 0% to 88% and such studies in the UK showed an isolation rate of 2.2% in the south-west of England and 2.16% in the south-east.

PROGNOSIS

The prognosis is good, but owners should be made aware of the disease's zoonotic potential, and the costs and the time involved in achieving a cure. Mycological cure can be achieved even in cattery situations.

TREATMENT OPTIONS

Although dermatophytosis is a self-limiting disease, it should be treated because of its zoonotic potential, especially to children and immunocompromised persons. Treatment also reduces the time it takes to resolve the condition and, in addition, it reduces the consequent environmental contamination, an important factor in the pathogenesis of the disease. Pet animals with dermatophytosis should be treated topically and systemically. In addition, measures to reduce the environmental contamination should be taken. Many of the antifungal agents mentioned here do not have a veterinary licence in the UK and therefore their use in the UK requires the owner's informed consent.

Systemic treatment

Systemic medication is recommended in all cases of dermatophytosis in small animals. Several different drugs are available for systemic use; itraconazole is the only one licensed for cats at present.

One of the difficulties in treating dermatophytosis is defining the end point of treatment. This is because there will be clinical resolution of lesions before the fungus has been eliminated from the skin and it is important to continue treatment until mycological cure is achieved. This is defined as two negative fungal cultures with an interval of a month between the tests.

Itraconazole: Itraconazole, a triazole antifungal agent, is the treatment of choice. It is administered with food, for improved absorption, at 5–10 mg/kg, once daily. The treatment should be pulsed, one week on and one week off, over 6 weeks or until mycological cure. Vomiting is a rare side-effect and it is generally better tolerated than ketoconazole. It exerts its effect by inhibiting the demethylation of lanosterol, a precursor sterol in the synthesis of ergosterol, which is a component of the fungal cell wall. It is available as a liquid formulation of 10 mg/ml.

Griseofulvin: Griseofulvin inhibits the growth of various species of *Microsporum*, *Trichophyton* and *Epidermophyton*. It is available in two formulations, a micro-size and an ultra-micro-size. The latter is commonly used for small animals at the dose of 10–15 mg/kg daily, with a fatty meal to enhance absorption. Therapy should be continued until two consecutive negative mycological cultures are obtained. Griseofulvin inhibits fungal cell mitosis by disruption of the mitotic spindle; it may also inhibit chitin synthesis. Adverse effects are not uncommon. The most common side-effects are vomiting, diarrhoea and anorexia. In cats, especially those with FIV, bone marrow suppression resulting in anaemia and leucopenia may occur. It is also teratogenic in humans and animals, and must not be used in very young or pregnant animals. Women of child-bearing age must wear gloves when handling the medication. It is no longer available as a licensed treatment for small animals in the UK.

Ketoconazole: Ketoconazole, an imidazole, is effective against dermatophyte infections. It is better absorbed at an acid pH, and so antacids and H2 receptor antagonists, such as cimetidine, should not be used concurrently. Ketoconazole is administered at the dose of 5–10 mg/kg orally s.i.d. Adverse effects include anorexia, increased liver enzymes and it may also suppress basal cortisol levels. Its mode of action is the same as itraconazole.

Terbinafine: Terbinafine is an allylamine antifungal, which is effective against dermatophytosis. The suggested dose is 20–30 mg/kg orally, once daily. Terbinafine blocks the synthesis of ergosterol by inhibiting the enzyme squalene epoxidase in the membrane. Potential side-effects include anorexia, raised liver enzymes and GIT disturbances. It is not licensed for veterinary use in the UK, and its use requires consideration of the prescribing cascade and informed written consent.

Lufenuron: The use of lufenuron, a chitin synthase inhibitor, remains controversial. Following the initial case report of good efficacy when administering lufenuron at 50–60 mg/kg, several further studies have reported much less encouraging results. Lufenuron failed to prevent infection, or alter the course of infection, in two blinded studies. In addition, lufenuron has failed to exhibit any antifungal activity in *in vitro* studies, and therefore at present its use for control or treatment of dermatophytosis is not recommended.

Vaccine: A killed *M. canis* vaccine is licensed for use in the USA and some European countries. It does not prevent infection, but is known to reduce the severity of the lesions after infection by *M. canis*. If the vaccine is used following infection, it hastens the resolution of clinical lesions, but not mycological cure. It may be of some value in cattery situations.

Topical treatment

Topical antifungal preparations containing miconazole, clotrimazole and enilconazole are available as shampoos, lotions, creams or rinses.

- *Shampoo*: a 2% miconazole/2% chlorhexidine shampoo is licensed for topical antifungal treatment in small animals. It is used as an adjunct to systemic therapy, and one study suggested that removal of the spores by shampoo reduced both environmental contamination and duration of treatment.
- *Creams and lotions*: 1% clotrimazole is available as cream or lotion and may be of some use on very focal lesions, where the hair has been clipped.
- *Rinses*: enilconazole diluted to a 0.2% emulsion can be applied topically. It is licensed for use in cattle, horses and dogs. Natamycin prepared as a 0.01% suspension is licensed for topical use in cattle and horses. Sodium hypochlorite (household bleach) diluted 1 : 10 in water is used by some dermatologists. It should not be used on black cats.

Clipping

Long-haired animals, especially Persian cats, or animals with generalized lesions should be clipped before application. Preferably this should be performed in an isolated area that can be easily decontaminated. To clip or not to clip is controversial; however, with due care, clipping removes the spores found in the hair coat and thereby reduces the load on the animal and further environmental contamination. Additionally, it makes it easier to apply topical therapies.

Environmental control

Environmental decontamination is an important adjunct to clinical treatment, since fungal spores can survive for prolonged periods away from the animal. Furthermore, spores can become airborne and are then spread by air currents. The number of animals infected, as well as the number of recurrent infections in the same animal, is directly related to the levels of spores in the environment. It is therefore easier to deal with infections in single-animal households. In multi-cat households and catteries, or kennels, additional measures are required.

The recommended procedures to control environmental contamination include:

- Confine the infected animal(s) to an area, such as a utility room, which can be easily decontaminated every day.
- Vacuum carpets and soft furnishings, and burn the vacuum cleaner bag every day (for bagless cleaners, disinfect the dust box).
- Disinfect surfaces with household bleach diluted 1 : 10 in water wherever possible (avoid in areas where discoloration could occur). Detergent–peroxide-based products (Virkon S®) and enilconazole sprays or foggers are also effective.
- Disinfect grooming implements.
- Do not introduce new animals to the house while treatment continues.
- Decontamination should be continued until two or three negative mycological cultures have been obtained from the affected animal(s).

The environmental decontamination of an infection involving kennels or a cattery is involved and expensive. The aim in such situations is long-term eradication, and detailed protocols for such situations are beyond the scope of this case report (see Further reading).

Treatment in this case

This case was treated with griseofulvin at the dose of 30 mg/kg orally given with a fatty meal. The affected area was washed in chlorhexidine/miconazole shampoo every day and a full body wash was done once a week (N.B. this cat was treated prior to the availability of itraconazole, the current licensed treatment for dermatophytosis in cats in the UK). The cat in this case was confined to the utility room to limit contamination, and it was an area that could be easily wiped with household bleach diluted 1 : 10.

The treatment was continued until 2 weeks after the second successive toothbrush sample tested negative for fungal culture. In total, the cat was treated for 7 weeks.

NURSING ASPECTS

Barrier nursing and disinfection at the surgery premises should be paramount, as with any infectious disease, especially if the cat is clipped in the practice.

CLINICAL TIPS

- Clinically, this condition can mimic almost any dermatosis, so always confirm the diagnosis with culture and species identification.
- Recognize the pitfalls in making the diagnosis, especially when using in-house methods.
- Environmental decontamination can be challenging and is heavily reliant on owner input. Every effort should be made to involve the owners when formulating the programme in order to maximize compliance.
- Always treat not just beyond clinical cure, but also mycological cure.

FOLLOW-UP

The cat in this case recovered completely and there were no recurrences up to the time of routine annual vaccination a year later.

Alopecia areata

INITIAL PRESENTATION

Multifocal, non-inflammatory alopecia and leucotrichia in a Labrador retriever.

INTRODUCTION

Alopecia is a frequent presentation in the dog. The most common causes include hair loss due to pruritus and self-trauma, infectious causes of folliculitis such as pyoderma, demodicosis and dermatophytosis, and hair growth cycle disorders resulting in inactive hair follicles. This case report describes a rare cause of multifocal alopecia in the dog resulting from an autoimmune folliculitis. Distinguishing features in this case include leucotrichia and non-inflammatory alopecia. This dog also had symptoms consistent with mild atopic dermatitis.

CASE PRESENTING SIGNS

A 7-year-old female, spayed, black Labrador retriever was presented with multifocal alopecia and leucotrichia.

CASE HISTORY

Although this is a rare disease and the number of reported cases is limited, most dogs first present with focal or multifocal patches of non-inflammatory alopecia over the face, and around a quarter of cases may also develop leucotrichia. The facial lesions are predominantly symmetrical in distribution. In multicoloured dogs, hair loss may be restricted to hair of one colour.

- The initial signs of disease had first appeared 15 months earlier with the onset of leucotrichia and subsequently non-inflammatory alopecia affecting the face region.
- Over the past few months, the shoulder regions and limbs had become similarly affected.
- In addition to alopecia, there was a history of aural, facial, ventral and pedal pruritus from around 1 year of age.
- There was no history suggestive of systemic involvement.
- There had been intermittent applications of fipronil and selamectin spot-on flea preparations.
- One other animal in the household, a cat, was unaffected and there was no evidence of zoonosis.
- Diet consisted of a combination of tinned food and biscuit mixer, along with scraps and leftovers, dog biscuits and chews.

CLINICAL EXAMINATION

The significant clinical findings in this case were:
- The physical examination was unremarkable.
- There were well-demarcated patches of complete, non-inflammatory alopecia over the face, pinnae, dorsal shoulders, limbs and perivulval area (Figs 29.1 and 29.2).
- Within and surrounding the areas of alopecia there were numerous white hairs.
- All the nails were short and dystrophic (Fig. 29.3).

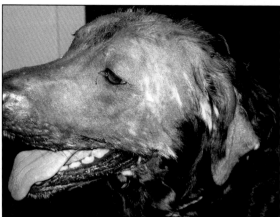

Figure 29.1 Well-demarcated, non-inflammatory alopecia and leucotrichia over the face and head.

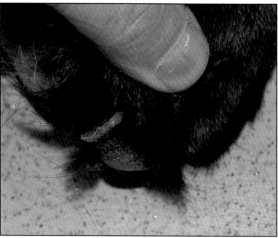

Figure 29.3 Dystrophic nail.

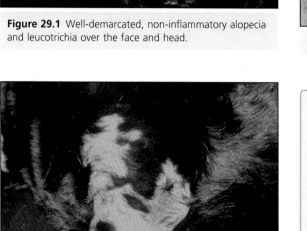

Figure 29.2 Alopecia and leucotrichia over the elbow.

DIFFERENTIAL DIAGNOSES

There were two clinical presentations to consider: alopecia and pruritus. Historical and clinical evidence indicated that these symptoms were unconnected. This hypothesis was based largely on the history:

- The pruritus had been evident for some years prior to the relatively rapid onset of alopecia.
- There was no historical evidence of increased self-trauma to explain the hair loss.
- The leucotrichia preceded the onset of alopecia.
- The alopecia appeared to be non-inflammatory.

The pattern of gradually spreading, well-demarcated, multifocal alopecia was consistent with a folliculitis. Demodicosis, staphylococcal infections and dermatophytosis are the most common causes of canine folliculitis, but generally result in an obviously inflammatory disease. Autoimmune causes of folliculitis, such as alopecia areata, result in non-inflammatory alopecia and may also involve the nails. Therefore, the differential diagnoses for the alopecia in this case were:

- Alopecia areata
- Pseudopelade
- Bacterial folliculitis
- Demodicosis
- Dermatophytosis.
  The main differentials for the pruritus were:
- Atopic dermatitis
- Cutaneous adverse food reaction.

CASE WORK-UP

The diagnosis of alopecia areata is dependent on the histopathological demonstration of a characteristic lymphocytic bulbitis but, prior to taking skin samples, other basic diagnostic procedures were indicated.

The following diagnostic tests were performed:

- Examination of multiple deep skin scrapes from areas of alopecia, which showed no evidence of demodicosis.

- Fungal cultures of material collected and submitted using a MacKenzie toothbrush technique, as well as hairs plucked from around the margin of lesions and material collected by superficial skin scraping, which were all negative.
- Histopathological examination of five skin samples, harvested under sedation and local anaesthesia using a 6-mm biopsy punch, which showed a mild, superficial perivascular dermatitis and a lymphocytic bulbitis affecting anagen hair bulbs.

DIAGNOSIS

The history, clinical signs and histopathology findings were consistent with a diagnosis of alopecia areata.

PROGNOSIS

Canine alopecia areata is benign and primarily of cosmetic importance although this does not detract from the concern experienced by owners. The course of the disease generally waxes and wanes, which can make response to treatment difficult to interpret. In both dogs and horses, hair regrowth may be spontaneous, commonly with initial regrowth being white, although normal pigmentation may return in subsequent hair cycles.

The symptoms of mild facial pruritus were not considered severe enough for further investigation and resolved with treatment for the alopecia.

ANATOMY AND PHYSIOLOGY REFRESHER

The hair follicle is divided into three anatomical regions (Fig. 29.4). The inferior portion extends from the insertion of the arrector pili muscle to the base of the follicle and, in an actively growing hair, the inferior portion contains the hair bulb. The isthmus extends from the insertion of the arrector pili muscle to the sebaceous gland duct. The infundibulum extends from the insertion of the sebaceous gland duct to the opening of the hair follicle on the skin surface.

The hair cycle is divided into three phases: anagen, catagen and telogen. Anagen is the active growth phase of the hair follicle associated with massive proliferation of hair bulb keratinocytes. In the transitional catagen phase the hair follicle is involuting due to keratinocyte apoptosis, and in the resting telogen phase the hair follicle is inactive. Telogen hair shafts are generally retained until the onset of the next anagen phase of the cycle (see Chapter 20).

AETIOPATHOGENESIS OF ALOPECIA AREATA

Alopecia areata affects hair follicles in the anagen phase of the cycle. Clinically, as in this case, it results in a benign, non-scarring alopecia. In man, there is a genetic association with both the susceptibility to and the severity of alopecia areata, but it is not known whether such genetic susceptibility exists in dogs.

There is a strong body of evidence in alopecia areata for an autoimmune aetiology causing selective and reversible damage to anagen hair follicles. Histopathologically, there is infiltration of the hair bulb and surrounding dermis by lymphocytes, macrophages, plasma cells and small numbers of polymorphs. In dogs with alopecia areata, the inflammatory cells consist mainly of CD8+ (cytotoxic) T lymphocytes, CD4+ (helper) T lymphocytes and dendritic antigen-presenting cells.

Direct immunofluorescence demonstrates the presence of IgG targeting the inner root sheath, the outer

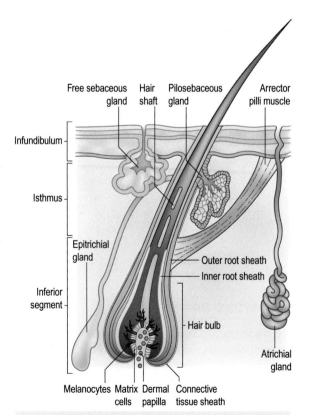

Figure 29.4 Diagrammatic representation of hair follicle and adnexal structures. (Source: Anita Patel.)

root sheath, the hair matrix and the dermal papilla. Indirect immunofluorescence and immunoblotting studies have demonstrated autoantibodies to trichohyalin. Trichohyalin is a protein found at the level of the hair bulb. Its importance lies in the fact that it promotes the correct alignment and aggregation of parallel bundles of intermediate filaments (keratin fibres), and thus a loss of trichohyalin is likely to lead to dysplastic hair shafts. There is also the possibility that melanocytes may be targeted in canine alopecia areata, which has been reported in humans. Evidence for this targeting includes the fact that persistent leucotrichia is a feature of alopecia areata in dogs.

Pseudopelade is another, very rare, immune-mediated folliculitis resulting in mainly non-inflammatory alopecia, which has a similar proposed pathogenesis to alopecia areata, but that targets the hair follicle isthmus rather than the hair bulb. The disease has been reported in both the dog and the cat.

EPIDEMIOLOGY

Alopecia areata is an uncommon to rare disease in man, dogs and horses, and is rare in the cat. It has also been described in cows and donkeys. In one study of 25 dogs with the disease, 19 out of the 25 were pure bred dogs; of this sample, four were German shepherds, three dachshunds, two beagles and two Labrador retrievers. The age of onset of disease varied from 1 to 11 years, but only four of the 25 dogs had developed the disease by 2 years old.

TREATMENT OPTIONS/SUGGESTIONS

In man, because this is an autoimmune disease, a variety of immunomodulatory and other therapies have been used, including glucocorticoids, PUVA, contact sensitizers and minoxidil. Successful therapy of canine alopecia areata has been reported using ciclosporin, and glucocorticoids may also be useful in some cases. As this is a cosmetic disease that does not affect the animal's quality of life, the use of potent immunosuppressive treatments in veterinary species is ethically questionable; however, the concern experienced by some owners may justify the use of such treatments, but not before counselling and a discussion of the implications of therapy.

In this case, following discussion, the owner elected to start treatment with ciclosporin. The initial dosage was 5 mg/kg s.i.d., given with food. As this was an off-label use of this product, informed consent was obtained

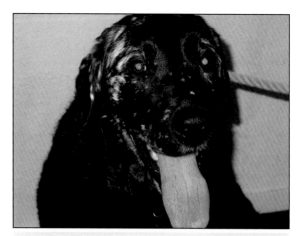

Figure 29.5 The same dog as in Fig. 29.1, after 3 months of ciclosporin therapy.

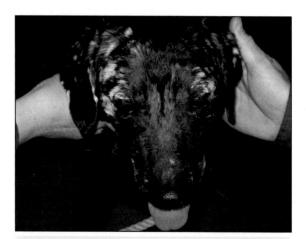

Figure 29.6 The same dog as in Fig. 29.5, 6 weeks after discontinuation of ciclosporin therapy.

prior to starting treatment, and blood and urine samples were obtained for routine haematological and biochemical examinations. These tests were repeated every 3 months during the first year of treatment.

After 3 months of therapy, there was regrowth of hair over all affected areas, although leucotrichia persisted (Fig. 29.5).

Ciclosporin was continued at the same dosage for a further 4 weeks and then discontinued. Within 6 weeks, there had been a recurrence of the facial alopecia (Fig. 29.6). Reinstituting ciclosporin therapy at the previous dosage resulted in regrowth of hair.

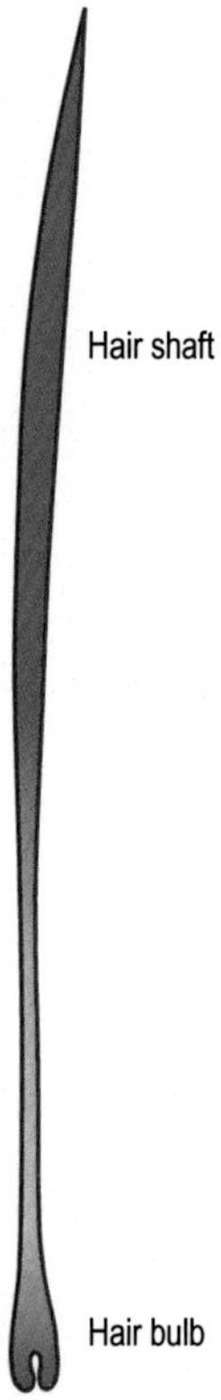

Hair shaft

Hair bulb

Figure 29.7 Diagrammatic representation of 'exclamation mark' hair shaft as seen in alopecia areata.

FOLLOW-UP

For the past 3 years, treatment has been continued, but at the reduced dosage of 5 mg/kg twice weekly, and this has been effective in preventing recurrence of alopecia.

Trichography

Although not applied in this case, trichographic examination has been reported to be helpful in the diagnosis of canine alopecia areata and may reveal hair shafts that taper towards the proximal end of the hair shaft; so-called 'exclamation mark' hairs (Fig. 29.7).

Skin biopsy

In cases where alopecia areata is suspected, it is advisable to take multiple specimens with a biopsy punch from the centre of the lesion and radiating outwards. Samples should be taken from the centre of an area of hair loss, the margins and even unaffected sites. In alopecia areata, the characteristic 'swarm of bees', representing the lymphocytic infiltrate into the hair bulb, is more likely to be identified on samples taken from the advancing margin of the affected area. In contrast, with conditions such as cyclical flank alopecia when the diagnosis is more likely to be made on samples taken from the centre of the area. Affected hair bulbs are sometimes very difficult to find on histopathological examination and further tissue may need to be examined. If the initial report indicates that the diagnosis has not been made, the clinician should request that further sections are cut and examined, if this has not already been done.

30 Lymphoma in a hamster

INITIAL PRESENTATION

Progressive hair loss and pruritus in a Syrian hamster.

INTRODUCTION

Alopecia, coat abnormalities and skin problems are non-specific and common presentations of hamsters in general practice. Often, these pets belong to children and are brought to the surgery only after clinical signs of illness have been present for some time.

In the past, it has often been the case that these pets are euthanized without further diagnostics due to a combination of welfare issues, short lifespan, financial considerations and a poor prognosis. This case discussion aims to challenge that approach, and where appropriate will try to encourage investigation, accurate diagnosis and even specific treatment of these sick hamsters.

CASE PRESENTING SIGNS

An 18-month-old Syrian hamster (*Mesocricetus auratus*) was presented with a history of progressive hair loss and, more recently, increased itching.

CASE HISTORY

As mentioned with the other exotics cases, a thorough history is an important first step in reaching an accurate diagnosis. Sometimes this can be challenging in the small mammals. Hamsters are predominantly nocturnal so are not normally seen at their most active; also, food

is often taken and buried, so food intake may not correlate with the amount being fed. Because hamsters are often children's pets, it may be better to ask the child about the husbandry, remembering to ask carefully and sympathetically, since they are likely to be worried by what you are going to suggest.

The hamster was a gift from a family friend (who had their own litter of hamsters) approximately 15 months ago. He was housed in a large plastic hamster cage with several 'add-on' tubes and tunnels. The substrate was sawdust, with some shredded paper for bedding material. Its diet was a standard commercial hamster mix, with some fruit and vegetable treats provided fresh daily. He was handled frequently by the family, seemed bright and alert, and was acting normally. The patient had a 3-week history of hair loss with some pruritus, mainly affecting the back and head. Otherwise, the hamster was reported to be well; no change in thirst or appetite had been noted.

CLINICAL EXAMINATION

The hamster was lively, alert and responsive during examination. He weighed 126 g and general clinical examination was unremarkable.

Dermatological examination revealed generalised erythema with multifocal areas of alopecia over the head and dorsum (Figs 30.1 and 30.2). There was also increased scaling of the skin in many areas. In addition, some erosions and excoriations were present on the face (Fig. 30.3).

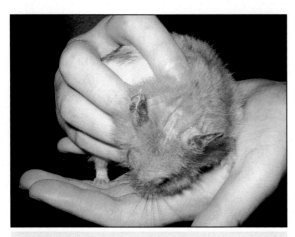

Figure 30.1 Alopecia and scaling on the head and neck. (Courtesy of N. Perrins.)

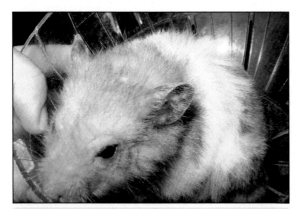

Figure 30.2 Periocular scaling and alopecia. (Courtesy of N. Perrins.)

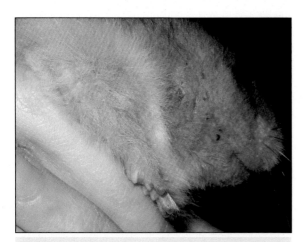

Figure 30.3 Facial alopecia, erythema and excoriation present on initial examination. (Courtesy of N. Perrins.)

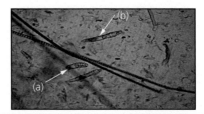

Figure 30.4 The two types of *Demodex* spp. that commonly infect hamsters – *D. criceti* (a) and *D. aurati* (b).

DIFFERENTIAL DIAGNOSES

- Demodicosis
- Cutaneous epitheliotropic lymphoma
- Dermatophytosis
- Hyperadrenocorticism
- Systemic illness (i.e. renal or liver disease)
- Bedding or environmental abrasions
- Stress- or husbandry-related problems
- Dietary protein deficiency.

Alopecia and rough hair coat are non-specific signs associated with multiple disease and husbandry problems. Chronic, non-pruritic, generalized alopecia with scaling and crusting around the ears and feet can be associated with any of the differential diagnoses listed above. Hairlessness can even have a hereditary predisposition. Therefore, diagnosis is important to provide the right treatment. Some of the other main differential diagnoses are considered briefly here:

Demodicosis

Demodex is the most common ectoparasite of hamsters. They are susceptible to five different species, with *D. aurati* (in hair follicles) and *D. criceti* (in keratin and pits of the epidermal surface) being the most common (Fig. 30.4). Approximately 50% of hamsters may be asymptomatic carriers, so demonstration of mites in scrapings from healthy skin does not necessarily indicate disease. Clinical signs of demodicosis include alopecia, hyperkeratinization and scaling over the back, legs and abdomen. Pruritus is not usually a feature unless the infestation is complicated with a secondary infection. The presence of clinical signs invariably suggests an underlying disease, immunosuppression, stress or ageing. Diagnosis is made with skin scrapes, examined with light microscopy. The most effective treatment is amitraz (Aludex; Intervet) diluted to 100 ppm once weekly until 4 weeks after negative skin scrapes, although toxicity is a risk due to their small size and the difficulty of preventing grooming. Ivermectin injections (Panomec; Meriel) are useful (0.4 mg/kg subcutaneously) but will need repeating three or four times, or there is topical ivermectin (Xeno 450; Genetrix).

Dermatophytosis

This is relatively uncommon in the UK, but hamsters can be clinically affected, or asymptomatic carriers. The most common dermatophytes isolated are usually *Trichophyton mentagrophytes* or sometimes *Microsporum canis*; therefore, the disease is potentially zoonotic. Clinical signs include dry circular alopecic skin lesions, usually affecting the thoracic and abdominal areas, with the clinical disease often complicated by pyoderma. Diagnosis is made with standard fungal culture techniques (see the guinea-pig case in Chapter 10). Treatment is also very similar to other pets, although it can be challenging to stop the hamster licking after using topical antifungal drugs. Regular cleaning of the cage and use of proper bedding (avoid wood shavings – e.g. allergic dermatitis attributed to pine or cedar wood shavings has been reported) helps prevent this disease.

Pyoderma

Staphylococcal pyoderma (primary or secondary) is relatively common in hamsters. Lesions include moist dermatitis, ulcerated sores and abscesses. Treatment includes correcting any husbandry problems, replacing any abrasive bedding material with newspaper and/or paper towels, and removal of any aggressive animals. Antibiotics should be selected based on culture and sensitivity, and restricted to those safe to use in hamsters. Enrofloxacin or marbofloxacin should be effective, but penicillins, cephalosporins and aminoglycosides should be avoided. Even some trimethoprim–sulpha combinations have been associated with death in hamsters.

Hyperadrenocorticism

Hyperadrenocorticism may be caused by hyperplasia, adenomas or carcinomas of the adrenal glands. It is more common in male hamsters and generally occurs in older animals. Clinical signs include bilateral and symmetrical alopecia, hyperpigmentation and thinning of the skin, polyuria, polydipsia and polyphagia. Whenever possible, diagnosis is made by demonstrating elevated plasma cortisol levels (normal range 13.8–27.6 nmol/l). Treatment is often not attempted, but metyrapone (8 mg orally once daily for 4 weeks) was effective in one hamster.

CASE WORK-UP

Given the presenting signs and age of the hamster, the main differential diagnoses were demodicosis, epitheliotropic lymphoma and dermatophytosis, with secondary pyoderma. Investigation was aimed at ruling out some of these diseases first.

Skin/hair scrapes: Multiple skin scrapes were taken from the lesions using a scalpel blade and liquid paraffin. They were then mounted on a slide, covered with a coverslip and examined under low power at ×40 magnification, using a light microscope. No ectoparasites were found. This does not entirely rule out ectoparasites, but since *Demodex* mites are usually quite common in hamsters, demodicosis was unlikely to be causing the clinical signs.

Cytology: Cytology was performed using Scotch® tape applied repeatedly to affected areas of skin. The tape was then stained using Diff Quik® stain, placed on a microscope slide. The sample was initially examined under low power and then under the oil immersion, at ×1000 magnification, using a light microscope. Large numbers of intra- and extracellular coccoid bacteria and neutrophils were seen. Cytological examination of samples from lesions (see Chapter 2), either tape strips or impression smears, is often underused in veterinary practice. It is a simple, inexpensive, non-invasive technique that often gives significant information about the lesions. In this case it confirmed the suspected pyoderma although this was not thought to be the primary problem.

Fungal culture: Hair pluck samples were taken from the periphery of the lesions and a toothbrush coat brushing was also collected. These samples were submitted to a commercial laboratory for fungal culture. The samples were inoculated onto Sabouraud's dextrose agar and incubated at 26°C for 4 weeks. No dermatophytes were isolated.

Whist waiting for the fungal culture results, empirical treatment was attempted (see 'Treatment' section) prior to further investigation. There was slight improvement in the pyoderma but there was no significant improvement of the lesions.

Skin biopsies: Two months after initial presentation (Fig. 30.5), the next step was to take skin biopsies since the other negative results made epitheliotropic lymphoma more likely. The hamster was anaesthetized with sevoflurane via a small induction chamber. Sevoflurane is less of an irritant than isoflurane for mask/chamber induction, so it is preferable for small mammal gaseous induction. In addition, it has a lower solubility than isoflurane making for shorter induction and recovery times with sevoflurane.

Under general anaesthesia, three skin samples were taken from the affected areas and submitted for histopathology. This revealed pleomorphic atypical lymphocytes infiltrating the superficial dermis and microabscesses in the follicular epithelium consistent with a diagnosis of epitheliotropic lymphoma.

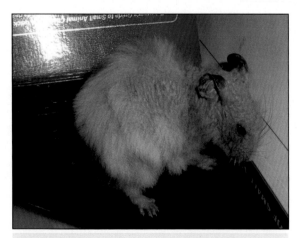

Figure 30.5 The hamster 2 months after initial presentation. Note the more generalized exfoliative erythroderma and alopecia.

Blood sampling: If the skin biopsy had not been diagnostic, then blood sampling may have been useful. Haematology and biochemistry could have been assessed for systemic illness and cortisol levels checked in the case of hyperadrenocorticism. However, obtaining blood is difficult in hamsters and only small quantities can be taken. The circulating blood volume is 7–8 ml/kg and up to 10% can be taken from a healthy hamster. In this case, 0.98 ml is the maximum volume that can be taken safely. Collection sites include the cephalic and saphenous veins (with a 25- to 27-gauge needle and capillary tube) or, for larger volumes, the cranial vena cava. Patients should be anaesthetized for sampling, especially for the vena cava!

DIAGNOSIS

Epitheliotropic lymphoma was diagnosed based on the histopathological findings in the skin biopsy samples.

PROGNOSIS

Prognosis for epitheliotropic lymphoma is poor. Despite the promising initial response to steroids, this patient became more alopecic and marked exfoliative dermatitis (erythroderma) extended over the whole body.

ANATOMY AND PHYSIOLOGY REFRESHER

The most popular pet hamster is the Syrian hamster (*Mesocricetus auratus*). All pet hamsters in the world originated from a family founded in Aleppo in 1930, giving rise to their name. Although the most common fur colour is golden, this species may also be seen in cinnamon, honey, brown, grey, silver, black, white band, piebald and albino. The eye colour may be black, red or unpigmented in albinos.

General husbandry: Syrian hamsters are solitary and should not be housed with others under any circumstances. Many have been injured and killed when littermates have been kept together past sexual maturity. An escape-proof cage is a necessity as hamsters can gnaw through wood, plastic and soft metals, and a secure lid must be provided. A nesting or hide box with deep litter for burrowing is suggested. Optimal nesting material is undyed, unscented toilet tissue, but paper or hay can also be used. This area should be cleaned regularly as hamsters tend to hoard food. The hamster will instinctively manipulate the litter to simulate the burrow, and it helps the hamster control temperature. Commercial nesting materials are not recommended because they are made from fibrous substances, which may lead to intestinal blockages or strangulated limbs.

Diet: In the wild, hamsters are omnivores, hoard their food and are coprophagic (eat certain types of faecal material). Pet hamsters are usually fed a commercial hamster mix, which should be supplemented with fruits, vegetables and nuts. Adults should consume 5–10 g of food per day. Breeding females should have the food provided on the cage floor, so the young are not neglected. Treats may include such items as tiny bits of apple (no seeds or skin), raisins and walnuts. Fresh water should be provided each day by sipper bottles and they usually drink 100 ml/kg per day.

EPIDEMIOLOGY

Aged hamsters often present with clinical signs consistent with skin neoplasia. Unfortunately, a combination of age, cost and poor prognosis often means no diagnostics are carried out and hamsters are euthanized without a specific diagnosis, meaning we cannot be certain of the true aetiology of these cases.

Older literature proposes lymphoma as the most common tumour of hamsters, but recent literature suggests adrenal tumours are more common. There are three reported presentations of lymphoma in the hamster: a haemopoietic form; an epizootic form caused by hamster polyomavirus; and a skin form, cutaneous or epitheliotropic lymphoma. This variation of lymphoma resembles mycosis fungoides, which is an epidermotropic T-cell lymphoma seen in humans. Often, the two terms epitheliotropic lymphoma and mycosis fungoides are used interchangeably, but the latter only really applies to humans.

With respect to skin tumours in hamsters, melanomas and melanocytomas are the most common, with cutaneous lymphoma being the second most common. There is a paucity of literature concerning treatment and prognosis of cutaneous lymphoma in hamsters, but in one study the mean survival time from presentation to euthanasia was reported as less than 10 months. However, this time does approximate to 6–9% of a hamster's expected lifespan and one of the hamsters in the study survived for 24 weeks. This was a case series of only six hamsters, and five of them progressed to a generalized exfoliative erythroderma over a variable time period of 4–20 weeks.

TREATMENT

Husbandry: Husbandry was fully reviewed and the owner received advice on making sure there were no environmental factors contributing to the disease.

Antibiosis: Prior to taking skin biopsies, in this case treatment with a broad-spectrum antibiotic that should be both effective against staphylococcal pyoderma and safe for use in hamster was initiated. Enrofloxacin (Baytril oral 2.5%; Bayer) was chosen at 10 mg/kg orally twice daily for 3 weeks. In-water medication is rarely effective due to low water intake.

Acaricidal therapy: Despite the negative skin scrapes, and while waiting for the fungal culture results, trial acaricidal therapy with three treatments of ivermectin (0.2 mg/kg s.c., 10 days apart) was given.

Topical therapy: A moisturizer (Lacticare; Stiefel) was advised, which markedly reduced the scaling and eased the hamster's discomfort.

Glucocorticoids: Once a diagnosis of lymphoma was made, treatment options were considered. The hamster was still deemed by the owner to have a reasonable quality of life and so euthanasia was declined. The owner was not keen to try a full chemotherapy protocol, but elected to trial palliative treatment with steroids. Initially, dexamethasone was administered subcutaneously at 2 mg/kg. This produced a temporary improvement in the clinical signs, so prednisolone was prescribed at 1 mg/kg twice daily by mouth (Fig. 30.6). This treatment, along with continued moisturizers, provided good palliative treatment for 10 months; much longer than the reported survival time for epitheliotropic lymphoma.

TREATMENT OPTIONS

There is currently no recognized treatment for cutaneous lymphoma. In the past, treatment has not been recommended and euthanasia carried out when the disease has progressed sufficiently to cause suffering.

Chemotherapy: There is limited information about chemotherapy protocols and therefore survival times are impossible to predict. Chemotherapy treatment has been described or protocols may be extrapolated from published dog protocols. Chemotherapy in dogs and cats using drugs like vincristine sulphate or doxorubicin

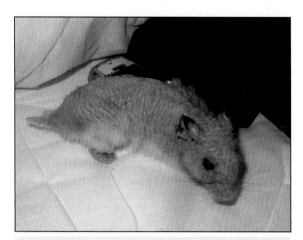

Figure 30.6 The hamster 5 months after the onset of clinical signs. There is a continued progression of the alopecia and erythroderma. Despite his appearance, he is lively, eating well and maintaining weight.

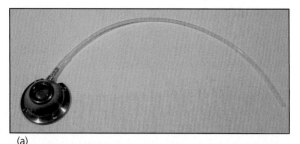

(a)

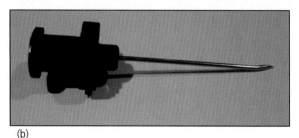

(b)

Figure 30.7

(a) Venus access port.

(b) Huber needle.

may be difficult to administer in hamsters due to the need for repeated intravenous access. Also, drugs such as cyclophosphamide may be difficult to dose down to the low level that would be required for a hamster. With the more recent use of venous access ports (VAPs) in animals, perhaps intravenous protocols may also be of use.

A VAP consists of a port with a septum that accepts a predetermined number of punctures. The port is surgically implanted under the skin, attached to a long catheter placed in the jugular vein (Fig. 30.7a). Then, the port can be accessed percutaneously using a specially designed non-coring 'Huber' point needle (Fig. 30.7b). These instruments are more expensive than normal needles and can be reused on the same patient several times. After using the port, it needs to be 'locked' with a 100 IU/ml heparin solution to fill the port and line, so it remains patent for the next time. Unfortunately, cost (£200–500 per port) is likely to limit their use.

Prednisolone: Prednisolone therapy has been attempted by this author as a palliative measure (1 mg/kg p.o., q12 h), but the relatively small numbers treated do not allow for statistical analysis.

Interferon alpha: It has been suggested that interferon alpha may have some application in these cases. A dose of 1 500 000–2 000 000 units/m^2 two or three times per week has been recommended, but has not been evaluated clinically.

Isotretinoin and prednisolone: Epitheliotropic lymphoma in a ferret was treated with isotretinoin (2 mg/kg once daily) and prednisolone (1.1 mg/kg twice daily), which appeared to slow progression of the disease.

CLINICAL TIPS

Often, when presented with a very sick hamster, especially if older than 1 year, case discussion can revert to considering the purchase price of the pet compared to the cost of diagnostics. Certainly, a different 'new' hamster can be purchased for less than £10 (which is probably even less than the consultation fee), but this viewpoint represents a failure to see that having a pet is about devotion and commitment to caring for a living creature, whether an expensive thoroughbred racehorse or a cherished hamster.

This author (SS) believes that veterinary surgeons can alter this view by example. By adopting the attitude that every pet matters, we can send a more positive message to members of the public who keep these pets. My personal response to the *purchase price vs. treatment price argument* when presented with a sick hamster is twofold. Firstly, dogs and cats can be obtained free from rescue centres; however, people are still willing to spend money on their treatment. Secondly, in Japan, where land is at a premium and cleanliness and tranquillity are treasured values in a pet, hamsters are considered to have the same status enjoyed by dogs and cats here.

In recent years, small mammal medicine has increased in both popularity and understanding. More veterinarians are specializing in the treatment of these pets, contributing to the advancement of diagnosis and treatment, and keeping up to date with the latest literature. The internet has also vastly changed the world of small animal breeding and care. Forums and mailing lists allow people of all ages to share experiences and, more importantly, differentiate anecdotal myths from hard evidence.

Euthanasia

Euthanasia with injectable barbiturates in the conscious hamster tends to be unpleasant and painful. The author prefers to mask-induce anaesthesia with sevoflurane (or isoflurane) and then administer intravenous barbiturate. Intra-hepatic or intra-cardiac injection would also be acceptable under anaesthesia.

NURSING ASPECTS

Handling

Confident and effective handling skills are required by vets and nurses if they are to administer medication effectively and even teach the owner how to handle their own pet.

Hamsters are often thought of as frequent biters, but if handled correctly without being startled then injury can be avoided. They should be gently lifted from their cage in cupped hands, and then, as necessary, restrained by grasping the skin over the neck and dorsum between thumb and fingers. An aggressive hamster will turn and bite if not enough skin is held, and startled hamsters may roll on their back, vocalizing and trying to bite.

Accurate weight

It is important to have weighing scales that weigh to the nearest 1 g, otherwise large dosing inaccuracies may occur.

FOLLOW-UP

The hamster died 10 months after the onset of clinical signs and was deemed by the owner to have enjoyed a good quality of life up to that point. This far exceeds the reported mean survival time of 9.6 weeks. The owner weighed the hamster weekly during treatment and it was noted to have lost a considerable amount of weight in the 2 weeks preceding his death.

31 Feline paraneoplastic alopecia

INITIAL PRESENTATION

Alopecia with shiny glistening skin and crusting in a cat.

INTRODUCTION

Feline paraneoplastic alopecia is a cutaneous marker for visceral neoplasia. This syndrome has been described in old cats in association with pancreatic adenocarcinomas and bile duct carcinomas, with or without metastases to the liver and/or other organs. A direct relationship between the neoplasm and the cutaneous lesions has been established by resolution of the skin lesions in response to surgical excision of the tumour, and their subsequent recurrence with metastatic disease in one reported case. However, often the condition progresses rapidly and affects the welfare of the cat. This report describes a case where there was sudden onset of skin lesions with rapid progression and poor health in association with hepatic neoplasia.

CASE PRESENTING SIGNS

A 15-year-old, neutered male domestic long-haired cat was presented with a short, sudden onset history of alopecia and crusting.

CASE HISTORY

Nearly all reported cases have a history of short duration and may show non-specific systemic signs such as polydipsia, polyuria, poor appetite, weight loss and lethargy. Pruritus is variable, ranging from none to excessive grooming. The affected cats may have no previous history of skin problems.

The history in this case was:

- Decreased appetite
- Weight loss from 7.4 to 5.5 kg in 8 weeks
- Polydipsia
- Lethargy
- Onset with erythema and pruritus on the medial aspects of the forelegs
- Rapidly progressing alopecia and pruritus involving the ventrum
- Poor response to antimicrobial therapy
- No response to glucocorticoids.

CLINICAL EXAMINATION

The cutaneous signs, which usually begin acutely, include a bilaterally symmetrical alopecia involving the ventrum and the limbs. As the lesions progress the characteristic shiny glistening appearance of the skin is seen, together with erythema, scaling and pigmentary macules. The hair is easily epilated. The footpads may be painful and become dry, with scaling and fissuring. Generally, affected cats show non-specific signs of weight loss with abdominal pain and distension. Abdominal palpation may reveal hepatomegaly, a mass and presence of fluid. Concurrent secondary bacterial and yeast infections are common.

In this case the significant findings were:
- Temperature and heart rate were within normal limits.
- There was evidence of weight loss.
- A mass was felt on hepatic palpation.
- There was bilateral, ceruminous otitis externa.

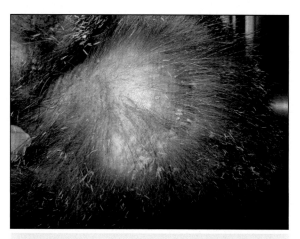

Figure 31.1 Focal alopecia, erythema and crusting on the dorsal neck.

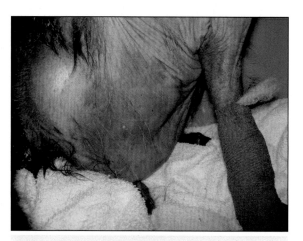

Figure 31.3 Erythematous patches, alopecia and glistening skin on the ventrum.

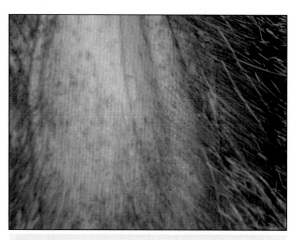

Figure 31.2 Alopecia, glistening skin and pigmented macules on the ventral neck.

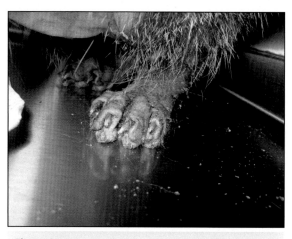

Figure 31.4 Keratosebaceous scale and paronychia on the distal limb.

- There were focal patches of alopecia with scaling and easily epilated hair on the dorsum (Fig. 31.1).
- The presence of alopecia, glistening skin surface, hyperpigmented macules, erythema, scaling and crusting on the ventral neck (Fig. 31.2), abdomen, axilla and inguinal regions (Fig. 31.3) extending to the feet.
- Brown keratosebaceous crusts were seen on nails and the distal feet (Fig. 31.4).
- The skin was inelastic, thin and greasy to the touch.
- The footpads were dry, fissured and painful on palpation.

DIFFERENTIAL DIAGNOSES

In this case the differentials were:
- Secondary bacterial and/or *Malassezia* dermatitis
- Paraneoplastic alopecia associated with hepatic and/or other visceral neoplasia
- Iatrogenic or spontaneous hyperadrenocorticism
- Telogen effluvium
- Metabolic epidermal necrosis
- Demodicosis.

CASE WORK-UP

Coat brushings and skin scrapings should be performed to rule out ectoparasitic conditions, with impression smears and tape-strip preparations to reveal secondary microbial colonization (bacterial and/or *Malassezia* spp.). Haematology and biochemistry usually reveal mild non-specific changes and generally give no indication of neoplasia.

Investigations into the localization and extent of the neoplasia may include survey abdominal radiography, ultrasonography and exploratory surgery. Ultrasound examination of the abdominal organs is recommended for identification and location of the tumour and any metastases. Ultrasound guided biopsies may help in identifying the origin and type of tumour.

The following tests were performed:

- **Trichography:** In this case, hair plucks from haired skin revealed telogen hairs.
- **Skin scrapes:** There was no evidence of ectoparasites on skin scrapings or coat brushings.
- **Cytology:** Tape-strip samples revealed a *Malassezia* overgrowth on the feet.
- **Blood tests:** Haematology and biochemistry were unremarkable.
- **Histology:** Skin biopsies revealed the histopathological change of marked atrophy of the follicular and adnexal structures, which is a typical finding in cats with paraneoplastic alopecia. In this case the epidermis was acanthotic, with apparent absence or thinning of the stratum corneum in places (Fig. 31.5a, b), whilst in other cases the epidermis may be atrophic. In addition, a superficial dermatitis, with mainly mast cells and few mononuclear cells, was present.
- **Ultrasonagraphy:** An ultrasound examination of the abdomen revealed a hyperechoic mass, 1.84 by 1.29 cm in size (Fig. 31.6), in the liver. Other abdominal organs appeared to be normal. Ultrasound guided biopsies could have been obtained to identify the type of tumour and provide a more accurate prognosis; however, the owner declined invasive procedures. In other cases exploratory laparotomy and direct examination of the organs may be indicated.

DIAGNOSIS

Malasseziosis and feline paraneoplastic alopecia.

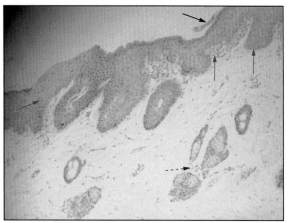

(a)

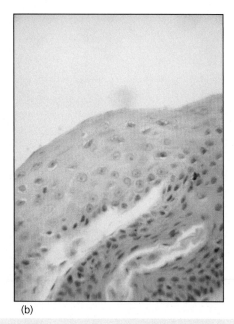

(b)

Figure 31.5

(a) Histological section showing parakeratosis (black arrow), epidermal acanthosis, (blue arrows) atrophic hair follicles and sebaceous glands (red arrow).

(b) Close-up view (almost absent stratum corneum).

PROGNOSIS

Prognosis is generally poor due to the aggressive nature of the tumour. Surgical excision may prolong the survival time, but the lesions can recur with metastatic disease. Most cats are reported to die within 1–3 months of diagnosis.

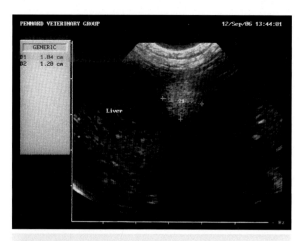

Figure 31.6 Ultrasound of the liver showing a hyperechoic nodule. (Courtesy of S. Aylward.)

ANATOMY AND PHYSIOLOGY REFRESHER

Although the relationship between the tumour and the cutaneous lesions has been suggested, the pathogenic mechanism for the marked follicular and adnexal atrophy is not known. Cytokines or other agents secreted by the neoplastic cells may be responsible for the effect on the hair follicle cycle.

EPIDEMIOLOGY

It is a rare condition seen mainly in cats above the age of 10 years. There is no reported sex or breed predisposition.

TREATMENT

There is no specific treatment; however, supportive treatment will improve the animal's quality of life. Antibiotic and antifungal treatments for bacterial and *Malassezia* dermatitis are recommended. Surgical excision of a solitary mass, where there is no evidence of metastasis, may increase longevity; however, most cases will have metastases to the liver, lungs and other visceral organs. If the owner decides to proceed with the surgical intervention the case is best referred to a surgical oncologist.

The owner opted for euthanasia in this case due to the cat's rapidly deteriorating condition.

NURSING ASPECTS

Nutritional support (enteral and parenteral), antimicrobial treatments and topical treatments may help relieve some of the discomfort in the short term. Intensive nursing will be required if the owners have opted for surgical intervention.

CLINICAL TIPS

This condition should be considered in any old cat presented with sudden onset of alopecia and with the characteristic shiny and glistening skin.

ULCERATIVE AND EROSIVE DERMATOSES

Introduction to ulcerative and erosive dermatoses

EROSIONS AND ULCERS

An erosion is a lesion involving loss of some or all of the layers of the epidermis, but without disruption of the basement membrane (Fig. 32.1). As a rule, these lesions do not bleed easily.

An ulcer is a lesion involving complete loss of the epidermis and also involving disruption of the basement membrane, leading to exposure of the underlying dermis (Fig. 32.2). Ulcers do tend to bleed easily. Ulcerated lesions also tend to crust due to the accumulation of blood and/or exudate on the skin surface. Clinically, it can sometimes be difficult to differentiate between deeper erosions and shallow ulcers. Features that may be helpful in determining the cause of ulcers and that should be considered when describing them include the site of the ulcer, the appearance of the border and base, any discharge and the nature of the surrounding skin.

Ulceration results in loss of the protection afforded by the epidermis, with leakage of fluids and electrolytes, and exposure of the underlying dermis to bacterial colonization, infection and potentially life-threatening sepsis. A more aggressive diagnostic approach is warranted in cases where there is significant ulceration.

AETIOLOGY

Extrinsic trauma and intrinsic disorders can both result in cutaneous erosions and ulcers.

Extrinsic trauma

The most common cause of erosive and ulcerative skin disease is from self-trauma due to an underlying pruritic skin disorder (Fig. 32.3). The distribution and appearance of the lesions in these cases will reflect the nature of the insult. Lesions in cases of self-trauma frequently have a linear distribution. Other external insults such as chemical or thermal burns will have varying morphologies depending on the agent involved.

Intrinsic disorders

There are many intrinsic skin diseases that may result in erosion or ulceration. Vesicular, pustular and bullous diseases can result in erosion or ulceration once the primary lesion has ruptured. The depth of the lesion depends on the level of disease within the skin and whether the epidermis, basement membrane zone or dermis is affected. Pustular diseases include pyoderma and pemphigus foliaceus, and vesicular and bullous diseases include pemphigus vulgaris, bullous pemphigoid, erythema multiforme, epidermolysis bullosa and vesicular cutaneous lupus erythematosus. Some vesicular or bullous diseases result in a positive Nikolsky sign, where rubbing of apparently normal skin adjacent to a lesion induces sloughing or separation of the epidermis, indicating a dermo-epidermal separation or clefting.

Loss of blood supply to the skin, due to a vasculitis or vasculopathy, can result in erosion or ulceration depending on the size and site of the blood vessel involved. Obstruction of a large dermal vessel will lead to necrosis of the area of skin supplied and a resulting circular 'punched out' ulcer (see Chapter 34). This appearance is characteristic of a vascular lesion. Blockage of smaller capillaries may not lead to frank ulceration, but may still produce an erosive or scaling presentation (Figs 32.4 and 32.5).

Severe inflammatory skin diseases such as viral infections (see Chapter 51) and lesions of the eosinophilic granuloma complex in cats (Fig. 32.6) can cause destruction of the epidermis and resulting erosion and ulceration. Similarly, neoplastic invasion can also result in epidermal destruction and ulceration (Fig. 32.7).

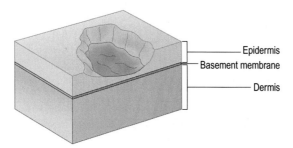

Figure 32.1 Diagrammatic representation of an erosion. The basement membrane remains intact.

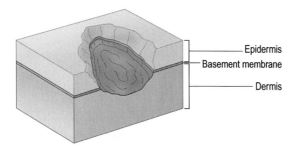

Figure 32.2 Diagrammatic representation of an ulcer. The basement membrane has been breached.

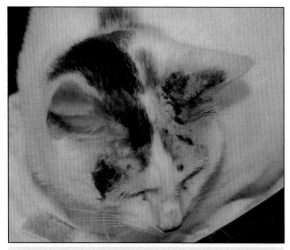

Figure 32.3 Crusted erosions and ulcers in a cat due to self-trauma as a result of pruritus.

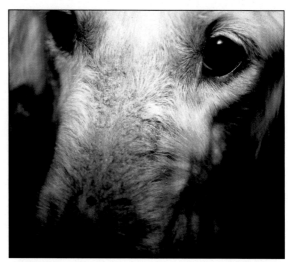

Figure 32.4 Scaling over the face of a golden retriever with small-vessel vasculitis due to a drug eruption.

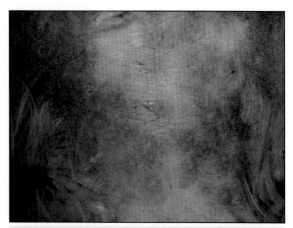

Figure 32.5 The ventral abdomen of the same dog as in Fig. 32.4 showing erythema and scaling with shallow erosions.

INVESTIGATION OF ULCERATIVE AND EROSIVE DISEASES

As with any dermatology case, a methodical approach involving thorough history taking, full physical and dermatological examinations, and diagnostic testing is required when investigating ulcerative and erosive disease.

Skin scrapings: Skin scrapings to rule out demodicosis, scabies and cheyletiellosis would be indicated in any pruritic erosive or ulcerative disease, particularly with evidence of pustules, alopecia or scaling.

Cytology: Cytology is always indicated, and may help to reveal the presence of bacterial or fungal infection, eosinophilic infiltrates, or acantholytic keratinocytes and

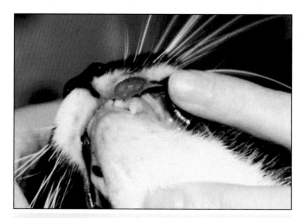

Figure 32.6 Deep ulceration of the upper lip in a cat with rodent ulcer.

non-toxic neutrophils in pemphigus foliaceus (see Chapter 2).

Histopathology: The diagnosis of an autoimmune cause of erosion or ulceration is dependent on ruling out the more common causes of ulceration, such as pyoderma and demodicosis, and histopathological examination of affected tissues for confirmation. Ideally, intact primary lesions should be sampled if the disease is vesicular, pustular or bullous. When sampling ulcerated lesions, a wedge biopsy should be taken that includes the margin of the ulcer (Fig. 32.7). It is advisable to resolve secondary bacterial infection prior to taking samples for histopathological examination and to take samples before initiating any immunosuppressive therapy. It is good practice to take multiple samples from representative lesions.

TREATMENT

If an autoimmune disease is suspected, it is inadvisable to institute immunosuppressive therapy without having

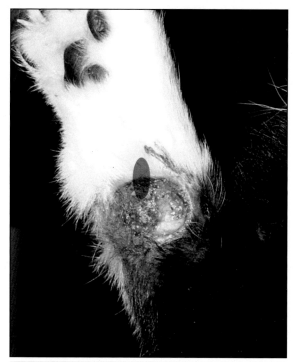

Figure 32.7 Full-thickness ulceration over the metatarsus in a cat due to a basal cell carcinoma. The ellipse shows the preferred excision site for scalpel biopsy.

a definitive diagnosis. In general, use the least potent drug or combination of drugs that will control the clinical signs of the disease and, when treating these diseases, it should not be assumed, just because signs recur, that this is a recurrence of the autoimmune disease – it may be a pyoderma or demodicosis. If in any doubt, consider referral to a dermatology specialist.

33 Erythema multiforme

INITIAL PRESENTATION

Oral, pinnal, footpad and truncal erosions and ulceration.

INTRODUCTION

Erythema multiforme is an immune-mediated, pleomorphic skin disease that frequently results in erosions and ulcerations over both skin and mucosal surfaces, but can also result in so-called 'target lesions' (see 'Aetiopathogenesis' section). Clinically, erythema multiforme is classified according to the extent of the skin lesions and mucosal involvement; however, confusion has arisen in the past because erythema multiforme is also a histopathological diagnosis, and the term is used by pathologists whenever the characteristic histological changes are present.

The aetiology is multifactorial and poorly understood. Recognized underlying causes include drug eruptions, infection and internal neoplasia, or disease may be idiopathic. This report describes a case of erythema multiforme, which was thought to have arisen as the result of a recent respiratory infection.

CASE PRESENTING SIGNS

A 4-year-old female, neutered Labrador retriever presented with oral, pinnal, footpad and truncal erosions and ulceration.

CASE HISTORY

This presentation was unusual and suggestive of an autoimmune or immune-mediated disease. In such cases a thorough history may provide valuable clues as to the underlying cause, if there is one. It is important to establish details such as recent drug therapy, symptoms of systemic illness and evidence of zoonosis or contagion.

The history in this case was as follows:

- One week after a recent stay in a boarding kennel, symptoms of lethargy, a serous ocular discharge and sneezing became apparent. Appetite remained unaffected.
- One week after the onset of these respiratory symptoms, skin lesions developed consisting of pinnal erythema and subsequently erosive, ulcerative and crusting lesions over the buccal mucosa, ventral trunk and feet.
- The respiratory symptoms resolved within a week of onset but the erosive lesions persisted.
- The dog had received annual routine vaccinations; the last vaccination had been 3 months previously when anthelmintic treatment had also been administered.
- At the time of examination, treatment consisted of oral clindamycin. Since the onset of skin lesions, the dog had also received treatment with ampicillin, carprofen and chlorpheniramine.
- One other dog in the household, the dam, was unaffected. There was no evidence of zoonosis and no history of travel abroad. There had been no recent changes to the house environment.
- The diet consisted of a commercial, complete dried dog food, a few scraps, vegetables but no supplements and water to drink.

CLINICAL EXAMINATION

Apart from target lesions, erythema multiforme can result in many other different skin and mucosal lesions. Skin lesions include erythematous annular and serpiginous configuration of plaques, papules, erosions, collarettes and, in more severe cases, areas of erosion and ulceration. Mucosal lesions consist of vesicles and bullae progressing to erosions and ulceration. The axillae and groin, the mucocutaneous junctions, the oral cavity, the pinnae and the footpads are reported to be the most frequently affected areas.

Clinical examination in this case revealed:
- Vesicles and bullae, erosions and ulcers over the oral mucosae involving both the hard and soft palates (Figs 33.1 and 33.2)
- Occasional epidermal collarettes and shallow crusting erosions over the glabrous abdominal skin and flank folds (Fig. 33.3)
- Erosions and crusting were evident over all the ungual folds and there were erosions and ulcers over the footpads and footpad margins on all four feet (Fig. 33.4).

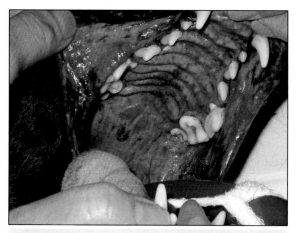

Figure 33.1 Erosions and ulceration over the hard and soft palates.

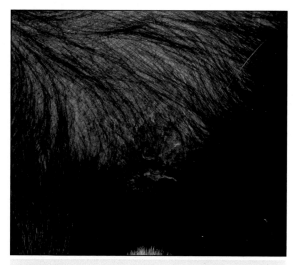

Figure 33.3 Epidermal collarette and crusting over one flank fold.

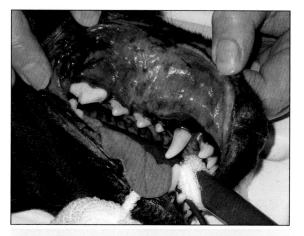

Figure 33.2 Macular erythema and erosions over the buccal mucosa. A bullous lesion is evident (arrowed).

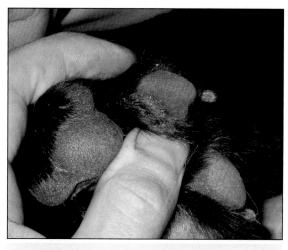

Figure 33.4 Ulceration over a footpad margin.

DIFFERENTIAL DIAGNOSES

The differential diagnoses for erythema multiforme are extensive due to the multiple lesions types that are encountered in this condition. They include urticaria, pyoderma, dermatophytosis, demodicosis and some of the bullous autoimmune diseases, such as pemphigus vulgaris, bullous pemphigoid and epidermolysis bullosa acquisita. More severe lesions with larger areas of erosion or ulceration would need to be differentiated from burns, toxic epidermal necrolysis and vasculitis.

The list of possible differential diagnoses in this case included:

- Erythema multiforme
- Pemphigus vulgaris
- Epidermolysis bullosa acquisita
- Bullous pemphigoid
- Mucous membrane pemphigoid
- Pyoderma.

CASE WORK-UP

Cytology: Cytological examination of impression smears from collarettes and erosions was indicated to look for evidence of bacterial infection and for the presence of acantholytic keratinocytes (see Chapter 17). Non-degenerate neutrophils and a small number of acantholytic keratinocytes were seen on examination of an impression smear from an erosion on the oral mucosa.

Histopathology: Histopathological examination is required to make a definitive diagnosis of erythema multiforme. Under general anaesthesia, an 8-mm biopsy punch was used to excise skin and mucosal samples. One sample was taken of an entire vesicle from the buccal mucosa and another of an earlier lesion consisting of macular erythema. The margin of one footpad erosion and an erythematous macule from the groin were also sampled. N.B. In order to keep the lesions intact, excisional biopsy is preferable when sampling large fragile vesicles, pustules and bullae.

In this case examination of the excised samples showed an interface dermatitis with keratinocyte apoptosis and lymphocyte satellitosis in all layers of the epidermis. Interface dermatitis is an inflammatory process that targets the dermo-epidermal junction, the junctional zone between the dermis and epidermis. There is usually

vacuolation of the basement membrane region, leading to a 'bubbly' appearance of this zone. Apoptotic keratinocytes show up as brightly eosinophilic and sometimes shrunken cells throughout all layers of the epidermis. Lymphocyte satellitosis is the term used to describe lymphocytes found in close apposition to keratinocytes. It is the interaction with the lymphocyte that induces keratinocyte apoptosis, a form of programmed cell death.

These changes are similar to those found in cutaneous or systemic lupus erythematosus, the principal differentiating feature being that keratinocyte apoptosis is more prominent in erythema multiforme and occurs throughout all layers of the epidermis, whereas in lupus erythematosus, the apoptosis is confined mainly to the basal layer of the epidermis.

DIAGNOSIS

The history, clinical signs and histopathology were consistent with a diagnosis of erythema multiforme minor (see 'Aetiopathogenesis' section below).

PROGNOSIS

The prognosis for erythema multiforme depends entirely on the underlying cause. If the cause is a drug eruption, then discontinuation of the drug treatment and supportive care should result in resolution of lesions within a few weeks. Similarly, if the cause is viral, with time and supportive care and if the viral infection resolves, the lesions should resolve. With underlying neoplasia or connective tissue diseases the prognosis is likely to be less favourable unless the disease process can be resolved. Similarly, idiopathic diseases carry an uncertain prognosis.

The prognosis is also less favourable if there are extensive areas of ulceration and care must be taken to prevent the onset of life-threatening infections of these areas.

In this case it was likely that the disease was the result of the recent, possibly viral, respiratory infection. The lesions were not severe, the dog not systemically affected and there was a likelihood of complete recovery.

AETIOPATHOGENESIS OF ERYTHEMA MULTIFORME

The aetiopathogenesis of erythema multiforme is still poorly understood but is considered to be a cellular hypersensitivity response directed at particular antigens. Antigens may be exogenous or endogenous and include infections, drugs, foods and proteins associated with neoplasia and connective tissue diseases. It is thought that mainly CD8+ lymphocytes interact with keratinocytes expressing the antigen on the cell surface, and the interaction induces keratinocyte apoptosis. This process is manifested histopathologically by the close apposition of lymphocytes to apoptotic keratinocytes, so-called 'lymphocyte satellitosis'.

Historically, the term erythema multiforme has been used in human clinical dermatology to describe skin lesions consisting of concentric rings of erythema or urticarial plaques, with areas of blistering and necrosis and/or resolution in a concentric array, so-called 'target lesions'. However, target lesions have only been identified in a small percentage of cases of canine erythema multiforme, and the diagnosis of erythema multiforme in animals has tended to be based on finding the characteristic histopathological changes and not on clinical presentation.

This reliance on histopathological diagnosis has led to confusion because erythema multiforme is part of a spectrum of diseases of varying clinical presentation and increasing severity that now includes erythema multiforme minor, erythema multiforme major, Stevens–Johnson syndrome (SJS), overlap syndrome (OVE) and toxic epidermal necrolysis (TEN). These diseases can, if biopsied at certain times, have very similar histopathological changes and thus misdiagnoses can be made.

It has recently been recommended that the diagnosis and differentiation of this group of diseases should be based on a set of clinical criteria, as well as finding the characteristic histopathological abnormalities. The new classification of the disease is based on a system adopted from human dermatology. Using this system, a clinical diagnosis is made according to the extent and severity of the lesions, and whether one or more mucosal surfaces are involved in addition to the skin (Table 33.1). Thus, this case could be diagnosed as erythema multiforme minor based on the histopathology and clinical presentation. The differentiation of these different diseases is of clinical importance, as one study has shown that cases of erythema multiforme are most frequently caused by viral infections and, at the other end of the spectrum, toxic epidermal necrolysis is most frequently the result of a drug reaction. In fact, a drug eruption was responsible for 92% of cases of Stevens–Johnson syndrome, overlap syndrome and toxic epidermal necrolysis, and only 19% of cases of erythema multiforme minor/major.

EPIDEMIOLOGY

This disease is uncommon in the dog and rare in the cat. One study reported that German shepherd dogs and Welsh Pembroke corgis are predisposed. A form of idiopathic erythema multiforme has been described in older dogs that tends to result in hyperkeratotic skin lesions, mainly involving the skin of the face and ears. In human dermatology, dermatoses classified clinically as erythema multiforme minor or major seem to be most commonly caused by viral (particularly herpes virus) infections, leading to lymphocyte-mediated keratinocyte apoptosis.

Table 33.1 Clinical characteristics of erythema multiforme (EM), Stevens–Johnson syndrome (SJS) and toxic epidermal necrolysis (TEN)

	EM major/minor	EM major/major	SJS	Overlap syndrome	TEN
Flat, raised, focal or multifocal polycyclic lesions	Yes	Yes	No	No	No
Number of mucosae involved	1	>1	>1	>1	>1
Erythematous or purpuric, macular or patchy eruption (% body surface)	<50	<50	<50	>50	>50
Epidermal detachment (% body surface)	<10	<10	<10	10–30	>30

After Hinn AC, Olivry T, Luther PB, et al. (1998): Erythema multiforme, Stevens–Johnson syndrome, and toxic epidermal necrolysis in the dog: clinical classification, drug exposure, and histopathological correlations. J Vet Allergy Clin Immunol 6 (1), 13–20, with permission from the Academy of Veterinary Allergy and Clinical Immunology.

TREATMENT OPTIONS

All drug treatment should be withdrawn and, most importantly, an attempt should be made to identify and correct the underlying cause of the disease. Any signs of systemic involvement should be thoroughly investigated and, where possible, systemic diseases should be treated and resolved.

Supportive care in the form of intravenous fluids or parenteral nutritional supplementation may be required if the animal is systemically unwell, or unable to eat or drink due to oral ulceration. Broad-spectrum antibacterial therapy may be indicated to prevent Gram-negative infection of areas of erosion and ulceration, using a chemically unrelated product if a drug reaction is suspected.

In more severely affected or idiopathic cases, where the lesions are unlikely to resolve spontaneously, immunosuppressive therapy may be indicated, although the use of such treatment in erythema multiforme is controversial and response tends to be variable. Prednisolone would be the first line of treatment and this could be combined with azathioprine or chlorambucil if there was an inadequate response. There is at least one report of successful therapy of a severe case of erythema multiforme (drug-induced Stevens–Johnson syndrome) with human intravenous immunoglobulin, and this treatment would be worth trying in more refractory or severely affected cases.

In this case as the dog's demeanour was unaffected and, as it seemed likely that the underlying cause was due to a recent viral infection, the decision was made to withdraw all treatment.

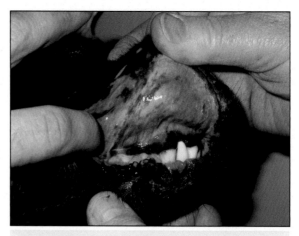

Figure 33.5 Three weeks after initial presentation, showing resolution of oral lesions.

(see Chapter 17), but they are also seen in cases of pyoderma and dermatophytosis and, potentially, they may be seen on impression smears from any erosive disease that will result in exposure of the underlying stratum spinosum.

The optimal samples to submit for histopathological examination in cases of erythema multiforme are early lesions consisting of erythematous macules. If a vesicle or bulla is to be submitted, then it is important to submit the margin of the lesion. Completely ulcerated samples are not helpful, as examination of epidermis and basement membrane is required to make the diagnosis. As with all autoimmune and immune-mediated diseases, it is advisable to try and take samples for histopathological examination prior to treatment with glucocorticoids, because such treatment will have a profound effect on the histopathological reaction pattern.

CLINICAL TIPS

A detailed history is essential when trying to ascertain the underlying cause in erythema multiforme. It is important to question the owner carefully about previous drug administration, including any routine treatment that the animal may have received, such as worming medication. Even an innocuous dietary supplement such as a multivitamin preparation could feasibly contain an additive that could result in the cutaneous eruption.

Acantholytic keratinocytes were evident on cytological examination. The presence of these cells may be associated with pemphigus foliaceus

FOLLOW-UP

Follow-up 3 weeks later revealed that there had been a gradual resolution of skin lesions. There were still erythematous macules over the buccal mucosae, but the vesicles, bullae and erosions had resolved (Fig. 33.5). The lesions subsequently completely resolved over a further 2-week period and follow-up after 2 years revealed no recurrence.

34 Vasculitis

INITIAL PRESENTATION

Severe ulceration over the caudal dorsal trunk.

INTRODUCTION

Vasculitis is an uncommon to rare cause of ulcerative skin disease in the dog. Direct inflammation of blood vessels, blood vessel damage and subsequent infarction results in a loss of blood supply to, and necrosis of, dependent tissues. The clinical presentation varies widely depending on the type, size and site of vessel involved. This report describes a case of vasculitis in a dog involving large dermal vessels resulting in severe cutaneous lesions. There was evidence in this case that a drug eruption may have triggered the disease.

CASE PRESENTING SIGNS

A 9-year-old, neutered male rough collie was presented because of severe ulceration over the caudal dorsal trunk.

CASE HISTORY

Vasculitis is not a specific diagnosis, but is usually a manifestation of some underlying disease process. There are many potential causes and this may be reflected in the history. As has been stated before in this book, a detailed history is essential to improve the chances of identifying and correcting the underlying cause.

The history in this case was as follows:
- The patient was initially presented for a dermatology referral with a 2-month history of full-thickness cutaneous ulcerations over the caudal dorsum and erythematous scaling lesions over the ventral trunk.

- Three months earlier, the dog had been presented for veterinary examination because of an inability to stand. Pyrexia (105°F) and lumbar pain had been evident on physical examination and discospondylitis was diagnosed on radiography. The dog was treated with a combination of carprofen and a 4-week course of cefalexin.
- A few days prior to completion of the initial course of cefalexin, the dog started to develop ventral skin lesions. The onset had been rapid, with development of large ulcerated areas of skin over a period of a few days.
- The skin lesions had been painful.
- Subsequent treatment with antibiotics, glucocorticoids and non-steroidal anti-inflammatory drugs had resulted in no clinical improvement in the appearance of the skin.
- There had been evidence of polyuria and polydipsia. This was probably associated with glucocorticoid administration as these symptoms were resolving with withdrawal of treatment.
- The dog had lost a moderate amount of weight since the onset of the skin lesions.
- There were no other animals in the house. There was no history suggestive of zoonosis and the dog had never been out of the UK.
- The diet consisted of a tinned dog food and biscuit mixer with additional scraps, with milk and water to drink.

CLINICAL EXAMINATION

Vasculitis can be associated with a wide variety of clinical signs. Damage to dermal and mucosal vessels results in leakage of contents and infarction. The signs of cutaneous vasculitis reflect this, and include petechiation, ecchymoses, purpura, subcutaneous oedema, scaling, alopecia, erosions, ulceration, necrosis and scarring. There may be substantial areas of necrotic tissue depending on the size of vessel involved. In addition, there are vasculitis syndromes in man and domestic animals involving vasculature of internal organs, and therefore many different systemic clinical signs can arise depending on the organ(s) involved. Clinical signs may also reflect an underlying disease process such as a connective tissue disease, infection or neoplasia. Systemic signs can include fever, anorexia, glomerulonephritis, polyarthropathies, myopathies, retinitis, uveitis, neuropathies, gastrointestinal signs, pancreatitis, epistaxis, and pleural and peritoneal effusions.

The clinical signs in this case were as follows:

- The patient was slightly obese and weighed 36 kg. Rectal temperature was 102.5°F and pulse rate was 136 bpm. Detectable abnormalities were otherwise confined to the skin.
- There were extensive, full-thickness, punched-out ulcerations with a symmetrical distribution over the caudal dorsum, with malodorous, necrotic debris within the ulcerated areas (Figs 34.1 and 34.2). In addition, there were coalescing, erythematous and scaling macules, patches and plaques over much of the ventrum, extending from the neck to the groin region (Fig. 34.3).

DIFFERENTIAL DIAGNOSES

The multifocal, full-thickness, punched-out ulceration was suggestive of a vasculitis or vasculopathy, but other possible differentials included:

- Deep pyoderma
- Other atypical bacterial infections
- Deep fungal infection
- Demodicosis
- Sterile panniculitis
- Vasculitis/vasculopathy

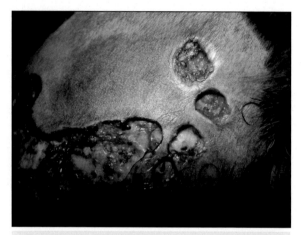

Figure 34.2 Cutaneous vasculitis at initial presentation. Full-thickness, punched-out ulcers with granulation can be seen over the caudal dorsum.

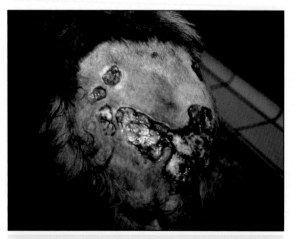

Figure 34.1 Cutaneous vasculitis at initial presentation. Full-thickness, punched-out ulcers with granulation are apparent over the caudal dorsum.

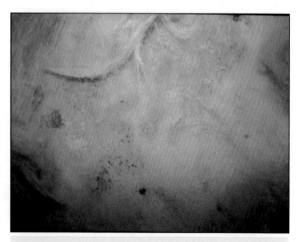

Figure 34.3 Cutaneous vasculitis at initial presentation. Erythematous and scaling macules and patches over the ventral trunk are apparent.

- Bullous pemphigoid
- Pemphigus vulgaris
- Erythema multiforme/Stevens–Johnson syndrome/toxic epidermal necrolysis
- Systemic lupus erythematosus
- Drug eruption
- Cutaneous T-cell lymphoma.

CASE WORK-UP

The skin lesions were severe to the point of being life threatening and an aggressive diagnostic approach was indicated. In addition to ruling out demodicosis and performing routine cytology, it was necessary to try and identify a possible underlying cause, including identification of any potential systemic involvement.

The following diagnostic tests were performed:
- Multiple deep skin scrapings, which were negative for *Demodex* mites.
- Cytological examination of smears from ulcerated areas, which showed degenerate neutrophils, activated macrophages, many cocci and a few rods.
- Routine haematological and biochemical examinations, which showed mild anaemia, thrombocytopenia (76 × 10⁹/l), mild neutrophilia, lymphopenia, hypoalbuminaemia (18.5 g/l; normal reference range 26–35 g/l) and hyperglobulinaemia. Alkaline phosphatase was moderately elevated (178 IU/l; normal reference range 38–108 IU/l). Antinuclear antibody titre was <1/8, well within the normal laboratory reference range.
- Urinalysis (collected by cystocentesis), which showed a specific gravity of 1.013 and a trace of haemolysed blood but was otherwise unremarkable.
- No abnormalities were detected on survey chest and abdominal radiographs.
- Skin biopsies were harvested and submitted for histopathological examination. Samples were taken from the ventral exfoliative lesions (8-mm biopsy punch), as well as the margins of ulcerated areas (excised using a scalpel). Histopathological examination showed varying changes, including vasculitis, panniculitis and diffuse granulomatous inflammation. It was considered that some, or possibly all, of the erosion and ulceration was ischaemic and due to vasculitis.
- At the same time, tissue samples were also submitted for bacterial and fungal culture, and further samples were sent to a mycobacterial reference laboratory for

culture. There was no bacterial, mycobacterial or fungal growth on tissue samples submitted.

DIAGNOSIS

The definitive diagnosis of vasculitis relies on histopathological demonstration of an inflammatory infiltrate targeting the blood vessel wall. The problem with cutaneous vasculitis is distinguishing true vasculitis from the physiological migration of leucocytes through vessel walls seen in any inflammatory response. There may be tissue changes associated with a vasculitis, but no evidence of blood vessel wall involvement. Many dermatopathologists use the term vasculopathy in this situation.

In this case, in multiple sections, there was evidence of vessels undergoing destructive inflammation and it was possible to make a definitive diagnosis of vasculitis. There was no obvious underlying systemic disease and, in view of the recent drug administration, a putative diagnosis of vasculitis due to a drug reaction to either cefalexin or carprofen was made.

PROGNOSIS

Provided the dog did not develop a life-threatening infection over the ulcerated areas of skin, and provided the underlying cause of the vasculitis could be corrected, there was a fair prognosis for recovery with treatment. However, some cases have an unpredictable or poor prognosis, especially where an underlying cause cannot be identified and resolved.

AETIOPATHOGENESIS OF VASCULITIS

Classification of vasculitis

It is important to be aware of the disease processes that may lead to vasculitis because this will have a bearing on the investigation and management of the case. The following useful classification of vasculitis in domestic animals has been proposed.

Primary classification:
1. Infectious vasculitis
2. Non-infectious vasculitis
   I. Immune mediated
      Exogenous antigen
      - drugs
      - vaccines (in particular, rabies vaccine)
      - food additives
      - infectious

Endogenous antigen
- neoplasia
- connective tissue disease

II. Idiopathic.

Subclassification:
1. First by vessel type, size, location
2. Second by inflammatory infiltrate.

Infectious vasculitis: Vasculitis may result from direct injury to endothelial cells caused by invasion of bacterial, viral, rickettsial or protozoal organisms. Rocky Mountain spotted fever caused by *Rickettsia rickettsii* is an example of an endotheliotrophic pathogen.

Immune-mediated causes: Antibodies may be produced against a wide range of antigens and form circulating immune complexes, which may become lodged in the basement membrane and collagen of blood vessel walls. This deposition is more likely to occur in blood vessels where there is a physiological outflow of fluid, such as in post-capillary venules, the glomeruli, synovial membranes and the choroid plexus. Hydrostatic forces in dependent areas such as the limbs and ventrum, and turbulent blood flow at blood vessel bifurcations, may also contribute to immune complex deposition. The presence of immune complexes within the vessel wall results in the activation of complement, recruitment of inflammatory cells and subsequent injury to the blood vessel. This is the basis of the Type III hypersensitivity reaction.

Exogenous antigens thought to cause immune-mediated vasculitis in small animals include drugs, vaccines, food additives and infections. Endogenous antigens may originate from connective tissue diseases such as systemic lupus erythematosus and rheumatoid arthritis.

There are similar immunological pathways operating in both the infectious and immune-mediated vasculitides, which result in up-regulation of inflammation and further tissue damage. Circulating neutrophils are drawn to the area by a chemical gradient of complement factors and chemokines produced by activated tissue macrophages and damaged or infected endothelial cells. Having reached the site of inflammation, neutrophils first adhere to the endothelial cell lining and then migrate through the blood vessel wall. They undergo a massive increase in oxygen consumption when they come into contact with foreign particles such as immune complexes. This results in the production of hyophalides and enzymes, both of which cause further, severe, tissue damage.

Relatively recently, in human medicine, the role of anti-neutrophil cytoplasmic antibodies (ANCAs) in the diagnosis and pathogenesis of some forms of vasculitis has been described. These are antibodies that are formed against neutrophil enzymes which are exposed to the immune system as a result of microbial infection. Anti-neutrophil cytoplasmic antibodies in the circulation do not react with unprimed neutrophils, because the target antigens are within the neutrophil cytoplasm. Infection causes the neutrophils to express the antigen at the cell surface, where they can react with the anti-neutrophil cytoplasmic antibodies. These activated neutrophils then adhere to endothelial cells, which results in injury to endothelial cells (and eventually underlying vessel wall structures) by release of granule enzymes and toxic oxygen metabolites. To date, anti-neutrophil cytoplasmic antibodies have not been described in small animals.

Idiopathic vasculitis: Several familial, idiopathic vasculitides involving medium to large blood vessels have been described in small animals. They include juvenile polyarteritis syndrome in beagles, idiopathic cutaneous and renal glomerular vasculopathy of greyhounds, and familial cutaneous vasculopathy in German shepherd dogs. Polyarteritis nodosa, with inflammation specifically involving arteries, is uncommon in small animals but has been described in the cat.

Canine dermatomyositis (see Chapter 35) causes a very subtle vasculitis affecting small arterioles of skin and skeletal muscle. A syndrome of cutaneous vasculitis involving small dermal vessels has been reported in Jack Russell terriers.

EPIDEMIOLOGY

Cutaneous vasculitis is an uncommon cause of skin disease in dogs and rare in cats. As already indicated, certain breeds may be predisposed to idiopathic disease, including German shepherds, greyhounds, dachshunds and Jack Russell terriers. There is no obvious sex predilection.

TREATMENT OPTIONS

Infectious causes of vasculitis

Infections may cause vasculitis either by direct invasion of endothelial cells or indirectly via hypersensitivity responses. Any infections should therefore be appropriately and thoroughly treated.

Immune-mediated vasculitis

Treatment of immune-mediated vasculitis is aimed at removing the antigenic stimulus, providing supportive care, reducing the immune response and reducing vessel wall inflammation.

Removal of antigenic stimulus: Drug administration should be discontinued in any case where a drug eruption is a possibility or, if available, a chemically unrelated compound should be substituted. It is particularly important not to substitute a cephalosporin with a penicillin or vice versa, as these are antigenically cross-reactive antibiotics. Underlying neoplastic or connective tissue disease should be treated.

Supportive care: Gentle antibacterial soaks are indicated where there is ulceration and crusting, to remove surface debris and eliminate surface microorganisms. Intravenous fluids and parenteral nutrition may be indicated to replace lost fluids, electrolytes and nutrients. Broad-spectrum antibacterial therapy is likely to be indicated to prevent Gram-negative infection of ulcerated areas, or if there is evidence of systemic infection.

Reducing the immune response:
Glucocorticoids: Glucocorticoids are extremely useful in the treatment of vasculitis. They decrease vascular permeability, inhibit neutrophil chemotaxis and migration, decrease antibody production, inhibit complement and inhibit the release of pro-inflammatory cytokines. Glucocorticoids are usually required in most idiopathic and immune-mediated vasculitides. Immunosuppressive doses are administered initially and gradually tapered once lesions start to resolve.

Pentoxifylline: Pentoxifylline is a methylxanthine derivative. It improves vascular perfusion by increasing fibrinolysis and erythrocyte and leucocyte membrane deformability, and by decreasing microvascular constriction, plasma fibrinogen levels and erythrocyte and platelet aggregation. Pentoxifylline has also been shown to have other useful anti-inflammatory effects on neutrophils, including reducing their adherence to endothelial cells and inhibiting degranulation. Doses of 10–15 mg/kg t.i.d. have been used to successfully treat vasculitis in the dog. This is a drug that can take 2–3 months to exert maximal effect and therefore should be used in conjunction with glucocorticoids in cases such as this one, where there was a potentially life-threatening disease. The use

of pentoxifylline may allow a reduction in the cumulative glucocorticoid dose used. Side-effects in man include nausea, vomiting, dizziness and headaches. This is an unlicensed drug in the dog, but clinical experience has shown this to be a safe treatment. Potential side-effects include gastrointestinal disturbance and an increased tendency to bleeding during surgery. Contraindications are hepatic and renal diseases.

Other immunosuppressive therapies: Other immunomodulatory or immunosuppressive therapies that may be used to treat vasculitis include azathioprine, chlorambucil, dapsone, a combination of oxytetracycline (or doxycycline) and nicotinamide, and large doses of vitamin E.

Treatment used in this case

In view of the possibility of a drug eruption, the decision was made to withdraw all treatment. The dog was hospitalized and bathed daily in a whirlpool bath in dilute povidone iodine.

He remained moderately pyrexic over the next week (temperature 102–103.4°F). After 1 week of daily whirlpool baths, the ulcerated areas had extended slightly and the decision was made to start systemic therapy. The following treatments were administered:
- Prednisolone (62.5 mg b.i.d.)
- Pentoxifylline (400 mg t.i.d.)
- Clindamycin (175 mg b.i.d.).

Within 48 hours of starting therapy, there had been an improvement with decreased erythema and no further increase in the size of the areas of ulceration. The patient was discharged from hospital.

On follow-up examination a week later, the dog was markedly polydipsic, polyphagic, polyuric and panting. Physical examination revealed a rectal temperature of 101.4°F and temporal muscle atrophy. There was oedema over the ventral thoracic wall caudal to the axillae. The ulcerated lesions had decreased in size and were crusted with underlying purulent exudate (Fig. 34.4). The ventral erythematous plaques had resolved. Repeat haematological and biochemical examinations showed mild anaemia (4.63×10^{12}/l) and marked leucocytosis (30.1×10^9/l) consisting of mainly segmented neutrophils (92%). ALT (570 IU/l), ALP (2230 IU/l), cholesterol (9 mmol/l) and bile acids (21.3 μmol/l) were all elevated and were a reflection of high-dose glucocorticoid therapy. Cytological examination of purulent material beneath crusts revealed large numbers of cocci and

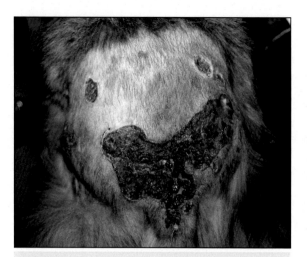

Figure 34.4 The same dog as in Fig. 34.1 after 1 week of immunosuppressive glucocorticoid therapy and pentoxifylline.

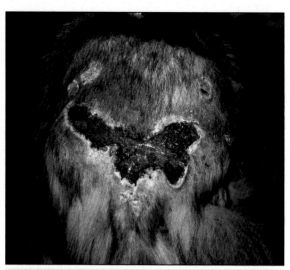

Figure 34.5 The same dog as in Fig. 34.1 after three and a half weeks of immunosuppressive glucocorticoid therapy and pentoxifylline.

rods. Systemic treatments were continued at the same dosage and the owner was instructed to soak the remaining crusted lesions in dilute povidone iodine on alternate days.

The patient was re-examined again after a further two and a half weeks. There were continued signs of glucocorticoid excess with abdominal enlargement, temporal muscle wastage and hyperextension of both carpal joints. The skin lesions were resolving with re-epithelialization of smaller ulcers over the caudal dorsum and healing around the margins of the large ulcerated areas (Fig. 34.5). The ventral lesions had mainly resolved. Haematological and biochemical examinations again showed similar changes consistent with glucocorticoid usage and chronic disease.

In the interests of trying to prevent further carpal hyperextension, the prednisolone dosage was reduced initially to 62.5 mg b.i.d. and 62.5 mg s.i.d. on alternate days for 1 week, and then 62.5 mg s.i.d. every day for the following week. Pentoxifylline was continued at the same dosage.

NURSING ASPECTS

This dog had a generalized crusting and ulcerative dermatitis. Daily immersion in a whirlpool bath containing dilute povidone iodine was of great benefit, and was a gentle, soothing, non-traumatic way of removing crust and microorganisms from the skin surface. If a whirlpool bath is not available, the use of a showerhead to gently wash off crust would be a good second choice, but standard shampoo therapy would have caused the dog considerable discomfort.

A soft bed that doesn't shed fibres or adhere to the open ulcerated lesions is essential. Bedding would need to be changed at least daily if soiled. An Elizabethan collar might be required to prevent self-trauma.

As with all dogs receiving glucocorticoid therapy, the common side-effects include increased appetite and thirst, weight gain and sometimes mood changes. Additional side-effects can include panting, diarrhoea, weight loss, skin and coat changes, urinary tract infections, and diabetes mellitus. Owners should be warned of these side-effects when treatment is dispensed, but may still require follow-up telephone counselling and reassurance. Food intake should be restricted to minimize weight gain and, if appropriate, a calorie-controlled diet should be instituted. It is much easier to prevent weight gain than to get the dog to lose weight. Water should always be available but should be regulated, so that large amounts are not consumed by the dog in one go.

CLINICAL TIPS

One aspect to highlight in this case was the clinical presentation. The lesions over the caudal dorsum looked as though they had been removed by a large biopsy punch. These punched-out lesions represent the area of skin supplied by the affected vessel and are characteristic of vasculitis. Scalding would perhaps be one other possible cause of this lesion distribution, but there was no history of this.

Excisional biopsies were taken of the margins of ulcerated lesions. It is helpful to provide the pathologist with the entire cross-section of the ulcer margin and a biopsy punch would be too small to accomplish this.

When deep bacterial or fungal infection is on the list of differential diagnoses, tissue should be taken for culture at the same time as histopathological examination. If a mycobacterial infection is suspected, skin samples may be wrapped in foil and placed in a deep freeze, and only submitted for culture if the histopathology suggests this aetiology.

FOLLOW-UP

The owner failed to attend subsequent follow-up appointments, but a follow-up phone call to the referring veterinary surgeon revealed that the skin lesions had healed uneventfully and the owner stopped treatment without further veterinary consultation. The dog lived for a further 4 years before being euthanized for unrelated reasons. Interestingly, further carprofen treatment was administered for treatment of suspected hip arthritis, without recurrence of further skin lesions.

35 Familial canine dermatomyositis

INITIAL PRESENTATION

Erosive ulcerations and alopecia.

INTRODUCTION

Familial canine dermatomyositis is an inflammatory disease affecting the skin, musculature and blood vessels. It is thought that compromised blood supply causing a low-grade cutaneous ischaemia leads to alopecia, erosions and at times ulceration of the skin. This report describes a case of dermatomyositis in a collie complicated by secondary pyoderma.

CASE PRESENTING SIGNS

A 2-year-old spayed female, lurcher cross collie was presented with multifocal patches of alopecia, erythema, crusting and scaling, and most recently more generalized papules and nodules.

CASE HISTORY

Typically, in cases of familial canine dermatomyositis, skin lesions first become apparent between 6 weeks and 6 months of age. The symptoms of myositis generally develop after the onset of skin lesions.

The history in this case was as follows:
- Scaling and crusting lesions over the bridge of the nose and pinnae that had first become apparent at 3–4 months of age.
- These lesions had waxed and waned since then and had shown improvement for variable periods of time following antibacterial therapy.

- Most recently, a papular and nodular eruption had developed over the skin on the trunk and limbs, and pruritus had been evident.
- The dog had shown intermittent hind limb lameness and had seemed stiff, particularly in the mornings. She had a tendency to 'shift' her weight from one hind limb to the other when affected in this way. The owners reported the hind limb abnormalities had appeared after the onset of skin lesions.
- There was no history of drug exposure prior to the onset of skin lesions.
- This was a house dog. There are no other pets in the household, no evidence of zoonosis and no history of travel abroad.
- The dog liked to sunbathe.
- The diet consisted of a proprietary, good quality, turkey and rice kibble with water to drink.

CLINICAL EXAMINATION

Lesions associated with dermatomyositis usually present as alopecia, erythema, scaling, ulceration and crusting. As with many vascular diseases, the extremities and prominences such as the face, tail, pinnae and limbs are mainly affected, so oral, footpad and nail lesions may all be present. Ulceration may develop in more severely affected cases that may also be hyper- or hypopigmented. In general, this is a non-pruritic disease unless there is secondary pyoderma. Temporal muscle atrophy is the most common initial symptom of myositis. Other signs of myositis include dysphagia, facial palsy, stiff gait and a generalized weakness.

Clinical findings in this case were:
- Rectal temperature was 102°F.
- The dog walked with a stiff-legged hind limb gait.
- Examination of the skin revealed focal, well-demarcated patches of shiny-appearing alopecia over the bridge of the nose, forehead (Fig. 35.1) and hindquarters (Fig. 35.2). There were two slightly crusted erosions over the convex aspect of the left pinna and a focal crusted erosion above the left eye (Fig. 35.1).

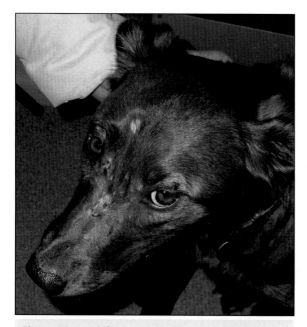

Figure 35.1 Multifocal, well-demarcated alopecia and crusting. Crusted erosion is seen above the left eye.

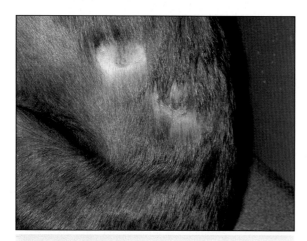

Figure 35.2 Focal alopecia and crusting exudative erosions over the hindquarters.

- Examination of the trunk revealed a generalized eruption consisting of focal alopecia, scaling, and crusted papules and erosions (Fig. 35.2).

DIFFERENTIAL DIAGNOSES

The list of possible differential diagnoses in this case was extensive. Patchy alopecia is suggestive of a folliculitis. The shiny appearance of the skin can be a feature of ischaemic, scarring dermatoses. There were lesions on the pinnae and over the face that were suggestive of a possible autoimmune aetiology. The differential diagnoses therefore included the following:
- Causes of folliculitis – demodicosis, pyoderma, dermatophytosis
- Autoimmune diseases – pemphigus foliaceus, cutaneous lupus erythematosus, systemic lupus erythematosus, epidermolysis bullosa, bullous pemphigoid
- Vascular disease – the age of onset, breed, appearance of the lesions and concurrent stiff gait were suggestive of dermatomyositis.

CASE WORK-UP

The initial requirement was to rule out the involvement of parasitic and infectious causes of folliculitis.
- No evidence of ectoparasitism was found on examination of three skin scrapes from affected areas.
- A pyogranulomatous inflammation with numerous phagocytosed cocci was evident on examination of impression smears from exudative lesions over the trunk.
- No dermatophytes were grown from material submitted for fungal culture, collected using the MacKenzie brush technique and by plucking hairs from around lesions.

There was evidence of pyoderma, which correlated well with the previous partial response to antibacterial therapy. The next step was to resolve the bacterial component and then to investigate the remaining symptoms. In a case such as this, treatment of the pyoderma can be regarded as a diagnostic tool.
- Initial treatment consisted of cefalexin at a dosage of 20 mg/kg b.i.d. for 3 weeks.

On re-examination 3 weeks later, there had been an obvious improvement with resolution of some skin lesions, and about a 50% reduction in the level of pruritus. However, there were still multifocal erythematous, scaling and partially alopecic macules and patches over the head and trunk (Figs 35.3 and 35.4). There were raised serpiginous, erythematous margins to the lesions.

The lesions had persisted despite treatment of the pyoderma and so histopathological investigation was indicated. Routine haematological and biochemical examinations, as well as urinalysis, were also indicated, partly because systemic lupus erythematosus was a differential and also because it might have been necessary to treat this case with immunosuppressive therapy.

- Four 6-mm punch biopsy samples were taken for histopathological examination under sedation and local anaesthesia. This revealed a superficial pustular dermatitis, a cell-poor interface dermatitis, and fading and atrophy of hair follicles.
- Apart from elevated serum creatine kinase, there were no other significant abnormalities on haematology, biochemistry and urinalysis.

Antibiotic treatment was continued pending the results of the histopathology.

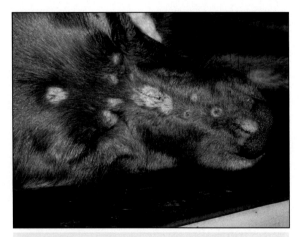

Figure 35.3 After 3 weeks of antibacterial therapy showing resolution of crusting. Scarring alopecia remains.

DIAGNOSIS

The history, clinical signs and histopathology were consistent with a diagnosis of dermatomyositis. Elevations of serum creatine kinase are a common finding in dermatomyositis and would be consistent with skeletal muscle damage.

Further investigation of the causes of the myositis was not performed, although histological examination of muscle tissue and electromyographic studies, when available, may also be of diagnostic significance.

PROGNOSIS

The prognosis in dermatomyositis is variable. In mildly affected cases there may be spontaneous resolution of lesions after a few months, although more severe disease is likely to persist throughout life.

In very severely affected animals the prognosis is poor, with stunted growth, difficulty in eating and drinking, development of aspiration pneumonia due to megaoesophagus and a shortened life expectancy. Severe secondary amyloidosis leading to renal failure has also been reported.

In most cases, the disease has a tendency to wax and wane. It is a scarring skin disease and, even in relatively mildly affected cases, permanent alopecia may result.

The patient in question was not severely affected, but the lesions had been present for 2 years and were unlikely to spontaneously resolve after this time. The owner was advised that the dog was likely to require lifelong treatment to control the lesions.

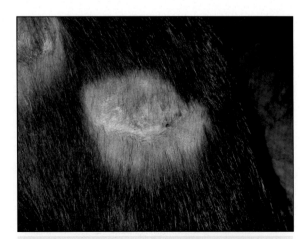

Figure 35.4 After 3 weeks of antibacterial therapy showing resolution of crusting. Scarring alopecia remains.

AETIOPATHOGENESIS
OF DERMATOMYOSITIS

Familial canine dermatomyositis is one of a group of diseases characterized by clinical and histopathological features very suggestive of an ischaemic dermatopathy. This group of diseases includes: canine familial dermatomyositis; dogs with juvenile-onset ischaemic dermatopathy similar to dermatomyositis but without proven breed predilection; post-rabies vaccination panniculitis; dogs with generalized post-rabies vaccination disease; and dogs with adult-onset generalized ischaemic dermatopathy without a history of rabies vaccination.

In addition to mild inflammation targeting the basal layer of the epidermis and the basement membrane zone ('cell-poor interface dermatitis'), a cell-poor vasculitis has been shown to be common to all these syndromes. It is thought that cutaneous hypoxia leads to the chronic skin changes of hair follicle atrophy and resulting alopecia, as well as erosions, ulcers and crusting. As with any vascular disease, bony prominences and extremities are mainly affected and scarring is a common sequela.

The disease may result in a myositis that usually appears after the onset of skin lesions. Electromyographic abnormalities include fibrillation potentials, positive sharp waves and bizarre high-frequency discharges.

The precise aetiology of familial canine dermatomyositis is not known but immunological abnormalities have been demonstrated, including elevated serum concentrations of IgG and circulating immune complexes. The IgG concentration increases around the time of development of the skin lesions and seems to correlate with the severity of disease. In severely affected animals, the serum IgG concentration continues to rise. Structures suggestive of picornaviruses have been identified in the endothelial cells of affected musculature, raising the possibility of a viral aetiology contributing to the pathogenesis of the disease. It has been speculated that exposure to a particular viral antigen triggers an inherited response that manifests as cutaneous disease. Molecular mimicry between host and viral epitopes is one possible explanation for the aetiopathogenesis.

EPIDEMIOLOGY

Familial canine dermatomyositis has been reported to occur in collies, Shetland sheepdogs and their crosses. It is only occasionally diagnosed in dogs with no collie or Shetland sheepdog ancestry. In collies, the disease appears to be inherited as an autosomal dominant trait with a variable degree of expression. There is no sex or coat colour predilection.

TREATMENT OPTIONS

Exposure to ultraviolet light trauma and oestrous are known to be exacerbating factors and should be avoided. Sun block should be used if ultraviolet exposure is unavoidable. Affected bitches should undergo ovariohysterctomy and entire males should be castrated. Apart from the consideration that oestrous may be an exacerbating factor, owners should be discouraged from breeding from affected animals because dermatomyositis is an inherited trait.

It may not be necessary to treat mildly affected dogs, as spontaneous resolution can be expected after a few months. At the opposite end of the spectrum, as very severely affected cases carry a poor prognosis and are difficult to manage, it may be appropriate to consider euthanasia. Although immunosuppressive glucocorticoid therapy may be beneficial for a time, unfortunately it can result in further muscle atrophy and compound the problems associated with the myositis.

In mild to moderately affected cases long-term therapy is required, but these dogs can have a reasonable quality of life. As in this case, secondary bacterial infections result in exacerbation of the skin lesions and increased pruritus, and should be thoroughly treated.

Vitamin E: Vitamin E, administered as α-tocopherol, has antioxidant and anti-inflammatory effects and may be of value in limiting the progression of lesions. The dosage is 10–20 IU/kg s.i.d., p.o. Vitamin E is usually given in conjunction with high-dosage omega-3 and omega-6 essential fatty acid supplementation.

Glucocorticoids: Intermittent treatment with prednisolone at doses of 1–2 mg/kg s.i.d. may be required to control flare-ups of skin disease that are not associated with pyoderma.

Pentoxifylline: As there is a vascular component to this disease, pentoxifylline administered at a dosage of 10–15 mg/kg t.i.d. (see Chapter 34) has also been reported to be of benefit, especially in early lesions. Pentoxifylline should be administered for 2–3 months before making any decision on efficacy. It may also be administered in conjunction with prednisolone for control of more severe lesions. Clinicians should be aware that the tendency for the disease to wax and wane can make it difficult to objectively assess the response to treatment.

Initial treatment in this case consisted of:
- A further 3 weeks of antibacterial therapy using cefalexin at a dosage of 20 mg/kg.
- Vitamin E at a dosage of 20 IU/kg s.i.d.
- An essential fatty acid supplement containing both omega-6 and omega-3 acids was administered, giving approximately 15 mg/kg s.i.d. γ-linolenic acid and 1.5 mg/kg s.i.d. eicosapentanoic acid
- The use of a factor 50 or 60 sun block applied to any alopecic areas was advised if sun exposure was unavoidable.

> ### CLINICAL TIPS
>
> Early alopecic lesions in conjunction with skin changes are the optimal sites to sample for histopathological examination. Sampling lesions with secondary bacterial infection or scarring is less likely to be diagnostic. In any case, where there is cytological evidence of bacterial infection, it is a good idea to treat infection prior to taking samples for histopathological examination. Firstly, there might be an excellent response to treatment and secondly, the inflammation resulting from the infection can mask more subtle changes associated with the underlying disease.

FOLLOW-UP

After 3 months of therapy, no new lesions had developed and the patient was no longer pruritic, although she still had a stiff legged gait at times. Physical examination revealed that all lesions, apart from those on the face, had resolved. Patches of alopecia and mild erythema with a slightly shiny appearance remained over the bridge of the nose and periocular skin, although there was no crusting (Fig. 35.5). The continued use of sun block was advised along with essential fatty acid supplementation and vitamin E at the same dosage.

Follow-up 3 years later revealed that there had been further episodes of pruritus, which had been associated

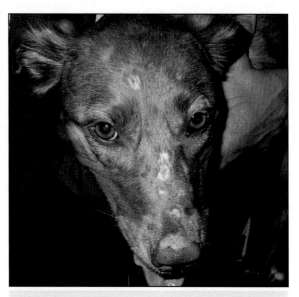

Figure 35.5 After 3 months of vitamin E and essential fatty acid supplementation. Focal alopecia remains.

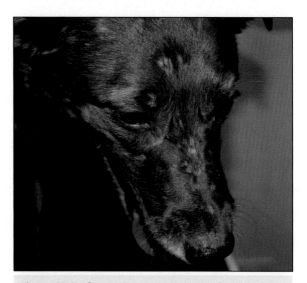

Figure 35.6 After 3 years. Occasional new focal patches of alopecia have developed but, overall, there has been little progression of disease.

with pyoderma. Patches of scarring alopecia remained over the face and occasional new lesions had appeared (Fig. 35.6). Symptoms of myositis were still evident but had not progressed. The owner felt that the dog had a reasonable quality of life.

36 Feline eosinophilic plaque

INITIAL PRESENTATION

Eroded raised plaques in a domestic short-haired cat with eosinophilic plaque.

INTRODUCTION

Eosinophilic granuloma complex represents a reaction pattern often seen in cats mostly with an allergic or ectoparasitic aetiology.

Eosinophilic granuloma complex includes three different entities – eosinophilic granuloma, indolent ulcer and eosinophilic plaque – which, although they have distinct clinical appearances, may have common aetiologies. It is not unusual to see more than one syndrome on the same animal, either at the same time or sequentially. In a small number of cases, cytological examination and a good response to antibacterial therapy confirms bacterial involvement.

CASE PRESENTING SIGNS

A 5-year-old, spayed domestic short-haired cat was presented with multiple raised plaques, with eroded, ulcerated and exudative surfaces on the medial aspect of the thigh.

CASE HISTORY

Given that eosinophilic granuloma complex is a reaction pattern rather than a diagnosis, a detailed history is invaluable in helping to determine the underlying cause. It is important, therefore, to take a full history, which includes the signalment, age of onset, management and any previous treatments.

In this case the relevant history was:
- The first sign of disease was 2 years previously and consisted of pruritic lesions over the groin and medial thighs. These lesions resolved with a single injection of a depot glucocorticoid, methylprednisolone acetate.
- Since then there had been further similar episodes, which also responded to depot glucocorticoid injections. However, the most recent episode had failed to respond despite multiple injections given at a higher dosage.
- The cat was polyphagic and polydipsic.
- The diet consisted of a variety of commercial foods.
- The cat received routine thorough flea control consisting of monthly applications of fipronil spot-on and the house environment had also been treated with a permethrin and pyriproxyfen spray twice in the last 3 months.
- There were no other animals in the household and the cat was allowed out during the day.
- There was no reported zoonosis.

CLINICAL EXAMINATION

In cats with eosinophilic plaque, the lesions are usually located on the ventral abdomen and medial aspects of the thighs. They appear as circular raised, eroded or ulcerated plaques, ranging from 1 to 2 cm in diameter, but they may coalesce into a large lesion several centimetres in length. Uncommonly, lesions may appear on the feet, which usually present with crusting, exudation, erythema and swelling of the plantar or the interdigital skin (Fig. 36.1).

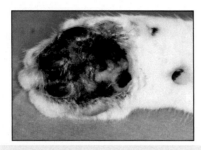

Figure 36.1 Erythema, crusting, exudation and swelling on the plantar aspect of the foot.

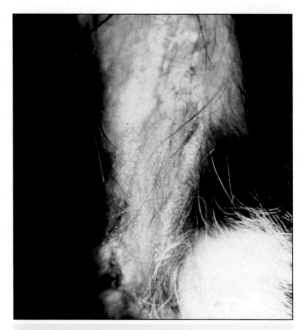

Figure 36.2 Linear granuloma on the caudal aspect of the thigh.

Other variants of the eosinophilic granuloma complex may be found on the same individual, e.g. 'linear granuloma', which is seen as a raised chord-like linear plaque, with a yellowish surface, on the caudal aspect of the thighs (Fig. 36.2). Indolent (rodent) ulcer may also be seen as an area of ulceration on the upper lip. Some individuals may also have lesions on the hard or soft palates.

Generally, affected cats do not show any signs of systemic illness, but they may have varying degrees of peripheral lymph node enlargement.

In this case the clinical examination revealed:

- Coalesced raised plaques, with erythematous, exudative, eroded surfaces (Fig. 36.3)
- Small satellite lesions of crusting on the skin surrounding the main lesion
- Moist skin surrounding the lesions, due to licking, and indicating pruritus
- Peripheral lymphadenopathy.

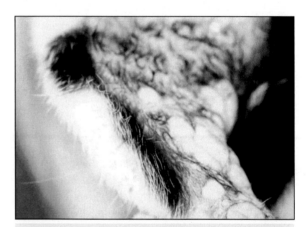

Figure 36.3 Raised plaque on the medial aspect of the thigh.

DIFFERENTIAL DIAGNOSES

- Eosinophilic granuloma complex with an underlying aetiology of:
  - Adverse food reaction
  - Atopic dermatitis
  - Contact hypersensitivity
  - Cheyletiellosis
  - Pediculosis
  - Demodicosis
  - Dermatophytosis
  - Secondary bacterial pyoderma
- Adverse drug reaction
- Viral infections (herpes virus, calicivirus, FIV, FeLV)
- Neoplasia
- Mast cell tumour
- Squamous cell carcinoma.

N.B. Flea allergy dermatitis was not included in this differential diagnosis in view of the previous thorough flea control.

CASE WORK-UP

It cannot be stressed enough that eosinophilic granuloma is not a diagnosis but a reaction pattern, and therefore the aim, particularly in cases such as this where the disease was recurrent, is to identify and correct the underlying cause. Amongst other tests, this usually involves therapeutic and diet trials to rule out the involvement of ectoparasitic and microbial diseases, and adverse food reactions. However, the clinician should be aware when undertaking such trials that despite correcting the underlying cause (e.g. avoidance of food allergens in a food allergic cat), the eosinophilic lesions may still not resolve. This is because the lesion is a source of cytokines and other factors (see 'Aetiopathogenesis') that not only cause tissue damage, but continue to stimulate eosinophil production in the bone marrow, recruit inflammatory cells to the damaged tissue, increase eosinophil survival time and perpetuate the lesion. Thus, it may be necessary to achieve resolution by therapeutic intervention in addition to investigation of the underlying cause. As might be expected, this complicates assessment of the response to therapeutic and diet trials. These are complex cases and it is important to warn the client at the outset of the time and commitment involved in making a definitive diagnosis.

In the first instance, the following investigations were carried out:

- An impression smear of the lesion, stained with modified Wright's stain, revealed a mixed inflammatory cell population, mainly of eosinophils and neutrophils. Extracellular and intracellular coccoid bacteria were also present (Fig. 36.4).
- A swab sample was cultured, which revealed coagulase-negative staphylococci (speciation was not carried out on the sample).
- Blood samples for routine haematological and biochemical parameters, which were within laboratory reference ranges.
- Skin scrapes, coat brushings and fungal culture from toothbrush combing, which were all negative for ectoparasites and dermatophytes.
- Three skin samples were taken by punch biopsy for histology, one from the centre of the lesion, one from the edge of the lesions and one from the surrounding skin. (The diagnosis of eosinophilic plaque may be made on clinical appearance and cytological examination alone but histopathological examination is indicated if there is any doubt about the diagnosis

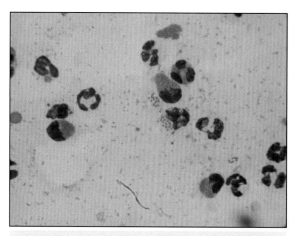

Figure 36.4 Eosinophils, neutrophils and intracellualr coccoid bacteria. (From August J (2005): Consultations in Feline Internal Medicine, 5th Edition. Saunders, Oxford, with permission of Elsevier.)

and in this case ruled out a number of the other differentials.)

The histological findings were:
- Epidermal acanthosis, crusting and ulceration
- Diffuse dense infiltrate in the dermis comprising macrophages, plasma cells, neutrophils and eosinophils
- Focal areas of amorphous eosinophilic material surrounded by macrophages and giant cells.

These changes were deemed to be consistent with eosinophilic granuloma and they ruled out any neoplasia.

The cytological evidence showed evidence of bacterial infection. Even though this was a coagulase-negative organism, and pending the results of the histopathological examination, 3 weeks of amoxicillin/clavulanate was prescribed at a dosage of 15 mg/kg b.i.d. Although following this treatment there was no evidence of bacterial infection on repeat cytology, the lesions showed no evidence of resolution.

The next step in the investigation was a restricted diet trial to rule out an adverse food reaction. For the reasons already described, the cat was prescribed medication to aid resolution of lesions, before starting the trial. This consisted of ciclosporin (5 mg/kg s.i.d.; see 'Treatment' section). Prior to starting treatment, further blood samples were taken for FIV, FeLV and toxoplasma serology, which were all negative. Ciclosporin therapy resulted in gradual resolution of lesions over a period of 4 weeks. Treatment was continued for a further 7 weeks, initially at 5 mg/kg every second day for 4 weeks and then for the last 3 weeks at 5 mg/kg twice weekly.

After 8 weeks of ciclosporin therapy and at the same time as reducing to twice weekly dosing, the cat was started on a restricted diet trial by feeding a chicken hydrolysate diet. This diet was fed for a total of 8 weeks. After 6 weeks of the diet (and 3 weeks after ciclosporin withdrawal), the cat started to vigorously overgroom the medial thighs once more. This ruled out an adverse food reaction as a cause of the eosinophilic lesions.

The final stage of the investigation was to perform intradermal testing, which gave positive wheal and flare reactions to house dust mites (*Dermatophagoides farinae* and *Dermatophagoides pteronyssinus*) and to one storage mite (*Tyrophagus putrescentiae*). There is no documented withdrawal time for ciclosporin prior to intradermal testing but the 3 weeks allowed in this case was sufficient.

In summary, the steps towards a final diagnosis in this case were:

- An initial work-up (cytology, skin scrapes, coat brushings, skin biopsies, bacterial and fungal culture), followed by
- Treatment of the secondary infection
- Treatment of the lesion
- Demonstration of lack of response to a restricted diet trial
- Intradermal testing.

DIAGNOSIS

The final diagnosis was eosinophilic plaque. The lack of response to the diet trial and ectoparasitic disease along with the positive intradermal test supported the likelihood that the eosinophilic lesions had arisen because of underlying atopic dermatitis.

PROGNOSIS

The prognosis for initial resolution of skin lesions of the eosinophilic granuloma complex is generally good. However, the longer term prognosis for this condition depends on whether the underlying condition can be identified and corrected or controlled. Many cases require some form of lifelong therapy, in this case therapy for atopic dermatitis.

AETIOPATHOGENESIS AND IMMUNOPATHOGENESIS

In cats, the response to pruritus is often eosinophil mediated, and can result in any of the lesions of the eosino-philic granuloma complex or simply self-induced alopecia, excoriations and ulcerations. The exact mechanism by which lesions of the eosinophilic granuloma complex arise is not clear; whether the lesions are a primary eruption or the result of the cat licking the area is yet to be elucidated.

Both haematological and histological evidence suggests that, in cats, eosinophil infiltration, inflammation and consequent tissue damage are important factors in sustaining pruritus, although mast cells and other mononuclear cells also contribute to the damage.

Eosinophils are produced by the bone marrow. Only small numbers are present in the circulation, and most are found in tissues such as the gut, lung and urinary tract. One important role for eosinophils is as a defence mechanism in ectoparasitic and endoparasitic infestations. On activation they release toxic granule proteins and free radicals, which can kill microorganisms and parasites, but in allergic reactions are responsible for tissue damage. They also induce the synthesis of chemical mediators such as prostaglandins, leucotrienes and cytokines. In turn, these mediators amplify the inflammatory response by activating epithelial cells and recruiting and activating more eosinophils.

The activation and degranulation of eosinophils is normally strictly regulated as inappropriate activation is harmful to the individual, so very few eosinophils are produced in the absence of infection or other immune stimulus. However, in cats, both infection and allergic skin disease activate Th2 lymphocytes, resulting in increased secretion of IL-5, which stimulates the bone marrow to increase the production of eosinophils. A second set of controls then regulates their infiltration into the tissue (eosinophil chemotaxis is controlled by eotaxin-1 (CCL11), eotaxin-2 (CCL24) and eotaxin-3 (CCL26); the eotaxin receptor (CCR3) on eosinophils is a member of the chemokine family of receptors, which can bind to other chemokines, and this binding can also activate eosinophils).

Recent studies support that the damage caused by eosinophils is associated with enzymes, toxic proteins and cytokines, and not collagenolysis as was previously thought. In fact, collagen microfibrils are unaffected. Eosinophils produce enzymes, toxins and cytokines such as:

- Eosinophil peroxidase (triggers histamine release by mast cells) and eosinophil collagenase (remodels connective tissue)
- Major basic protein (toxic to parasites and mammalian cells, and triggers release of histamine), eosin-

ophil cationic protein (toxic to parasites) and eosinophil-derived neurotoxin
- IL-3, IL-5 and GM-CSF (increase production and activation of the eosinophils), and IL-8 (promotes influx of leucocytes).

Eosinophils also secrete lipid mediators such as leucotrienes (causing smooth muscle contraction, increased vascular permeability and increased mucus secretion) and platelet-activating factor (attracts leucocytes, amplifies production of lipid mediators, and activates neutrophils, eosinophils and platelets).

EPIDEMIOLOGY

In one study on allergic disease in cats, about a third had eosinophilic granulomatous lesions. Although there is no age, sex or breed predilections, some cats may have a genetic predisposition to develop lesions of the eosinophilic granuloma complex. The seasonality and the incidence of the disease in individuals, or within a group, will depend on the causative underlying conditions.

TREATMENT AND TREATMENT OPTIONS

Most cats at the time of presentation have lesions resulting from the damage caused by the activation and degranulation of eosinophils. Whilst the diagnosis of the underlying condition is important in preventing and controlling the disease in the long term, resolving the damage caused by the eosinophils is more important in the short term.

The initial treatment should be symptomatic, aimed at limiting and resolving the eosinophil damage and any secondary infections. For the specific underlying aetiology, the treatment or management will depend on its cause, i.e. lifelong flea control in the case of FAD, food avoidance in case of adverse food reaction or allergen-specific immunotherapy in cases of atopic dermatitis.

Symptomatic treatments aimed at limiting and resolving the damage caused by eosinophil infiltration include glucocorticoids and cyclosporin.

Glucocorticoids

Glucocorticoids are the first-line treatment for lesions of the eosinophilic granuloma complex. In general, the long-term use of glucocorticoids should be avoided but they may be the most appropriate treatment for those cats with seasonal lesions or for those owners with limited financial resources.

Injectable glucocorticoids are commonly used in practice; in particular, methylprednisolone acetate is used at the dose of 5 mg/kg i.m., 2–4 weeks apart for a maximum of three injections. Careful patient monitoring is advisable during this period, due to the incidence of side-effects to depot glucocorticoids as there is the potential for serious adverse effects such as diabetes mellitus, iatrogenic hyperadrenocorticism and congestive cardiac failure.

For long-term therapy, an alternate-day glucocorticoid regimen is safer than daily treatment because it allows the hypothalamic–adrenal–pituitary axis to recover on the 'day off'. Thus, the shorter-acting, orally administered glucocorticoids, prednisolone or methylprednisolone, are the most appropriate drugs to use in this respect. Furthermore, in individuals where there is concern about adverse effects, they are preferred because they can be easily discontinued. Another incentive to use oral, rather than injectable, glucocorticoids is that in the authors' experience, apparent treatment failures with injectable preparations will often respond to oral therapy.

Oral dexamethasone or triamcinolone are alternatives to prednisolone for refractory lesions, but these steroids have a high potency and an increased risk of adverse effect.

Cats have fewer glucocorticoid receptors, are more resistant to side-effects of glucocorticoids and generally require higher dosages of glucocorticoids than dogs. Apparent treatment failures are commonly the result of inadequate dosing, particularly with lesions of the eosinophilic granuloma complex.

Initial suggested dosages to achieve remission of lesions are as follows:
- Prednisolone, 2–4 mg/kg divided b.i.d.
- Methylprednisolone, 1.6–3.2 mg/kg divided b.i.d.
- Triamcinolone, 0.2–0.4 mg/kg s.i.d.
- Dexamethasone, 0.1–0.2 mg/kg s.i.d.

Once lesions are in remission, the dosage should be gradually tapered to the lowest level that maintains remission (see Chapter 17). Aim to reduce the frequency of administration to alternate days if using prednisolone or methylprednisolone and perhaps every third day for dexamethasone or triamcinolone.

Ciclosporin

Ciclosporin (5 mg/kg orally once daily) is useful for intractable corticosteroid-resistant eosinophilic granuloma complex lesions; however, it is not licensed for use

Table 36.1 Commonly used antihistamines in cats

Antihistamine	Dosage and frequency	Side-effects (many of these are reported in humans but could occur in cats)
Chlorphenamine	2–4 mg total dose b.i.d.	Drowsiness, diarrhoea, vomiting and anorexia
Diphenhydramine	1–2 mg/kg b.i.d.–t.i.d.	Urine retention and sedation
Clemastine	0.05–0.01 mg/kg b.i.d.	Sedation
Hydroxyzine	1.0–2.0 mg/kg t.i.d.	Sedation
Amitriptyline	1.0–2.0 mg/kg b.i.d.	Sedation, dry mouth, diarrhoea, vomiting, excitability, hypotension, increased appetite and weight gain
Cyproheptadine	0.5–1.0 mg/kg t.i.d.	Sedation, polyphagia and weight gain

None of these drugs hold a veterinary licence and the owner's consent is needed for their use.

in cats and it requires the owner's written, informed consent. In addition, routine screening tests are advised (see 'Case work-up' section). An improvement with this drug is usually reasonably rapid, but, in the authors' experience, a few animals will have immediate side-effects, such as soft faeces and diarrhoea, and occasionally vomiting. Other longer-term side-effects may include gingival hyperplasia, papillomatosis, and the activation of latent viral and *Toxoplasma* infections.

Other immunosuppressive drugs

Chlorambucil (0.1–0.2 mg/kg every 24 hours) or gold salt aurothioglucose (0.1 mg/kg i.m., weekly) may help in recalcitrant cases. If one is not familiar with the use of these drugs, the monitoring required and their potential adverse effects, referral should be considered.

Megosterol and medroxyprogestrone

In the past, megosterol acetate and medroxyprogesterone have been used to manage eosinophilic granulomas. However, the risks of using these drugs outweigh their benefits and, with the increased availability of some of the newer immunomodulating drugs, they should not be used.

Antihistamines

Antihistamines may be valuable to control pruritus in some cases, but only after the eosinophilic tissue damage is resolved (see Table 36.1). They are extremely unlikely to be of any benefit in the face of active eosinophilic granuloma lesions.

Essential fatty acids

Omega N3 and N6 fatty acids are usually prescribed concurrently with antihistamines. Because different

manufacturers produce different concentrations, it is best to use their guidelines on dosing; however, higher dosages appear to increase efficacy.

Other therapies

Surgical excision, cryotherapy, laser therapy and radiotherapy have also been used with varying degrees of success; however, unless the underlying condition is successfully managed, the lesions have a tendency to recur either at the same or different sites.

Treatment in this case

In this case, the cat was treated with ciclosporin, as the lesion did not respond to increased doses and frequency of methylprednisolone acetate. The lesion had almost resolved after 4 weeks and entirely after 7 weeks (see 'Case work-up' section). Once the final diagnosis of atopic dermatitis had been made, long-term management with monthly injections of allergen-specific immunotherapy (see Chapter 6) was initiated.

NURSING ASPECTS

Although there are no specific nursing aspects, there may be an involvement in educating the owner on the proper use of an Elizabethan collar in the early stages of the treatment. If oral medication is prescribed, some owners may require instruction and/or help in administering the tablets.

CLINICAL TIPS

The role of secondary infection is often ignored in these cases. Cytology is a rapid, inexpensive and effective way of assessing whether there is an infection or not, but if the results are unclear a swab sample should be submitted for culture and sensitivity testing.

It is always important to bear in mind the role of the eosinophil. A frequent mistake is to assume that if an adverse food reaction is suspected, then a hypoallergenic diet alone will resolve the lesions, or in cases of atopic dermatitis allergen-specific therapy alone will suffice. The key to the successful management of this condition lies in limiting and resolving eosinophil damage prior to instituting long-term management.

FOLLOW-UP

Allergen-specific immunotherapy was successful in preventing further episodes of eosinophilic plaque over a follow-up period of 4 years.

37 Head and neck pruritus

INITIAL PRESENTATION

Ulcerative dermatitis due to head and neck pruritus in a cat.

INTRODUCTION

Pruritus, crusting and ulcerative dermatitis of the head and neck is a common reaction pattern in cats. This is a particularly distressing presentation for both the owner and cat, and is often fairly refractory to treatment. There are four recognized feline cutaneous reaction patterns that are essentially manifestations of pruritus. Head and neck pruritus is one such pattern, and the other three are symmetrical alopecia, miliary dermatitis and lesions of the eosinophilic granuloma complex (see Chapter 36). These reaction patterns are not diagnoses and common underlying causes include hypersensitivity disorders, ectoparasitic diseases and microbial infections, and a systematic approach is required to identify and correct the underlying disease. The diagnostic approach involves careful and thorough history taking, clinical examination and diagnostic investigations. The success of long-term management of the case will depend on the final diagnosis. In this case a staphylococcal infection and an adverse food reaction were found to be responsible for the ongoing self-induced lesions on the neck.

CASE PRESENTING SIGNS

Ulceration, excoriations, crusting, exudation, erythema and alopecia on the lateral aspect of the neck in a 5-year-old, neutered female domestic short-haired cat.

CASE HISTORY

Most cats with this condition are intensely pruritic and are able to cause severe self-excoriation within a short space of time. In first opinion practice, most cases are presented after a sudden spontaneous onset of pruritus, although there may be an association with a previous injection site or topical treatment.

History taking should establish evidence of systemic involvement, seasonality, contagion, zoonosis, diet, management and response to previous treatment, in particular antimicrobial or glucocorticoid therapy (see Chapter 1). Some conditions that affect the head and neck may not exhibit early pruritus, but it can occur as the condition progresses and other complications occur. Thus, it is helpful to know whether the condition initially started as pruritus with subsequent development of lesions or whether there were already skin lesions present before pruritus became evident suggesting a primary eruption.

The relevant history in this case was as follows:
- A long-standing history of non-seasonal facial and neck pruritus, which had started at an early age and which was gradually becoming more severe.
- Previous treatments (dexamethasone combined with clindamycin or potentiated amoxicillin) had been intermittent, because of the difficulty in medicating the cat with oral, and even topical, treatments. There had been only a partial response to these therapies.
- The cat had been injected with lufenuron every 6 months and over the past 4 weeks had received three applications of selamectin at fortnightly intervals.
- There was no history of zoonosis.

- A recently acquired, in-contact cat was unaffected.
- The cat had access to the outside and to all the rooms within the house.
- Both cats were fed on tuna, as well as a variety of commercial foods.
- An Elizabethan collar was ineffective in controlling the self-trauma.
- There was no history of the use of a flea collar.

CLINICAL EXAMINATION

The clinical signs on examination are generally non-specific and vary from case to case. The lesions may be localized to focal areas, or be more severe and involve the entire head and neck regions. The types of lesions include papules, crusting, alopecia, excoriations, erosions and ulceration. Some individuals may have concurrent signs of bilateral ceruminous otitis externa and/or conjunctivitis.

The relevant findings on examination in this case were:

- Ulceration, excoriations, crusting and self-induced alopecia were apparent on the left side of the neck (Fig. 37.1).
- A few papulocrustous lesions were present on the dorsal neck (Fig. 37.2).
- There were no other skin lesions elsewhere on the body.
- Full physical examination was unremarkable.

DIFFERENTIAL DIAGNOSES

The differentials in this case were:
- Secondary bacterial pyoderma
- Adverse food reaction
- Contact allergic dermatitis
- Atopic dermatitis
- Dermatophytosis
- Herpes virus-associated erythema multiforme
- Idiopathic sterile granuloma
- Feline ulcerative dermatitis with linear subepidermal fibrosis.

N.B. Flea allergy dermatitis, cheyletiellosis and otodectes would be important differentials in a case with this presentation but could be excluded on the basis of the previous antiparasitic therapy.

CASE WORK-UP

The following diagnostic tests were undertaken:
- Cytological examination of an impression smear from the neck lesion revealed erythrocytes and numerous neutrophils, some with intracellular coccoid bacteria consistent with a neutrophilic inflammation and secondary bacterial infection (Fig. 37.3).
- Skin scrapings and coat brushings failed to reveal any ectoparasites or flea dirt.
- A swab sample was taken, and *Staphylococcus aureus* was cultured, sensitive to all routinely used antibacterials except penicillin and ampicillin.

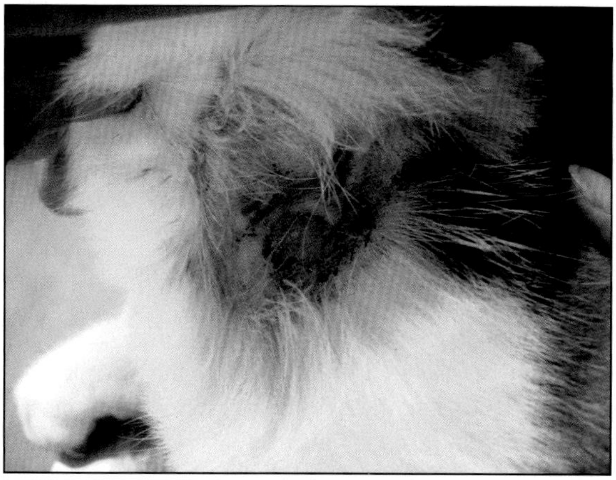

Figure 37.1 Self-induced excoriations, ulceration, erythema, crusting and alopecia on the lateral aspect of the neck.

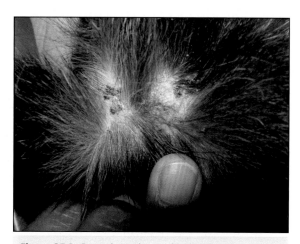

Figure 37.2 Crusted papules on the dorsal neck.

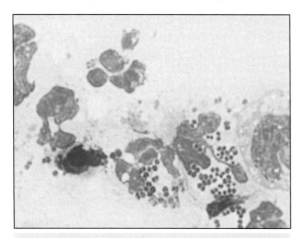

Figure 37.3 Neutrophils with intracellular and extracellular coccoid bacteria.

- No dermatophytes were grown from hair plucks and scrapings submitted for fungal culture.
- An allergen-specific IgE ELISA test, based on the FcEpsilon receptor technology, did not show significantly raised serum concentrations of IgE to environmental or insect allergens, and serological tests for FIV and FeLV were negative.

These tests indicated a bacterial infection. The first step was to resolve the bacterial component and the cat was treated with two injections of cefovecin (8 mg/kg s.c.) at fortnightly intervals. After 3 weeks of antibiotic treatment, most skin lesions were resolving but head and neck pruritus persisted. The next step was to rule out the involvement of an adverse food reaction. The cat was started on a diet trial consisting of a chicken hydrolysate and antibiotic treatment was continued for a further 2 weeks. Within 3 weeks of starting the diet, there was an obvious reduction in pruritus and all symptoms had completely resolved after 5 weeks. At this point, reintroduction of the original food resulted in recurrence of pruritus within 3 days which resolved once again within a week following re-institution of the hydrolysed diet. At this point sequential provocation with individual proteins was undertaken. Within 24 hours of feeding fish, the owner noted the cat was obviously pruritic again.

In this case, no further work-up was undertaken but histopathological examination would have been indicated if the lesions had persisted despite antibacterial therapy. Further tests, such as viral isolation or electron microscopy, would have been applicable if the histology had indicated a viral aetiology.

DIAGNOSIS

Head and neck pruritus resulting from an underlying adverse food reaction with secondary superficial pyoderma.

PROGNOSIS

The prognosis for head and neck pruritus is variable. Provided the underlying cause can be identified and corrected, as in this case, the prognosis is favourable. If not, long-term therapy is indicated, often requiring the use of glucocorticoids. It can be a challenge to control the pruritus in severely affected cases.

AETIOPATHOGENESIS

As already stated, head and neck pruritus is a cutaneous reaction pattern resulting from a wide variety of conditions and a detailed discussion of the aetiopathogenesis of all these disorders is beyond the scope of this chapter. Most commonly, hypersensitivity disorders such as flea allergy dermatitis, atopic dermatitis, adverse food reactions and mosquito bite hypersensitivity are implicated. These conditions can result in the other feline cutaneous reaction patterns (see Chapter 36) and it is not clear why, in one cat, an adverse food reaction can result in head and neck pruritus, and in another, symmetrical alopecia is the main presenting symptom.

There are a number of other skin diseases that do not fall into the category of hypersensitivity disorders but result in head and neck pruritus and cause broadly similar symptoms. These conditions include ectoparasitic disease (*Otodectes cynotis, Notoedres cati, Demodex cati*), pemphigus foliaceus, herpes and pox virus infections, and idiopathic facial dermatitis of Persians.

As in this case, many cases of head and neck pruritus are complicated by secondary bacterial infections that tend to result in increased pruritus. Management of these secondary infections may result in a marked clinical improvement. Skin infections in cats are usually the result of secondary invasion of a traumatized area by organisms from carriage sites, such as the nose and oral cavity, or from environmental contamination of the wound. Apart from cat bite abscess, feline bacterial skin infections, both primary and secondary, have been reported as being uncommon; however, their role as a secondary complication is being increasingly recognized. The infection in most cases is secondary to an underlying condition, such as flea allergic dermatitis, atopic dermatitis, adverse food reactions, ectoparasitic infestations and systemic diseases (neoplasia, diabetes mellitus or hyperthyroidism).

Staphylococcus aureus, *S. intermedius* and *S. felis* have all been cultured from cases of feline pyoderma. Staphylococci are capable of producing toxins, enzymes and other factors that aid their colonization and initiate, or perpetuate, the subsequent disease.

Ultimately, the significance of the organism and its role in the pathogenesis is assessed on the animal's response to antibacterial treatment. In this case there was a favourable response and, once identified, the management of the adverse food reaction resolved the pruritus completely. For the aetiopathogenesis of adverse food reactions, refer to Chapter 11.

EPIDEMIOLOGY

Although there is no specific age, sex or breed predilection, much depends on the actual aetiology and initial cause of the condition. For instance, *Otodectes* hypersensitivity is common in young cats, whereas flea allergic dermatitis and adverse food reactions may occur at any age.

TREATMENT OPTIONS

As already stated, the management of head and neck pruritus can be something of a challenge. Wherever possible, every effort should be made to identify and correct the underlying cause for the pruritus and the treatment in any individual cat will depend on the specific aetiology. Referral to a specialist dermatologist should be considered if a diagnosis cannot be made. As in this case, at the outset, many cases will require antibacterial therapy and in the longer term, if the pruritus is idiopathic, long-term symptomatic therapy.

Antibiotics

An antibiotic used to treat feline pyoderma should be effective against *Staphylococcus* spp. and ideally be based on culture and sensitivity testing, although in practice the choice is frequently made empirically. The individual should be treated with the optimum dose for 7–14 days beyond clinical cure. In this case, cefovecin (8 mg/kg s.c.) was given on two occasions, 2 weeks apart, which was beyond clinical cure (Fig. 37.4). There

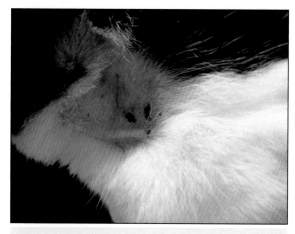

Figure 37.4 Lesions at 7 days after treatment.

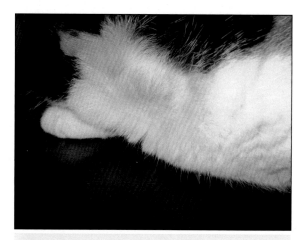

Figure 37.5 All lesions resolved by day 14.

was almost complete resolution of the skin lesions at day 14 (Fig. 37.5).

Glucocorticoids

Glucocorticoids should ideally be avoided when there is evidence of infection. The repeated use of glucocorticoids in the common belief that they are well tolerated by cats can result in immunosuppression and exacerbation and perpetuation of secondary bacterial infection as a complicating factor. Thus, it is imperative to thoroughly treat bacterial infection prior to the use of glucocorticoids and every effort should be made to investigate and identify the underlying cause of the pruritus and to manage that. Only in cases where, after exhaustive searching, a cause cannot be identified should glucocorticoids be considered for managing the pruritus. See Chapter 36 for drugs and drug dosages.

Ciclosporin: Ciclosporin may be helpful in the long-term management of feline head and neck pruritus due to atopic dermatitis. See Chapter 36 for further information.

Topicals: Cats in general tend not to tolerate topical treatment and therefore their use is very limited.

NURSING ASPECTS

If the lesions are confined to the face and ears, an Elizabethan collar is used to limit the self-trauma.

CLINICAL TIPS

- Staphylococcal resistance to both penicillin and amoxicillin is being reported in the USA and in the UK, and therefore they should not be used as first-line treatments.
- Unless the underlying cause of the head and neck pruritus is obvious, a full discussion should be held with the owners regarding the complex nature of this condition and the time and commitment required in making a diagnosis.
- In general, rule out ectoparasitic and microbial infections first before undertaking diet trials and allergy testing.
- When doing a diet trial, all the cats in the house may have to be fed the same food. To prevent scavenging, consideration should be given to keeping cats indoors, although inability or unwillingness to do this should not constitute a reason not to undertake a diet trial (the cat may be reactive to its own food).
- Impression smears are easily performed and can provide vital information at an early stage.

FOLLOW-UP

There have been no further episodes of pruritus for over a year. The owner has continued to feed both the cats on the chicken hydrolysate.

38 Fly strike in a rabbit (myiasis)

INITIAL PRESENTATION

Lethargy, inappetance and depression in an odiferous rabbit with maggots.

INTRODUCTION

Myiasis, or fly strike, is unfortunately a common problem with domestic rabbits, often with severe consequences. When attracted to the rabbit by certain conditions, flies will lay their eggs on the rabbit, which subsequently hatch into maggots (larvae). These maggots feed on the living tissue and undergo several moults, each time increasing their digestive capabilities.

The disease is very distressing for the owner, and will often go unnoticed for several days. More importantly, fly strike is extremely serious and painful for the rabbit, which not uncommonly necessitates euthanasia in advanced cases.

CASE PRESENTING SIGNS

A 7-year-old male, neutered English lop rabbit (*Oryctolagus cuniculus*), weighing 1.8 kg, was presented in mid-July as an emergency, with a 2- to 3-day history of lethargy, inappetance and generally not being himself. The owner had noticed an increased smell from his hutch and whilst cleaning him out saw he had a wet and dirty rear end. On closer examination live maggots were found.

CASE HISTORY

With the majority of sick rabbits, complete and thorough history taking is vital. The owners may not think the information is relevant to the presenting problem, but around three-quarters of problems in rabbits and other exotic pets are related to poor husbandry and the owners' lack of knowledge about proper diets, housing and healthcare requirements.

In this case the relevant history was:

- The rabbit was acquired at 1 year old as a pet for the children and was kept alone. There has been no known contact with other rabbits. The family also had a pet dog.
- The rabbit was housed in a standard-sized rabbit hutch (approx. 4 ft×1.5 ft×2 ft), with a separate area for urination and defaecation.
- Handling had initially been every day, but more recently the patient had been handled less frequently. Access to the garden was allowed two or three times per week.
- Vaccinations against myxomatosis and viral haemorrhagic disease were not continued since the original vaccination course with the previous owner. The owner was unaware they required boosting every 6 and 12 months respectively.
- No other preventative healthcare, such as blowfly strike prevention, was used.
- The diet offered was made up of commercial muesli-type mixed rabbit food fed ad lib. Each morning the owner would discard the leftover portions and refill the bowl with fresh food. Hay was offered daily, with a small amount being consumed. In addition, a selection of fresh or leftover vegetables was given once daily.
- The owner reported that the rabbit occasionally got a 'mucky bottom', which the owner cleaned as

required. There had been a slight reduction in appetite over the preceding few weeks, which the owner thought was due to the hot weather.

• The owner became concerned when her rabbit had become lethargic, with a reduced appetite, and on closer examination she noticed the maggots within the fur of the rear end. She did not attempt removal of the maggots, but sought emergency veterinary attention.

CLINICAL EXAMINATION

On presentation, the rabbit was quiet and depressed, but responsive to stimulus. Clinical examination revealed an elevated heart rate of 280 beats per minute and fast respiration (approx. 60 breaths per minute), both of which could have been related to stress at being examined or pain. There was a small amount of salivary staining around the mouth and on the forepaws, suggesting increased salivation. Abdominal palpation demonstrated mildly dilated, gas-filled loops of bowel with less ingesta than normal, consistent with the inappetence. Otoscopic examination of the oral cavity revealed subjectively elongated teeth, with several lingual spurs on the lower arcades.

Thorough examination of the perineal region revealed maggots and lesions consistent with fly strike. The skin around the perineum, inguinal area and tail base was grossly inflamed, moist and exudative (Fig. 38.1). There was faecal and urine contamination of the area, causing matting of the fur in places (Fig. 38.2). Stage L1–L3 maggots were seen, suggesting that initial egg laying occurred at least 40 hours ago (Table 38.1). Several skin wounds were found in the perineal and tail base area, with L2 and L3 stage maggots moving in and out of these wounds (Fig. 38.3).

Careful and systematic examination, particularly around the tail base, perineum and inguinal area, is required to avoid missing early cases of myiasis. A common site for maggots to feed is in the two deep folds of skin either side of the anal orifice. These are the inguinal glands and in the healthy rabbit are normally filled with a yellow–brown odiferous deposit. The L1 stage maggots are only a few millimetres in length and can be missed during a brief examination. These larvae only feed on skin debris and exudate, and so will cause mild inflammation, but not gross skin damage alone. Clumps of small eggs, looking like grains of rice, may be seen within the coat. In older cases of myiasis, larger

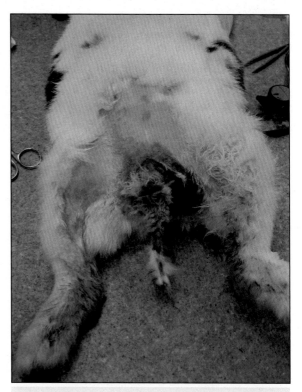

Figure 38.1 Extent of the damage caused by fly strike in this case. The fur has already been carefully clipped away in the anaesthetized rabbit.

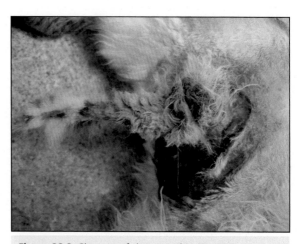

Figure 38.2 Close-up of the wound in Fig. 38.1.

Table 38.1 Development rate of *L. sericata* (hours) at three different temperatures

Temp. (°C)	Egg	Larva 1st instar	Larva 2nd instar	Larva 3rd instar	Pre-pupa	Pupa	Total time (days)
16	41	53	42	98	148	393	32
21	21	31	26	50	118	240	20
27	18	20	12	40	90	168	14

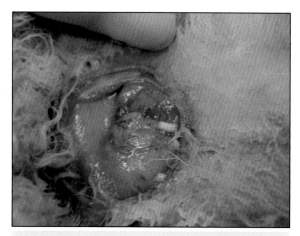

Figure 38.3 L3 maggots in the wound. Careful examination and removal are required to ensure none are missed.

second- and third-stage larvae will be present, which will be easier to see and are likely to be associated with more severe soft tissue damage.

The clinical signs encountered with a case of myiasis will depend on the duration of the disease. In the very early stages (up to 18 hours at 27°C), fly eggs will be present, but the eggs will not have hatched. This means no fly strike damage has yet occurred, but the rabbit may have been presented due to signs of the underlying disease, such as reduced appetite or perineal soiling. If fly eggs have already hatched, they will have begun attacking the epidermal tissues (to varying degrees depending on life stage) and the number of maggots will dictate the extent of lesions present. Environmental conditions of at least 60% humidity and 9–11°C are needed for larval development.

The perineum is a very sensitive area and conscious examination should be kept brief, simply to assess the degree of damage. For more detailed examination and treatment, sedation or general anaesthesia (Table 38.2) must be used.

Clinical signs of myiasis in rabbits include:
- Lethargy, depression, inappetance
- Soiling of the perineal region (with urine or caecotrophs)
- Soiling of the tail base area
- True diarrhoea (does occur but not so common)
- Dehydration
- Coat matting
- Skin erosions with varying degrees of severity
- Weight loss
- Presence of fly eggs or larvae
- Characteristic putrid odour.

Full assessment of the damage caused by the maggots is required to give the client an accurate prognosis. This assessment should to be carried out early in the investigation, using sedation or anaesthesia as appropriate. Where the larvae have attacked deeper tissues the prognosis is poor, and if they have entered the body cavity it becomes grave. Conversely, if larvae have not progressed beyond L1, or the damaged caused by L2 larvae is not yet severe or deep, then treatment may be initiated with reasonable hopes of success.

Candidates and criteria for considering euthanasia would include:
- Where the patient is seriously debilitated or badly injured, allowing blowfly strike to occur.
- Extensive soft tissue damage caused by maggot migration.
- Extension of fly strike into the body cavity, including testicles.
- Where there is extensive tissue necrosis or infection.
- If large wounds extend beyond the dermis into deeper tissues, such as muscle.
- If appropriate after-care cannot be provided by the client, either due to time or financial constraints. These cases are not resolved quickly, or cheaply, and investigation of the underlying cause is mandatory.

DIFFERENTIAL DIAGNOSES

There are no differential diagnoses for fly strike; however, determination of the underlying cause is necessary. Blowfly myiasis does not occur in the healthy rabbit. There is invariably a cause of perineal soiling or urine scalding that creates an appropriate environment for greenbottle flies to deposit their eggs.

Perineal soiling

This will be due to caecotroph accumulation or genuine diarrhoea. Often, the owner will get these two confused, but failure to ingest caecotrophs is more common.

Caecotrophy

Several hours after eating, mainly at night or early in the morning, soft, mucus-covered caecal pellets are produced and eaten directly from the anus (caecotrophy). Caecotroph production stimulates a reflex licking of the anus and ingestion of the caecotrophs, which are swallowed whole and not chewed. The mucus covering protects caecal pellet bacteria from the low pH of the stomach. Caecotrophs remain in the stomach for up to 6 hours with continued bacterial synthesis, and eventually the mucus layer dissolves and the bacteria are killed. This process of caecotrophy allows absorption of nutrients and bacterial fermentation products (amino acids, volatile fatty acids, and vitamins B and K), and the redigestion of previously undigested food. A food item can therefore pass through the digestive tract twice in 24 hours.

A rabbit will stop eating caecotrophs if pain prevents it reaching the back end, or if it cannot physically reach the anus. Therefore, caecotrophs may accumulate due to:
- Obesity – physically unable to reach the base of their tail for grooming
- Spinal disease – such as arthritis or encephalitozoonosis
- Dental disease and pain
- Other painful foci
- Reduced palatability of caecotrophs (excessive dietary fat).

Diarrhoea is less common, but anything that alters the complex hindgut flora may lead to loose faeces. The aetiology may be multifactorial and include:
- Lack of fibre in the diet (offering wrong food, or due to dental disease)
- Overfeeding of carbohydrates
- Coccidiosis (younger rabbits)
- Stress
- Antibiotic-associated diarrhoea (due to clostridial overgrowth)
- Enteritis
- Sudden dietary change.

Urine scalding

Urine scalding occurs when urine is allowed to come into frequent contact with the skin. It will occur with polyuria or other factors that alter urination, such as incontinence.

Possible causes of incontinence include:
- Lumbosacral vertebral fractures
- Spinal osteoarthritis
- *Encephalitozooan cuniculi* infection
- Neurological urinary dysfunction
- Urolithiasis.

The differential diagnoses for polyuria and pollakiuria are many, but include:
- Kidney disease
- Pyometra
- Cystitis
- Urolithiasis and hypercalciuria.

Other factors leading to urine scalding include:
- Arthritis
- Pododermatitis or weakness that leads to an incorrect stance for urination
- Obesity
- Pain on urination
- Long-haired coat.

It is also worth considering that rabbits are fastidious creatures, so if kept in a dirty environment, they will retain urine and void it abnormally.

Table 38.2 Anaesthetic protocols for fly-struck rabbits

Anaesthetic agent(s)	Dose	Notes
Fentanyl/fluanisone	0.2–0.3 ml/kg i.m.	• Provides *sedation* and good analgesia • General anaesthesia can subsequently be induced with midazolam (0.5–2 mg/kg i.v.) to effect, or isoflurane by mask • Long recovery (3–6 h) but can be shortened by antagonizing with buprenorphine (0.01–0.05 mg/kg i.m.) or butorphanol (0.1–0.5 mg/kg i.m.) • Schedule 2 drug so has to be recorded
Midazolam	0.5–2.0 mg/kg i.v.	• Can be used alone for *sedation* but only allows minor procedures
Medetomidine and ketamine	(M) 0.2 mg/kg i.m. followed by (K) 10–15 mg/kg i.v. to effect	• Allows approx. 20 min *anaesthesia* • Intubation can be performed
Medetomidine, ketamine and butorphanol	(M) 0.2 mg/kg (K) 10 mg/kg and (B) 0.5 mg/kg all given together s.c.	• Inhalational agent will be required for more painful or prolonged procedures • Medetomidine can be antagonized with atipamezole at 1–2 mg/kg i.m. • Allows easy i.v. catheter placement
Fentanyl/fluanisone and isoflurane (Isoflo; Abbots)	(F/F) 0.3 ml/kg i.m., then mask induction with isoflurane	• 10–20 min for fentanyl/fluanisone to be effective • Pre-oxygenation and slow incremental induction reduces the risks of breath holding
Fentanyl/fluanisone and midazolam	(F/F) 0.3 ml/kg i.m., then (M) 0.5–2 mg/kg i.v. 10–20 min later	• 30–45 min surgical *anaesthesia* • Avoids the need for anaesthetic equipment, other than oxygen if required • Allows easy i.v. catheter placement • Fentanyl/fluanisone can be antagonized as above
Isoflurane or sevoflurane only	Either starting on 1% and increasing by 0.5% every few minutes, or start with 5% for isoflurane or 8% for sevoflurane	• Used for *anaesthesia of critically ill* rabbits, who tend not to struggle or breath-hold with mask induction • Many will already have received an analgesic premedicant • Pre-oxygenate for several minutes • Sevoflurane is less irritant for mask induction • Incremental induction may be beneficial, but this author prefers the speed of rapid induction on 8% sevoflurane
Propofol	10 mg/kg IV	• As with other species, apnoea is common

CASE WORK-UP

The clinical signs with the presence of maggots is all the case work-up required to make the diagnosis; however, there is always an underlying reason for contamination of perineal fur, leading to the fly strike. Initially, the patient needs swift supportive treatment (see 'Treatment' and 'Treatment options' sections), but during stabilization, or when the rabbit's condition is less critical, the following further investigation can be considered:

Blood sampling: Bloods are important to evaluate for concurrent disease, particularly if there is polyuria con-tributing to urine scalding. Evaluation of renal function and *E. cuniculi* serology may be indicated.

A decrease in both albumin and globulin may be associated with haemorrhage or exudative skin lesions such as found with myiasis.

Faecal analysis: Faeces should be checked for intestinal coccidiosis (*Eimeria* spp.), other parasites (such as oxy-urids – but rare in pet rabbits), indigestible fibre and excessive carbohydrate.

Dental examination: Intra-oral assessment of the teeth is best performed under anaesthesia, otherwise the narrow oral cavity may prevent detection of problems in the back of the mouth. This can be done easily and quickly while the rabbit is anaesthetized, or sedated, for treatment of the fly strike.

Radiography: Radiographic evaluation of the lumbosacral spine is important in case of neurological problems predisposing to fly strike. In addition, one should consider skull radiographs to evaluate for dental disease and abdominal radiographs to check for bladder stones or other abdominal abnormalities.

Urinalysis: Specific gravity may be useful to aid in assessment of renal concentrating ability, but is often affected by minerals (normal specific gravity is reported as 1.003–1.036). In inflammatory diseases, blood or protein will be present in the sediment and hypercalciuria may be detected. If there is suspicion of infection, a sterile sample should be taken by cystocentesis for culture and sensitivity.

Ultrasound: Abdominal ultrasonography is useful to evaluate bladder and kidney structure, and to examine the reproductive tract for pyometra in entire females. However, gas in the gastrointestinal tract will often hinder further examination of the abdomen with ultrasound.

In this case, the dental abnormalities found on oral otoscopic examination were confirmed intra-orally and on skull radiography. The teeth were burred to remove the spikes and the exposed crowns were slightly reduced in height.

DIAGNOSIS

The diagnosis of myiasis was based on the clinical signs, and the presence of maggots on and under the skin. The underlying cause in this patient was found to be dental disease.

PROGNOSIS

Prognosis does depend on the severity and duration of the clinical signs; the criteria for euthanasia have been discussed earlier. The underlying cause will also have a bearing on prognosis and susceptibility to myiasis in subsequent seasons. In this case, the dental disease was easily managed, with regular dental treatment, and the prognosis was good. More recommendations on dental treatment are available in the suggested Further reading section.

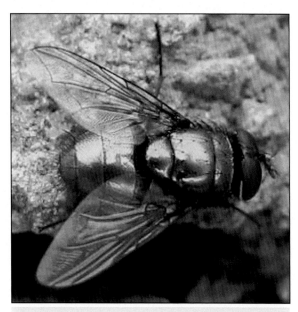

Figure 38.4 *Lucilia sericata*, otherwise known as the greenbottle fly due to its dramatic colour. These, along with bluebottles, are the commonest causes of fly strike in rabbits in the UK.

AETIOPATHOGENESIS OF MYIASIS (FLY STRIKE)

Fly strike, or myiasis, occurs when fly eggs are laid on wet and dirty areas of the skin or fur and then hatch into larvae, which develop by feeding on the tissue of the host. Many flies within the order Diptera are capable of attacking living and dead tissue. *Cochliomyia hominivorax* and *Chrysomya bezziana* are true screw-worms and will attack healthy living tissue, as will some flesh flies such as *Wohlfahrtia magnifica*. However, in the UK, the vast majority of cases of fly strike are attributed (anecdotally) to blowflies. Blowflies include greenbottles (*Lucilia* spp.) and bluebottles (*Calliphora* spp.), with *Lucilia sericata*, the greenbottle (Fig. 38.4), being considered the most common cause.

Whilst screw-worms and flesh flies are obligate parasites of living tissue, the majority of blowflies are opportunistic parasites and can complete their life cycle on dead tissue and other organic matter, as well as damp and damaged living tissue. Blowflies can be categorized as *primary flies* – capable of initiating myiasis – whereas *secondary flies* can only attack an area that is already struck or otherwise damaged.

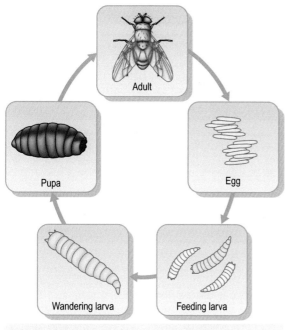

Figure 38.5 Schematic of the blowfly life cycle.

Blowflies can pick up faint traces of the odour of decay and can fly up to 20 km from their birthplace in search of a suitable place to lay their eggs. Female blowflies use their tongue-like mouthparts to feed on the protein secretions oozing from tissue, prior to laying their eggs through their ovipositor. Blowfly eggs are 2 mm long and laid in clumps that resemble miniature rice balls. A single female can lay nearly 2000 eggs during her life, and 5645 eggs have been counted from a small piece of meat (150 g) after 5 hours' exposure. The eggs hatch after 12–48 hours, depending on the temperature.

Blowfly larvae feed using their mouth-hooks and rapidly increase in size. They moult three times during their development (Fig. 38.5). Each stage of development is called an instar and the time it takes to develop between instars is fairly constant, although dependent upon temperature. The identification of larvae of a particular instar, combined with knowledge of recent weather conditions, allows forensic entomologists to determine the time of death in murder investigations.

When the third-instar larva has finished growing, it leaves the corpse and burrows into the ground, where it develops into a pupa, followed by an adult fly 14 days later.

EPIDEMIOLOGY

Fly strike commonly affects pet rabbits, but is seldom seen in their wild counterparts. During the warmer months (April to October), rabbits that are housed in hutches, or those that are unwell, can be affected by maggot infestation. The disease does not affect healthy individuals.

Sheep are the other species that commonly suffer from myiasis. In Europe, *Wohlfahrtia magnifica* and *L. sericata* are the most common causes, but other reported parasites include *Lucilia caesar* and *Protophormia terraenovae*. Blowfly myiasis is occasionally found in other animals such as tortoises, debilitated birds and other wild mammals such as hedgehogs; in these cases, *L. sericata* is usually involved.

Another cutaneous parasite that can affect rabbits in the USA is *Cutebra* spp., causing fistulous nodules in the skin that require individual removal.

TREATMENT

Many rabbits presented with myiasis will be in circulatory shock and require prompt veterinary attention. Initial treatment in this case was aimed at treating shock and providing analgesia to reduce the pain that the rabbit must have been suffering. Some people believe that maggots release a local anaesthetic so that infestation is not painful; however, with large skin defects, scalding and infection, pain is likely to be present.

Fluid therapy: A catheter was placed in the marginal ear vein to deliver intravenous fluids. In healthy rabbits they can be very jumpy for catheter placement in this site; pre-placement of lidocaine–prilocaine anaesthetic cream (EMLA cream; AstraZeneca) 20 minutes before catheter placement eliminates this reaction (Figs 38.6 and 38.7). Depending on the rabbit's size, cephalic or saphenous veins may also be used for intravenous fluid therapy, and may be better tolerated for prolonged placement than ear catheters.

Any standard isotonic fluid can be used for fluid therapy in the rabbit. Initial shock doses may be given at 90 ml/kg/h, but the rabbit should be carefully monitored during this time for signs of fluid overload, such as pulmonary oedema. Because of the large skin wounds, fluid losses will continue, so maintenance rates for cases of fly strike should be 5–10 ml/kg/h until the rabbit is drinking.

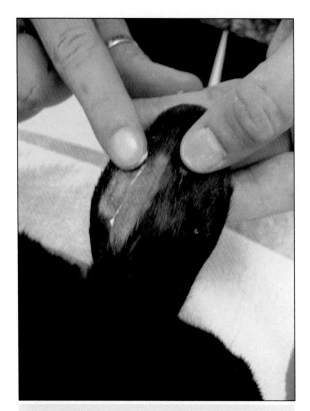

Figure 38.6 Preparation of the ear using EMLA cream to provide local anaesthesia for easy catheter placement in the marginal ear vein for fluid therapy.

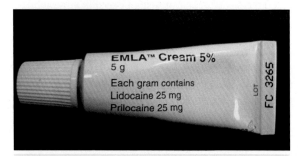

Figure 38.7 EMLA cream.

Analgesia: Multi-modal analgesia is indicated to prevent pain and suffering. A combination of opioids, such as buprenorphine, and non-steroidal anti-inflammatory drugs, such as carprofen or meloxicam should be used. In this case meloxicam was given s.c. at 0.2 mg/kg and buprenorphine i.v. at 0.03 mg/kg.

Antibiotics: Blowflies are likely to contaminate the skin and wounds with many different bacteria. Therefore,

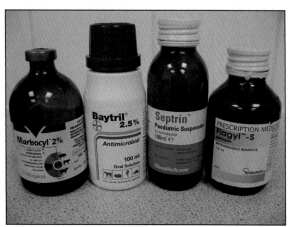

Figure 38.8 Safe antibiotics for use in rabbits.

even without culture and sensitivity testing, a broad-spectrum antibiotic is indicated in cases of fly strike. Secondary clostridial infection is also possible, and is often cited as the cause of death in rabbits that appear to have responded well to initial stabilization. Enrofloxacin (10 mg/kg p.o., b.i.d.) and sulphamethoxazole-trimethoprim (30 mg/kg p.o., b.i.d.) are both safe broad-spectrum antibiotics for use in the rabbit (Fig. 38.8). Several authors routinely use penicillin drugs parenterally as first-line treatment. Whilst often effective, these drugs can cause fatal antibiotic-associated diarrhoea and in this author's opinion should be reserved for refractory cases, or where sensitivity testing indicates it is the best, or only, choice.

Removal of eggs and larvae: Cleaning was attempted soon after presentation, once the rabbit had received fluids and analgesia and was more stable. Anaesthesia was induced with medetomidine (0.2 mg/kg i.m.), followed by ketamine (7.5–10 mg/kg i.v.) to effect 5 minutes later. The patient was intubated and maintained on oxygen, adding isoflurane as required. The medetomidine was antagonized with atipamezole (same volume as medetomidine) at the end of the procedure.

Owing to the pain and discomfort of this condition, removal of maggots should not be attempted on a conscious rabbit. The procedure will cause considerable pain and distress to the patient, and a conscious animal is unlikely to allow a detailed enough examination to ensure removal of all the maggots. Sedation may be carried out with intravenous midazolam or diazepam with buprenorphine in the very sick rabbit. In mild cases of fly strike, fentanyl/fluanisone also provides good sedation with analgesia.

Options for inducing anaesthesia include mask induction of a previously sedated rabbit. The animal should be pre-oxygenated for several minutes and then anaesthesia induced via the mask with isoflurane or sevoflurane, the latter being slightly less irritant and marginally faster acting. Alternatively, general anaesthesia can be induced with injectable agents such as medetomidine and ketamine, midazolam and ketamine, or propofol. In all anaesthetized patients, an endotracheal tube should be placed to allow delivery of oxygen and inhalational agent if required (Table 38.2).

General anaesthesia is likely to be more appropriate for the initial assessment, treatment and removal of maggots. It will allow thorough wound exploration and retrieval of maggots from deeper tissue with forceps. Maggots may also be removed by inserting a tube deeper into the wound and flushing them out. Second- and third-stage larvae are the most destructive, so should be removed first. Then, where possible, an attempt should be made to remove all first-stage larvae and the eggs, to prevent the development of the more damaging life stages. Eggs are easily removed with a flea comb and a hair dryer may encourage the smaller stages out of the wounds, since they are attracted to heat. If the fur has been washed to remove faeces and urine, drying is important to remove excess humidity (which will aid egg and larval development) and reduce the attraction for further fly egg laying.

Ivermectin was injected subcutaneously at 0.4 mg/kg to kill any remaining maggots. Avermectins act on the γ-aminobutyric acid (GABA) receptors throughout the body to cause insect paralysis and death. Selamectin at 6–18 mg/kg should also be effective, although it has not been evaluated by clinical studies.

Wound management: Certain proteases released by *L. sericata* are able to degrade the extracellular matrix in the skin and have been used in humans for the debridement of non-healing wounds. Rabbits' skin is very susceptible to these proteases and appears not to be able to inactivate them, as is the case with human skin. Therefore, *L. sericata* larvae are able to penetrate rabbit skin, causing a primary myiasis and leaving 'enzymatic burns' that require careful wound management.

In this case, the wounds were cleaned with warm water and dilute povidone–iodine lavage, under anaesthesia, to remove all the debris, faecal material and urine contamination. The wounds were debrided to remove

necrotic tissue and any remaining maggots or eggs. Appropriate disinfectant such as povidone–iodine or chlorhexidine should be used, since these wounds are contaminated. Insecticidal washes are available to kill the maggots, but may prove toxic due to increased systemic uptake in an inflamed area. Manual maggot removal remains the safest option.

Once cleaned, the deep wounds were covered with a hydrogel (Intrasite; Smith & Nephew) and a permeable dressing to allow excess moisture to escape. Hydrogels are bacteriostatic, maintain wound hydration and have been shown to slow larval development. The wound was checked every 4–6 hours for emergence of undetected larvae, but none further were found in this case. Once satisfied that the wound is clean, a more permanent hydrocolloid dressing (Granuflex; BMS) can be applied, and either bandaged or sutured in place. This should be changed every 2–3 days initially, and then less frequently depending on progress. The wound then has to be managed as with any open wound to heal by second intention. Topical creams such as silver sulphadiazine are useful to help debride further necrotic tissue.

TREATMENT OPTIONS

When presented with a case of myiasis in the rabbit, supportive care and treatment should be approached in the following order of priority, as with this case:

- Intravenous fluid therapy
- Analgesia and antibiosis
- Supportive nutritional care (prior to anaesthesia if inappetant for an extended period)
- Diligent removal of larvae and eggs under sedation or anaesthesia
- Treatment to prevent further development of remaining larvae
- Wound management
- Investigation and specific management of underlying cause.

During fluid therapy it is often beneficial to add duphalyte (1 part duphalyte to 4 parts isotonic solution) to the fluids to aid with parenteral nutrition, while the rabbit is critical. It is important to remember to warm the fluids to body temperature, prior to administration, to prevent chilling of the patient.

Analgesia doses:

- Carprofen, 2–4 mg/kg s.c., q24 h; 1.5–2 mg/kg p.o., q12 h

- Meloxicam, 0.2 mg/kg s.c., q24 h; 0.1–0.2 mg/kg p.o., q24 h
- Buprenorphine, 0.01–0.05 mg/kg i.m./i.v., q6–8 h
- Butorphanol, 0.1–0.5 mg/kg s.c./i.m./i.v., q2–4 h
- Pethidine (Arnolds Dechra), 5–10 mg/kg s.c./i.m.
- Tramadol (Zydol Grünenthal), 10 mg/kg p.o., q24 h.

Products to prevent fly strike or inhibit larval development

There are several medications marketed to prevent or treat myiasis in the rabbit.

Cyromazine: The only licensed POM-V product available in the UK is cyromazine. Contrary to a common misconception, it does not repel flies, but is an insect growth regulator. Blowflies will still deposit their eggs, but the product prevents larval development beyond the L1 stage, before the more destructive L2 and L3 stages develop. Therefore, fly eggs and L1 larvae can still be found if the conditions are right, but serious myiasis should not occur. The drug should be *painted* on and around the rabbit's rump and is active for 10 weeks after application, although the active period may be reduced if the rabbit is bathed often. Cyromazine should not be applied to broken skin, so cannot be used on affected areas during treatment of myiasis, only as prevention. If the product is licked shortly after application, transient inappetance may occur.

Avermectins: Avermectins such as ivermectin (0.4 mg/kg s.c., i.m. or topically 1:10 in propylene glycol) and selamectin (6–18 mg/kg topically) have been used in the treatment of myiasis to kill any remaining larvae. An ivermectin product (Xeno450; Genitrix) has recently been marketed for rabbits under the Small Animal Exemption Scheme (SAES; see Chapter 16).

Permethrins: Permethrin and cypermethrin cause larval paralysis and can be indicated in fly strike. Xenex Ultra Spot-on (Genitrix) contains permethrin and is licensed in the UK (under the SAES) for preventing myiasis. There is also a new product being developed, combining F10 (Health and Hygiene), a quaternary ammonium and biguanidine disinfectant, cypermethrin and piperonyl. This has not been fully evaluated at the time of going to press, but is promising in that it will provide safe and effective wound disinfection with larvicidal action. Permethrins penetrate poorly beyond the sebaceous layer of the skin, so may only act superficially.

Fipronil: Fipronil is effective at killing *L. sericata* larvae, but has a *specific licensed contraindication* for use in rabbits in the UK. Therefore, despite claims on its usefulness in myiasis cases, it is not justifiable under the veterinary cascade.

Nitenpyram: Nitenpyram has been anecdotally used to treat fly strike, but is not licensed in rabbits.

Topical wound medications: Topical medications used safely in larger species have been associated with toxicity in rabbits. This may be due to thinner skin, ingestion while grooming, hypersensitivity to the vehicle or overdosing. Organophosphate wound powders (e.g. Negasunt; Bayer) were used to kill larvae in horses' wounds. Many practices still have stocks remaining, but it should not be used in rabbits. It has an oral lethal dose (LD50) in rabbits of 80 mg/kg and a dermal LD50 of 500 mg/kg, and is likely to cause organophosphate toxicity.

Fly repellents: Reducing the number of flies near the rabbit is an obvious way to prevent fly strike. Xenex (Genitrix) is a plant-based repellent containing octanoic and decanoic acids. Old-fashioned sticky papers (available from DIY stores and garden centres) may be used in the home or shed, providing they are kept out of reach of the rabbit. Use of a fly screen may be beneficial. A number of plants are also said to repel insects and flies:

- Citronella is a natural, widely available repellent.
- The dried flowers of pyrethrum deter mosquitoes and flies.
- Pennyroyal is a low-growing mint with tiny spikes of mauve flowers in summer and a strong peppermint scent.
- Nigella (love in a mist) is a pretty annual flower and a good fly and midge repellent.
- Many herbs are said to repel flies – for example, balm, camomile, hemp, agrimony, lavender, mugwort, rosemary, rue, peppermint, santalina (Cotton Lavender), basil, shofly.
- Green oregano's pungent smell repels just about everything in the way of insects.

The use of such products does not, however, eliminated the need to treat the predisposing cause of the fly strike.

NURSING ASPECTS

Maggot removal

This is very important, and plenty of time and patience must be spent exploring wounds repeatedly for the presence of maggots. They will tend to move in and out of wounds, so a previously clear area may have several maggots upon reinspection. The use of a hair dryer will help dry the damp fur and will also attract maggots out of wounds towards the heat. Initially, this process is carried out with the rabbit anaesthetized. Subsequent checking for maggots over the following days should be just as thorough, but can usually be carried out in the conscious rabbit. In order to monitor closely for further larvae, it is advisable to hospitalize fly-struck rabbits for several days after presentation.

Clipping fur

See the case of 'Cheyletiellosis in a rabbit' (Chapter 16) for recommendations about clipping rabbits' fur. In fly strike cases, the fur is often matted and caked in faeces or other dirt. Often, it is best to clip away some of the fur before attempting to wash the affected area.

Postoperative nutritional support

Rabbits with myiasis are often debilitated, inappetant and painful; therefore, early nutritional support is essential. Their metabolism usually receives a continuous supply of nutrients from the gut, so anorexia can have dire consequences. Nutritional support will provide much needed calories, fluids and electrolytes, as well as aiding early return to normal digestive function.

In most cases, nutrition can be provided by syringe feeding three to six times per day. An approximate guide for volume is 10–20 ml/kg, but will depend on the type of food offered. Options include baby foods, puréed vegetable and cereal products, moistened and mashed pelleted rabbit food, or specifically marketed food such as Critical Care for Herbivores (Oxbow Pet Products) or Science Recovery (Supreme Pet Foods).

The most important aspects of syringe feeding are time and patience. Rabbits may be slow or reluctant to swallow, and attempting to syringe feed 20 ml in a few minutes during a busy morning surgery is likely to result in aspiration pneumonia. Adequate time must be allowed for syringe feeding, and the person doing the feeding must be adequately trained and patient.

CLINICAL TIPS

Choice of anaesthetics/sedation

There are a number of options for sedation or anaesthesia of the fly-struck rabbit. The protocol selected may depend on the veterinary surgeon's familiarity of a particular technique or the availability of anaesthetic drugs within the practice. Some sedation/anaesthetic protocols are listed in Table 38.2, but for more detailed explanations, the reader is referred to the Further reading.

Gastrointestinal hypomotility

Rabbits with maggot infestation, skin wounds and infection are likely to be in considerable pain and stress. This will lead to generalized adrenergic stimulation, which will inhibit gut motility, leading to gut stasis or ileus. This can be prevented by judicious use of multi-modal analgesia, as mentioned earlier. It is frustrating to treat the myiasis, then have the rabbit die from gut stasis due to inadequate pain relief.

Wound management

Rabbit hutches are particularly dusty, so this should be considered while the wounds are being treated. It is advisable to bed the rabbit on clean newspaper and provide plenty of fibre in the form of dust-free hay.

Owner education

Prior to embarking upon treatment of these cases, ensure the client is fully informed. They need to know that treatment will be long, require time and patience from them, that there will be significant after-care and that cost may be a factor. The owner also has to appreciate that the underlying cause of the fly strike needs to be established as part of the investigation and treatment. Euthanasia is the preferred option by a proportion of clients.

SECTION 5

PIGMENTARY DISORDERS

39 Introduction to skin and hair pigmentation

Skin and hair colour is genetically determined and is mainly due to the presence of melanin pigment. Melanin is produced by melanocytes, cells present in the epidermis and hair follicles, in a highly organized multiple-step process. Within melanocytes, melanin is synthesized in intracellular cell organelles called melanosomes.

Melanocytes are derived from melanoblasts, precursor cells, which originate in the neural crest and under the control of a number of growth factors, migrate to the skin, eyes, meninges and inner ear during embryonic development. Melanocytes are dendritic cells and in the skin are found mainly in the basal layer of the epidermis and hair follicle. Each melanocyte interacts with a number of keratinocytes by way of dendritic processes. The 'epidermal melanin unit' consists of one melanocyte interacting with around 36 keratinocytes. In a 'follicular melanin unit', one melanocyte interacts with around five hair follicle keratinocytes.

The melanosome is the principal product of melanocytes and is a highly organized, membrane-bound organelle within which melanin synthesis takes place. The initial steps (Fig. 39.1) of melanin synthesis are under the control of the enzyme tyrosinase, which oxidizes tyrosine to DOPA and then to dopaquinone. This undergoes a series of further complex reactions, involving cyclization and oxidative polymerization, to form the different types of melanins. The process of melanin transfer to surrounding keratinocytes involves transport of melanosomes to the tips of the dendrites and then subsequent transfer across to keratinocytes (Fig. 39.2). The transfer of melanosomes to neighbouring cells occurs by a combination of phagocytosis and diffusion through cell membranes, and is known as cytocrinia. As keratinocytes ascend through the epidermis and undergo differentiation, transferred melanins are released from melanosomes by lysosomal acid hydrolases. The visible skin colour depends on the stage of melanosome transfer, the size of the melanosomes and on how widely they are dispersed.

Hair pigment is derived from melanocytes found in the hair bulb. The melanocytes in the hair bulb are active only during the anagen (active growth) phase of the hair cycle. Hair coloration is predetermined, but the mechanisms controlling hair pigmentation are not known.

There are two basic types of melanins which are responsible for four basic pigments. *Eumelanins* are responsible for black and brown pigment, and *pheomelanins* are responsible for yellow and red pigments. Although the pigmentation is genetically determined and controlled by several enzymatic steps, other factors such as ultraviolet radiation, and hormones including melanocyte-stimulating hormone (MSH) and adrenocorticotrophic hormone (ACTH) acting in both endocrine and paracrine modes, can influence the degree of pigmentation. Keratinocytes are important sources of MSH and ACTH, and this may partially explain the focal hyper- and hypopigmentation seen in some inflammatory skin disorders.

Melanin has many functions in addition to protection from ultraviolet light.

Functions of melanins:
- Sun screening by direct absorption of ultraviolet light
- Scavenging of free radicals
- Camouflage and adornment

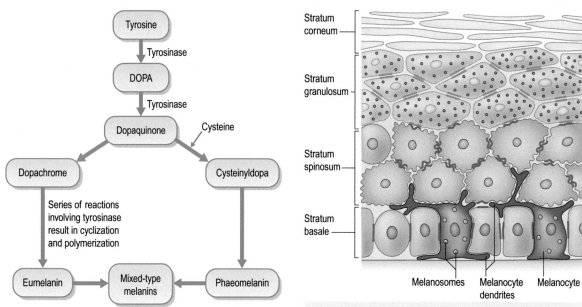

Figure 39.1 Major steps in the multi-step pathway in the synthesis of melanins.

Figure 39.2 Diagrammatic presentation of melanocytes. (Source: Anita Patel.)

Table 39.1 Conditions where hypopigmentation is the main presenting sign

Condition	Disorder	Stage involved	Clinical phenotype
The Waardenburg syndrome	Genetic	Defect in melanoblast migration and differentiation	Deafness, white coat colour, blue or heterochromic irides. Described in Dalmatians, Great Danes, collies, bull terriers and cats
Vitiligo	Heritable Acquired	Destruction of melanocytes	Hypopigmented macules at mucocutaneous sites, depigmentation of footpads, nails and hair. Seen in Dobermanns, Rottweilers, German shepherds, Siamese cats
Oculocutaneous albinism type 1	Genetic	Mutation of tyrosinase gene	White hair and skin and translucent irides with severe photophobia
Temperature-sensitive oculocutaneous albinism	Genetic	Mutation of tyrosinase gene resulting in temperature-dependent activity	Cats such as Siamese Himalayans and Birmans bred for colour points at the extremities which are cooler and also have ocular abnormalities such as absence of binocular vision, lack of pigment in the choroid and retinal epithelia and decreased visual acuity
Chediak–Higashi syndrome	Genetic	Mutation of gene encoding for a protein involved in organellogenesis	Hypopigmentation, bleeding disorders and increased susceptibility to infections reported in Persian cats
Canine cyclic haematopoesis	Genetic	Lethal autosomal recessive disorder	Silver–grey hair coat, weak at birth and predisposed to infections, and affected dogs die early in life. Seen in collies
Piebaldism	Genetic	As above	White spotting accepted as normal in animals
Uveodermatological syndrome	Acquired	Post-inflammatory	Nasal depigmentation and uveitis reported in several breeds, but akitas, samoyeds and Siberian huskies are predisposed

Table 39.2 Conditions where hyperpigmentation is the main presenting sign

Condition	Disorder	Stage involved	Clinical phenotype
Canine lentigo	Genetic	Increased number of melanocytes and melanin	Hyperpigmented macules reported in pugs
Lentigo simplex	Genetic	As above	Affects lips, eyelids, gums, nose and pinna in ginger cats
Secondary to any allergic, endocrine or infectious skin disease	Acquired	Increased melanocytes and melanin production in response to various inflammatory mediators and/or hormones	Diffuse hypigmentation at affected sites

- Regulation of vitamin D3 biosynthesis by influencing the penetration of UV light through the skin
- Displays of aggressive behaviour
- Thermoregulation
- Detoxification by binding to certain organic molecules, drugs and heavy metals.

PIGMENTARY DISORDERS

The whole process of melanocyte development and differentiation, and melanin pigment production and transfer, is highly regulated. Any disruption involving the migration of melanoblasts to the skin, failure of differentiation of melanoblasts into melanocytes, or failure of survival and proliferation of melanocytes, results in the absence of melanocytes and a group of *melanocytopenic* disorders which are sometimes associated with hearing, ocular, enteric or limb abnormalities. Failure of melanocytes to synthesize or deliver the pigment to epidermal or follicular keratinocytes results in decreased pigmentation and so-called *melanopenic* disorders.

Pigmentary abnormalities can be presented as either hypopigmentation or hyperpigmentation. The hypopigmentary disorders (Table 39.1) are either genetic or acquired. The genetic disorders are either due to a defect in the multi-step pathway that leads to melanin production, or to the transfer of melanin to the epidermal or follicular keratinocytes. Acquired hypopigmentation in small animals is mainly a post-inflammatory condition, which is caused by the destruction of melanocytes during skin inflammation.

Similarly, hyperpigmentation (Table 39.2) can be genetic, or acquired following inflammation, or due to hormonal imbalances, or due to pigmentary neoplasia. Many of the genetic conditions have no treatment and animals known to possess the gene should not be bred from, if the condition affects the animal's well-being. In the majority of cases the defect will only be of aesthetic importance and the owners will not be concerned; however, a minority may seek advice. The case reports in this section demonstrate an approach to investigating and dealing with pigmentary disorders.

40 Vitiligo in two dogs

INTRODUCTION

Vitiligo is a specific, acquired disorder, characterized by well-circumscribed depigmented patches and macules and leucoderma that result from a complete absence of melanocytes in affected areas of skin. This case report describes two cases, one in a Labrador and the other in a Rottweiler.

CASE PRESENTING SIGNS

One case involved a 13-month-old, spayed female Labrador retriever that was presented because of progressive depigmentation of the nasal planum.

The second case was a 4-year-old, entire male Rottweiler with depigmentation of the nasal planum and extensive leucotrichia.

The two dogs were from separate households and were examined on different occasions.

CASE HISTORY

Vitiligo typically starts in young adult dogs and results in progressive multifocal depigmented macules, or patches, over the nasal planum, lips, face, buccal mucosa and footpads. The hair and nails may also be affected. Affected animals have no history suggestive of systemic disease and the disease is non-pruritic.

In the case of the Labrador the history was:
- A 4- to 5-month history, initially of loss of pigment and then slight crusting over the nasal planum.
- The dog had no other history of skin disease.
- There was no history suggestive of systemic involvement.

- The dog had never been outside the UK.
- There were no other animals in the household.
- There was no evidence of zoonosis.
- Diet consisted of a proprietary complete dried chicken- and rice-based food.
- The dog received vaccinations as a puppy, but had not been vaccinated since then. There had been no routine anthelmintic treatment over the past 6 months.

The history of the Rottweiler was:
- A 3-month history of progressive depigmentation, initially around the eyes, with later involvement of the lips, nasal planum, pads, nails and over the trunk. There was no evidence of pruritus.
- Recently, there had been some repigmentation over the nasal planum and footpads.
- There was no other history of skin disease.
- There was no history suggestive of systemic involvement.
- There was no history of drug administration prior to the onset of depigmentation.
- There was no contagion and no zoonosis
- The dog had been fed a tinned dog food and biscuit mixer.

CLINICAL EXAMINATION

Examination of the Labrador revealed well-demarcated depigmentation over the nasal planum and a depigmented macule over the pad of digit 5 on the left fore foot, with another on the central tarsal pad of the left hind foot (Figs 40.1, 40.2 and 40.3). The buccal mucosa over the hard and soft palates also showed evidence of macular depigmentation. There was mild crusting over

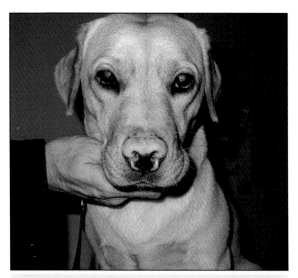

Figure 40.1 Well-demarcated depigmentation over the Labrador's nasal planum.

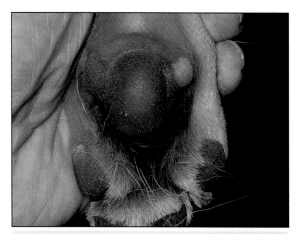

Figure 40.3 Depigmented macules over the Labrador's footpads.

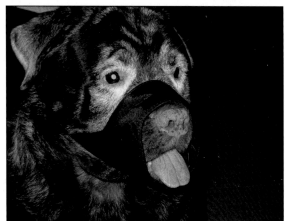

Figure 40.4 Leucotrichia and nasal depigmentation in the Rottweiler.

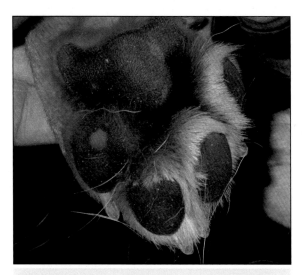

Figure 40.2 Depigmented macules over the Labrador's footpads.

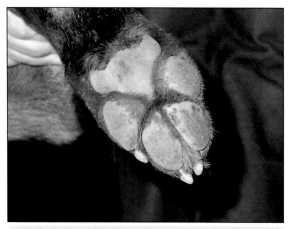

Figure 40.5 Footpad depigmentation in the Rottweiler.

the dorsal aspect of the affected nasal planum, but the footpad areas and the rostral nasal planum were neither inflamed nor crusted.

Examination of the Rottweiler revealed a generalized but variable leucotrichia of most of the hair coat. There was patchy depigmentation of the nasal planum and footpads, and depigmentation of the proximal nails (Figs 40.4, 40.5 and 40.6).

Neither dog had any abnormality on general physical examination.

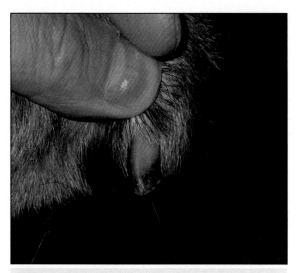

Figure 40.6 Depigmentation of a nail in the Rottweiler.

DIFFERENTIAL DIAGNOSES

There are many potential causes for depigmentation of the nasal planum, including infection, autoimmune and neoplastic diseases. The distinguishing feature of both these cases was the well-demarcated nature of the depigmentation and, with the exception of slight crusting in the case of the Labrador, the almost complete absence of any inflammation. These findings were highly suggestive of vitiligo. However, the differential diagnoses for depigmentation are extensive and include:

- Vitiligo
- Uveodermatological syndrome
- Nasal depigmentation ('snow' or 'Dudley' nose)
- Mucocutaneous pyoderma
- Autoimmune skin diseases such as cutaneous lupus erythematosus and the pemphigus complex of diseases
- Leishmaniosis
- Epitheliotropic lymphoma.

CASE WORK-UP

The definitive diagnosis of vitiligo is made by the demonstration of a complete absence of melanocytes on histological examination of affected areas. In the case of the Labrador, samples were taken from the nasal planum and central tarsal footpad under general anaesthesia using a 6-mm biopsy punch. Samples were taken from the junctional zone between the depigmented and normally pigmented skin. Histopathological examination of the samples from the Labrador retriever showed a complete absence of melanocytes in the depigmented areas, confirming the diagnosis of vitiligo. There was mild surface serocellular crusting in the samples from the nasal planum, and a mild superficial lymphocytic and plasmacytic perivascular dermatitis.

Histopathological examination was recommended to the owner of the Rottweiler, but was declined.

DIAGNOSIS

A definitive diagnosis of vitiligo was made in the case of the Labrador based on history, clinical signs and confirmed by histology. A definitive diagnosis was not made in the case of the Rottweiler but, clinically, the lesions were consistent with a diagnosis of vitiligo.

PROGNOSIS

In most cases, the full extent of the depigmentation will occur within 6 months of disease onset. Vitiligo is a cosmetic disease that does not generally affect the animal's quality of life. The depigmentation is usually permanent but, in some cases, spontaneous repigmentation does occur.

AETIOPATHOGENESIS OF VITILIGO

Vitiligo arises because of a complete loss of melanocytes from the lesional skin, with the consequent complete loss of pigment. The precise aetiology remains unknown, but there are three hypotheses to explain vitiligo: the neural hypothesis, the self-destruction hypothesis and the autoimmunization hypothesis.

Neural hypothesis: The neural hypothesis is that a melanotoxic neurochemical is released from nearby nerve endings that results in destruction of melanocytes. Support for this in humans stems from the fact that vitiligo may arise in skin that has been neurologically compromised; vitiligo may spare paralysed limbs and numerous neurotransmitter abnormalities have been identified in affected, as compared to healthy, skin.

Self-destruction hypothesis: The self-destruction hypothesis is that certain melanin precursors (tyrosine analogues and intermediates) are known to be toxic to melanocytes. Melanocytes appear to have an intrinsic protective mechanism and dysfunction of this mechanism in affected cells results in cellular destruction.

Autoimmunization: The third hypothesis is that autoimmunization against one or more components of the melanogenic system results in the formation of toxic autoantibodies, or in a cell-mediated destruction of melanocytes.

It is likely that multiple mechanisms could be responsible for the same phenotypic appearance.

EPIDEMIOLOGY

Vitiligo has been described in a number of breeds, including the Belgian tervuren, German shepherd, Newfoundland, German short-haired pointer, Rottweiler, Old English sheepdog and Siamese cats. There is a predilection for young animals, with most cases under 3 years of age at onset.

TREATMENT OPTIONS

Owners should be counselled as to the benign and cosmetic nature of vitiligo. Avoidance of ultraviolet light exposure is important in dogs with lesions on sun-exposed skin and the use of sunblock is advisable to protect vulnerable areas.

There is no effective treatment for vitiligo that results in permanent repigmentation of affected areas. Various treatments are used in people with vitiligo, when it may be appropriate to try and induce repigmentation. Treatment modalities include topical glucocorticoids, psoralen photochemotherapy (PUVA) and treatment with the plant extract *Polypodium leucotomos*. To date, these treatments have not been used in animals with vitiligo.

CLINICAL TIPS

It is likely that the slight crusting over the dorsal aspect of the nasal planum in the case of the Labrador was the result of sun exposure, but a striking characteristic of vitiligo is non-inflammatory depigmentation. A thorough history and full physical examination are important to rule out systemic and other inflammatory skin diseases. Full haematological and biochemical examinations and urinalysis should be performed if there is any evidence suggestive of systemic involvement.

Early skin biopsy is recommended, and the ideal sites to sample are the junctional zones between normally pigmented and affected areas, because the striking difference between the two zones is a diagnostic feature. Although a 6-mm biopsy punch was used in this case, it might be advisable where possible to use an 8-mm punch or consider taking an elliptical incision across the margin between the affected and non-affected zones.

FOLLOW-UP

A follow-up phone call to the owner of the Rottweiler revealed that, over a period of a year, there was complete repigmentation of the footpads and partial repigmentation of the nasal planum. The hair coat colour darkened, although some leucotrichia remained.

The Labrador was lost to follow-up.

INITIAL PRESENTATION

Depigmentation, crusting, scaling and alopecia on the nose.

INTRODUCTION

Uveodermatological syndrome is a rare condition characterized by ocular and cutaneous signs in dogs. The ocular signs include uveitis, glaucoma, conjunctivitis, blepharospasm and photophobia. The cutaneous signs include depigmentation of the skin and hair, crusting, erythema and ulceration, usually at the mucocutaneous sites. The condition is similar to Vogt–Koyanagi–Harada syndrome described in people. Vogt–Koyanagi–Harada syndrome is progressive, starting with a meningoencephalitis phase, followed by an ophthalmic–auditory phase, which progresses to a convalescent stage, where the ocular signs subside, but the cutaneous changes occur and remain. During the early phase of the disease the clinical signs include fever, malaise, headaches, nausea and vomiting. The ocular signs and deafness are followed by poliosis, alopecia and leucoderma during the convalescent stage. In contrast, in dogs, ocular signs are usually acute and precede the cutaneous signs. Ophthalmic assessment is essential in dogs, even when there are no obvious ocular signs. This chapter describes a case where the cutaneous signs preceded ocular signs, and where early recognition and treatment for ocular disease allowed early intervention.

CASE PRESENTING SIGNS

A 5-year-old, castrated Japanese akita was presented with depigmentation, crusting and alopecia on the nose.

CASE HISTORY

Ocular signs are the usual reason for presentation of these cases. The owner may present the dog because it has ocular discharge, conjunctivitis, oedema, photophobia or blindness. Depigmentation of skin and hair may be evident, and may be accompanied by erythema, ulceration and alopecia. The relevant history in this case was:

- Onset of depigmentation and alopecia on the nose, with duration of about 1 year.
- General health was unaffected.
- The nasal condition was non-pruritic.
- The dog had travelled to northern France, but the condition started before going abroad.
- Familial history was unknown and no zoonosis was reported.
- The dog was up to date with routine vaccination and endoparasitic and ectoparasitic control.
- Only after close questioning did the owner report that the dog was uncomfortable in sunlight.
- There was no previous history of eye problems, and the nasal lesions were poorly responsive to topical treatment with fusidic acid- and betamethasone-containing ointment.

CLINICAL EXAMINATION

This is a condition where physical examination should include a detailed ophthalmic examination. Ocular signs include conjunctivitis, blepharospasm, anterior and posterior uveitis, retinal haemorrhage and/or detachment. The main cutaneous sign is depigmentation of the nasal planum, eyelids, scrotum, vulva and paw pads. Crusting,

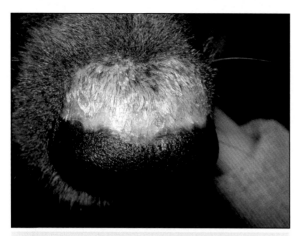

Figure 41.1 Scaling, crusting, depigmentation and alopecia on the bridge of the nose.

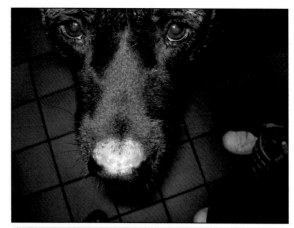

Figure 41.3 Focal depigmented macules on the medial canthi.

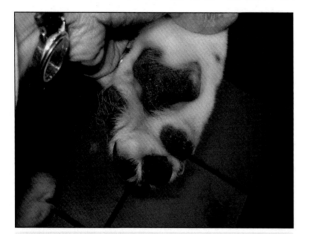

Figure 41.2 Depigmentation of the footpads.

The following differential diagnoses were considered:

- Uveodermatological syndrome
- Discoid (cutaneous) lupus erythematosus
- Pemphigus foliaceus
- Pemphigus erythematosus
- Leishmaniosis
- Vitiligo
- Mucocutaneous pyoderma
- Epitheliotropic lymphoma
- Fungal infections
- Actinic dermatitis
- Contact irritant or allergic reactions.

ulceration, erythema and alopecia are likely to be present in advanced cases. Oral ulceration may also be observed in chronic, untreated cases.

In this case the relevant findings on dermatological examination were:

- Crusting, scaling, erythema and alopecia on the nose at the junction of the nasal planum and the haired skin (Fig. 41.1)
- Depigmentation of the lip margins
- Depigmentation of several pads on the feet (Fig. 41.2)
- Mild crusting at the medial canthi and few depigmented macules of only 1–2 mm in size on the lower eyelids (Fig. 41.3)
- There was no obvious evidence of uveitis, but an ophthalmic referral was arranged.

CASE WORK-UP

Many of the conditions on the differential list are confirmed on histopathology. In this case the following diagnostic tests were performed:

- Hair plucks and tape-strip preparations ruled out demodicosis.
- There was not sufficient exudation to make an impression smear but stained tape-strip preparations failed to reveal any microorganisms. Where possible, direct impressions should be made to demonstrate the type of inflammatory infiltrate and the presence or absence of acantholytic keratinocytes.

- Routine haematology and biochemistry were within normal laboratory reference ranges, and an antinuclear antibody (ANA) test was also negative.
- Fungal culture from hair plucks and scrapings was negative after 3 weeks of incubation on Sabouraud's dextrose agar.
- Skin biopsies were obtained under general anaesthesia (because of the site involved), induced using propofol and maintained with isoflurane. The main histopathological findings were multinodular to diffuse inflammation, predominantly composed of macrophages in the mid and upper dermis (Fig. 41.4) consistent with uveodermatological syndrome. These findings were not typical of discoid lupus erythematosus, where the pattern is of interface dermatitis with predominantly lymphocytic infiltrate. Acantholysis and subcorneal pustules, the main features of pemphigus complex, were absent in this case. *Leishmania* amastigotes were not evident within the macrophages.

- Because of the travel history, further exclusion testing for leishmania was carried out: PCR, which was negative; serology, which was negative; and immunostaining of skin biopsy sections with *Leishmania* antibody, which was also negative. Neoplasia was also ruled out.

Two days before presentation to the eye clinic, the dog developed a red eye.

The ophthalmological findings were:
- Poor menace responses and sluggish papillary light reflexes
- Mild episcleral congestion and corneal oedema in the left eye, with posterior synechia and slight swelling of the iris
- Retinal vessel attenuation and multiple depigmented patches on the non-tapetal fundus (Fig. 41.5).

DIAGNOSIS

The ophthalmic and dermatological changes were consistent with uveodermatological syndrome in this case.

PROGNOSIS

The prognosis for the ocular disease is guarded, as the condition is progressive and can lead to glaucoma and eventually blindness. The dermatological signs may cause aesthetic problems or localized lesions, which are not life threatening. It is therefore very important to involve an ophthalmologist at an early stage, even if obvious uveitis and other ocular signs are absent.

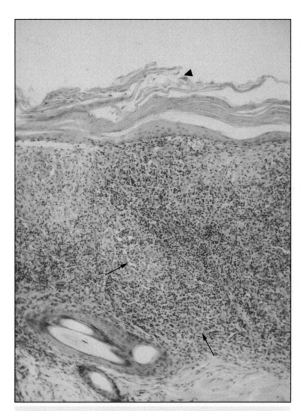

Figure 41.4 Histological section showing parakeratosis (arrowhead) and diffuse inflammatory infiltrate (arrows) at the interface and the upper dermis.

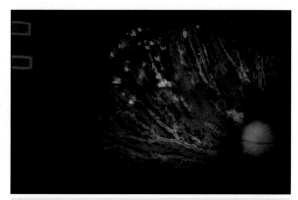

Figure 41.5 Depigmentation of the fundus. (Courtesy of S. Turner.)

AETIOPATHOGENESIS OF UVEODERMATOLOGICAL SYNDROME

During embryonic development, pigment-producing precursor cells migrate from the neural crest to the retina, choroid, skin, meninges and inner ear. These cells develop into specialized cells at the various sites. In the skin, melanoblasts, the precursor cells, differentiate into melanocytes.

The precise pathogenesis of uveodermatological syndrome in dogs is not known, but is thought to be an immune-mediated cellular response against melanin and melanocytes; hence, the clinical signs involve sites where there are pigment-producing cells. The cellular response in people is primarily T-lymphocyte mediated and predominantly made up of CD 4+ type cells. A recent report on the immunohistochemical study of uveodermatological syndrome in dogs suggests that the cutaneous lesions are T-cell and macrophage mediated, whereas the ocular lesions are B-cell and macrophage mediated.

EPIDEMIOLOGY

The condition is rare and is mainly seen in Nordic breeds such as akitas, samoyeds, Siberian huskies, chow-chows and Alaskan malmutes and their crosses. It is also seen in other breeds such as golden retrievers, German shepherd dogs, Australian shepherd dogs, Shetland sheepdogs, Old English sheepdogs, Irish setters, dachshunds and standard poodles. There is no sex predisposition and the onset can be seen as early as 6 months, up to 6 years of age.

TREATMENT

Treatment should include topical and systemic immunosuppressive drugs, targeted to the treatment of both the ocular and cutaneous lesions. Because the treatment of the ocular lesions may need to be aggressive, an ophthalmologist should be involved. In more advanced cases, systemic treatment with immunosuppressive doses of prednisolone (2 mg/kg every 24 h) or azathioprine (2 mg/kg every 24 h) should be considered. The ophthalmologist should advise on when the prednisolone dose can be reduced to alternate days and then tapered to the minimum dose required to keep the disease under control. Likewise, the azathioprine dose should also be reduced to every 48 hours and eventually tapered down to 0.5–1 mg/kg every alternate day. Regular haematology and biochemistry are performed when these drugs

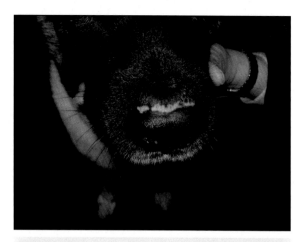

Figure 41.6 Repigmentation and hair regrowth at most of the previously affected site, 4 weeks after treatment.

are used, due to their potential adverse effects, and the cases require regular eye check-ups.

Treatment in this case

In this case, because of the early ocular signs, topical treatment with 1% prednisolone eye drops was started. On re-examination the uveitis had improved; however, there were early signs of a secondary glaucoma in the left eye. Brinzolamide topical drops were added to the ongoing treatment with 1% prednisolone eye drops.

The nasal lesions were treated with 0.1% tacrolimus ointment twice daily. Tacrolimus has immunomodulating properties (see Chapter 6 under 'Treatment'). The response to it in this case was favourable, and within 4 weeks there was hair regrowth and repigmentation of the affected site (Fig. 41.6).

> ### CLINICAL TIPS
>
> - Definitive diagnosis and ophthalmic assessment are a must in dogs with this condition.
> - When to intervene with aggressive systemic treatment should be determined by the ophthalmologist.
> - The condition requires regular monitoring by an ophthalmologist.
> - Owners should be warned of the long-term prognosis and the likely costs involved in long-term monitoring.

- Owners need to be warned of potential adverse effects of immunosuppressive drugs and that in some cases these adverse effects could be life threatening.
- Owners need to be dedicated, as the treatment and management are time- and labour-intensive.
- Euthanasia should be considered in dogs with irreversible severe glaucoma, pain and blindness.

FOLLOW-UP

This case was monitored monthly by the ophthalmologist, with the view that early aggressive intervention would probably be required. The dermatological monitoring was 3-monthly.

At the time of writing the dog was being maintained on topical ocular treatment and 0.1% tacrolimus ointment every other day on the nose.

42 Lentigo simplex

INITIAL PRESENTATION

Hyperpigmented macules on the nasal planum and lip margins in a cat.

INTRODUCTION

Hyperpigmentation (also referred to as melanoderma or hypermelanosis) is an increase in the cutaneous pigment melanin. This increase may be genetic or acquired (post-inflammatory, endocrine), or neoplastic. Lentigo (plural lentigenes) is a flat brown–black pigmented macule that is circumscribed and well demarcated. In dogs, lentigenes may be more visible on the glabrous skin of the ventrum, although they can be present anywhere. They are seen mainly in adult dogs, where they increase in size and number over a period of months and then remain static. An inherited form, referred to as lentiginosis profusa, is reported in pugs.

A genetic hypermelanosis, 'lentigo simplex', is recognized in ginger cats. This type of hypermelanosis is only cosmetic in nature, but some owners who are concerned about an apparent disease may seek advice. It is important that clinicians are aware of it, and this report describes such a case in a cat.

CASE PRESENTING SIGNS

A 2-year-old castrated cat was presented with hyperpigmented macules on the nasal planum and the lip margins.

CASE HISTORY

Lentigo simplex is not associated with any systemic signs. The hyperpigmentation usually appears in young ginger or tortoiseshell cats. The condition becomes static over time and is unaffected by the seasons. The main reason for presentation is the owner's concern over the appearance of these spots.

In this case the relevant history was:
- An increase in the number of pigmented spots on the lips over the past few months.
- The condition was non-pruritic.
- The cat was otherwise healthy.

CLINICAL EXAMINATION

The lesions appear on the lips as small spots which gradually increase in number and size, varying from 1 mm to several millimetres in diameter. The lesions are intensely black in colour, and are well circumscribed and demarcated from the surrounding unpigmented skin. In some cats they are visible on the eyelids, pinna and nasal planum.

In this case the relevant findings on clinical examination were:
- Flat, multiple hypermelanotic macules on the lower lips (Fig. 42.1) and nasal planum (Fig. 42.2), varying in size from about 3 mm in diameter to several centimetres in length, where a number of them had coalesced.
- No other abnormalities were detected in this case.

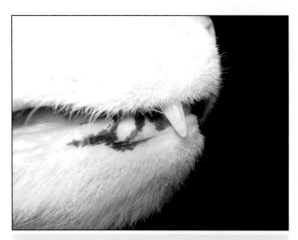

Figure 42.1 Hyperpigmented macules which have coalesced to form linear patches.

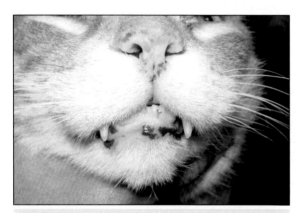

Figure 42.2 Hyperpigmented macules on the nasal planum. Note the onset of depigmentation on the upper aspect.

DIFFERENTIAL DIAGNOSES

The history, clinical examination and colour of the cat are usually enough to make a diagnosis. In this case the differentials were:
- Lentigo simplex
- Melanomas (similar, but usually raised, lesions occur in older cats and tend to also involve other sites, such as eyes).

CASE WORK-UP

The clinical appearance of the lesions is usually sufficient to make a diagnosis; however, if required, it can be differentiated from neoplastic conditions on histology.

Biopsies of both affected and unaffected skin should be taken. The histopathological finding is of increased melanocytes and melanin in the basal layer of the macule, compared to the unaffected skin.

In this case, the diagnosis was made on clinical examination alone, because it was deemed unnecessary to subject the cat to unnecessary investigations.

DIAGNOSIS

A diagnosis of lentigo simplex was made based on history and clinical examination.

PROGNOSIS

Good.

ANATOMY AND PHYSIOLOGY REFRESHER

Melanocytes are found mainly in the basal layer of the epidermis, where they produce pigment (melanin; see Chapter 39). Increased numbers of melanocytes, due to hyperplasia, are responsible for the lentigenes. The pathogenesis of this condition is not known, but because it is mainly seen in ginger or tortoiseshell cats, a genetic mode of inheritance is suspected.

EPIDEMIOLOGY

This condition is seen in ginger or tortoiseshell cats of either sex. It usually starts at a young age and is slowly progressive; the rate of progress slows, becoming static in time.

TREATMENT

No treatment is advised, as this is purely a cosmetic problem.

CLINICAL TIPS

Clients that seek advice for this condition normally just require reassurance and education. It is not essential to subject the cat to tests in most cases, unless there is genuine risk of it being a melanoma.

43 Hyperpigmentation due to hypothyroidism

INITIAL PRESENTATION

Marked ventral hyperpigmentation in a cross-bred dog.

INTRODUCTION

Hyperpigmentation is a frequent presentation in canine skin disease and is most commonly the result of inflammation, due to parasitic, bacterial, fungal or allergic skin disease. Hormones also exert an effect on the pigmentary system, although their mode of action is not well understood. This report describes a case of hypothyroidism that resulted in marked ventral hyperpigmentation.

CASE PRESENTING SIGNS

A 5-year-old neutered male, cross-bred dog was presented with ventral hyperpigmentation and poor hair coat.

CASE HISTORY

- Initial signs of skin disease had first appeared 10 months previously, and consisted of ventral erythema and hyperpigmentation, teat enlargement, dorsal pruritus, alopecia and greasiness of the hair coat. More recently, pedal pruritus had been evident.
- There was no history suggestive of systemic involvement.
- Fleas had not been observed and no flea prevention was used.
- There were two other dogs in the household, neither of which had skin disease.
- There was no history suggestive of zoonosis.
- The dog was kennelled with the other two dogs in a garage with no access to the house.
- The diet consisted of a proprietary tinned food, biscuit mixer and food scraps, with just water to drink.
- Previous treatment 2 months earlier with a trimethoprim/sulphonamide antibacterial, weekly benzoyl peroxide shampoos and glucocorticoid therapy had resulted in reduced pruritus and erythema, but had not affected the pigmentation and the hair coat had not improved in quality. Discontinuation of therapy resulted in recurrence of erythema and pruritus within 2 weeks.

CLINICAL EXAMINATION

- The patient was afebrile and mildly obese. There was mild generalized peripheral lymphadenopathy.
- Examination of the skin revealed erythema, hyperpigmentation and alopecia over the bridge of the nose and periocular skin (Fig. 43.1).
- The presence of patchy, poorly demarcated, bilaterally symmetrical dorsal alopecia with comedones, papules, pustules and yellow greasy scaling was noted (Fig. 43.2).
- The glabrous skin over the groin and axillae was markedly hyperpigmented and lichenified, with erythema and papules evident around the margins of the hyperpigmented areas. The teats were enlarged (Fig. 43.3).

255

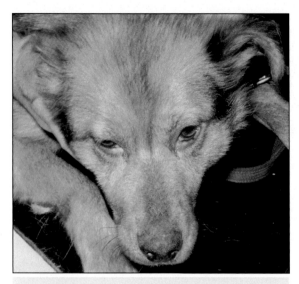

Figure 43.1 Alopecia and hyperpigmentation over the bridge of the nose and periocular skin.

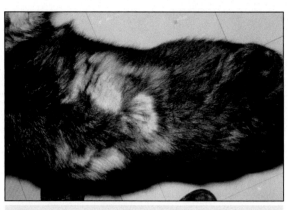

Figure 43.2 Bilaterally symmetrical alopecia, scaling and papule formation over the dorsal trunk.

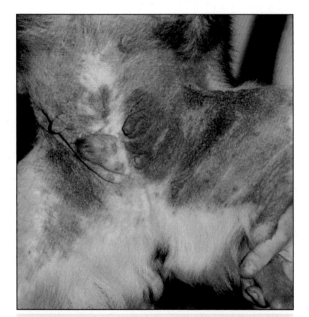

Figure 43.3 Diffuse hyperpigmentation and lichenification over the groin with erythema and papule formation. Note teat enlargement.

DIFFERENTIAL DIAGNOSES

Overall, the history of pruritus and signs of papules, scaling, erythema, lichenification and hyperpigmentation were most suggestive of an inflammatory skin disease. Ventral hyperpigmentation is a common presentation in hypersensitivity disorders. The multifocal dorsal alopecia could have been due to a staphylococcal folliculitis, or perhaps self-trauma that the owners were unaware of. However, the hair loss had a bilaterally symmetrical pattern suggestive of an endocrinopathy, which can also be a factor in the development of hyperpigmentation. There was no historical evidence of signs suggestive of hyperadrenocorticism and hypothyroidism was considered the most likely endocrinopathy to be involved. Therefore, the differential diagnoses included the following:

- Flea allergy dermatitis
- Cheyletiellosis
- Demodicosis
- Pyoderma
- *Malassezia* dermatitis
- Dermatophytosis
- Atopic dermatitis
- Cutaneous adverse food reaction
- Hypothyroidism.

CASE WORK-UP

The first stage in this case was to rule out the involvement of ectoparasitic and infectious causes of alopecia and pruritus, before investigating the other possibilities.

- There was no evidence of ectoparasitism on microscopic examination of scale from the dorsal trunk, nor on multiple superficial and deep skin scrapes from the affected areas.
- Cytological examination of tape-strip preparations from the groin revealed the presence of moderate numbers of *Malassezia* organisms and coccoid bacteria.
- There was no evidence of dermatophytosis on Wood's lamp examination of affected areas.
- Routine haematological and biochemical examinations were unremarkable. Basal thyroxine concentration was 11.9 nmol/l, just below the laboratory reference range.

Demodicosis could be ruled out on the negative skin scrapes, but trial therapy was required before flea allergy dermatitis and cheyletiellosis could be excluded. There was evidence of pyoderma and a *Malassezia* dermatitis that required treatment. A therapeutic antiparasitic and antimicrobial trial was indicated. The slightly depressed basal thyroxine concentration could have been due to genuine hypothyroidism, recent sulphonamide and/or glucocorticoid therapy, or euthyroid sick syndrome.

TRIAL THERAPY

- Initial treatment consisted of fortnightly applications of selamectin to all three dogs, and treatment of the garage and car environments with a permethrin and pyriproxyfen spray.
- Antimicrobial therapy consisted of three times weekly chlorhexidine and miconazole shampoos and clindamycin (10 mg/kg s.i.d.) for 4 weeks.

Re-examination after 4 weeks revealed that there was still marked erythema and hyperpigmentation over the groin, but the pyoderma had resolved. No *Malassezia* organisms were seen on repeat cytology from the groin. There was no evidence of hair regrowth over the dorsal patches of alopecia. The level of pruritus was reduced but not completely resolved.

The lack of hair regrowth over the dorsum tended to rule out the involvement of a staphylococcal pyoderma, but was supportive of a hair growth cycle disorder. Further investigation of hypothyroidism was indicated. A TSH stimulation test was performed using the recombi-

nant human TSH that is now available (see Chapter 22 for further information on diagnostic testing).

- The TSH stimulation test gave the following results: pre-TSH serum T4 concentration, 13.9 nmol/l; post-TSH serum T4 concentration, 13.2 nmol/l.

DIAGNOSIS

The history, clinical signs and results of the TSH stimulation test were consistent with a diagnosis of hypothyroidism.

PROGNOSIS

In general, the prognosis for hypothyroidism is good, with complete resolution of clinical signs following levothyroxine supplementation. In this case, it was not certain whether all the skin signs would improve with treatment. Further investigation of a possible hypersensitivity disorder would have been required if the pruritus had not resolved.

AETIOLOGICAL AND PATHOPHYSIOLOGICAL ASPECTS

The production of melanin within the skin is regulated qualitatively and quantitatively by many different factors. The mechanism of action of various hormones on the pigmentary system is not well understood, but the proopiomelanocortin (POMC) peptides, α-MSH and ACTH, are known to be important regulators of melanogenesis. POMC peptides interact with a cell surface receptor on melanocytes (MC1R) to switch on melanin production. Thus, the hyperpigmentation seen in *hyperadrenocorticism* can in part be explained by the excess production of POMC peptides such as ACTH. However, although hyperpigmentation is a relatively frequent finding in cases of hypothyroidism, the effect of thyroid hormones on the pigmentary unit is not clear, as hyperpigmentation is associated with hyperthyroidism in man, whereas it is associated with hypothyroidism in dogs.

There is evidence of paracrine regulation of melanogenesis by UVR-exposed keratinocytes that secrete several stimulatory (PGE2, α-MSH, ACTH, endothelin-1 and nitric oxide), as well as inhibitory (TNF-α, IL-1α), factors that act on melanocytes. Thus, it is possible that keratinocytes may play a central role in fine-tuning melanocyte growth and differentiation. The post-inflammatory hyperpigmentation commonly seen in pyodermas and *Malassezia* dermatitis is thought to arise from paracrine regulation of melanogenesis by activated keratinocytes. Over 50% of biopsy specimens from hypothyroid dogs' skin show variable degrees of inflammation, reflecting the common occurrence of secondary bacterial and yeast infection and seborrhoea, and this may explain the hyperpigmentation seen in hypothyroidism. Another possibility is that hyperpigmentation in canine hypothyroidism could be associated with tanning of UVR-exposed areas of alopecic skin. However, this dog presented with marked hyperpigmentation of the ventral areas that didn't respond to treatment of pyoderma and *Malassezia* dermatitis, but only resolved following levothyroxine supplementation, which might suggest a more direct role of thyroid hormones in the regulation of melanogenesis.

EPIDEMIOLOGY

Several breeds are reported to be at increased risk for hypothyroidism, including Irish setters, Dobermann pinschers, giant schnauzers, miniature schnauzers, Airedale terriers, golden retrievers, Afghan hounds, Shar Pei and chow-chows. Unlike hyperadrenocorticism, hypothyroidism can affect any age of dog and may be seen in giant breeds less than 2 years of age. However, the majority of cases occur in dogs between 6 and 10 years of age. There is no sex predilection. Spontaneously occurring hypothyroidism is extremely rare in cats.

TREATMENT

(For a full discussion of the treatment of hypothyroidism, see Chapter 22.) The dog was started on levothyroxine supplementation at a dosage of 0.02 mg/kg b.i.d. To prevent recurrence of further *Malassezia* dermatitis during the early stages of therapy, it was bathed weekly with a chlorhexidine/miconazole shampoo.

CLINICAL TIPS

As in this case, hypothyroidism can present as a strikingly inflammatory disease, with very few of the signs classically associated with hypothyroidism, such as weight gain, lethargy, heat seeking and mental dullness. Interestingly, it is often only after treatment that owners remark how the dog is now brighter and more active. The common cutaneous signs in hypothyroidism are: a poor coat quality with symmetrical alopecia; lightening of the hair coat in some breeds due to bleaching of retained telogen hairs; hyperpigmentation and lichenification; and secondary *Malassezia* dermatitis and pyoderma. Alopecia over the bridge of the nose, as seen in this case, is strongly suggestive of hypothyroidism.

If samples are to be taken for histopathological examination from suspected hypothyroid animals, take samples from areas of advanced hair loss and avoid areas where there is secondary pyoderma or, better still, treat the pyoderma before taking the samples.

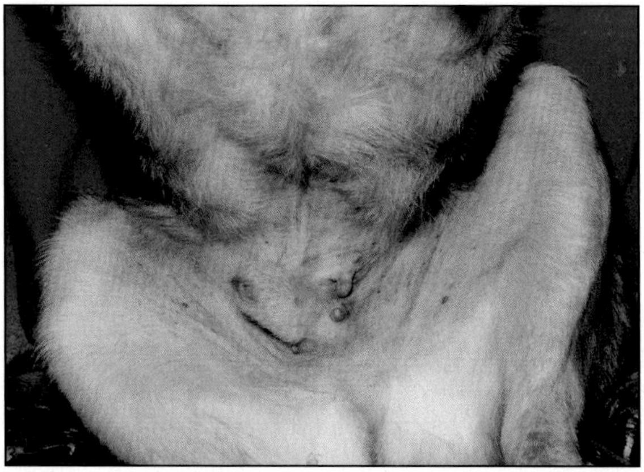

Figure 43.4 The same dog as in Fig. 43.3 after 2 months of thyroid hormone replacement therapy.

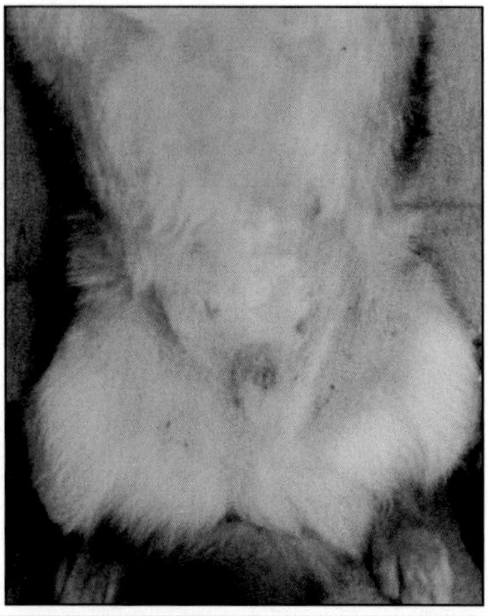

Figure 43.5 Complete resolution of clinical signs after 6 months of thyroid hormone replacement.

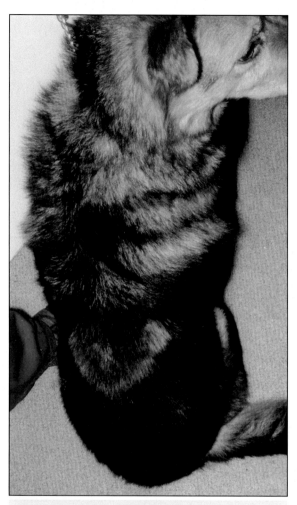

Figure 43.6 Complete resolution of clinical signs after 6 months of thyroid hormone replacement.

FOLLOW-UP

Reinspection 8 weeks later revealed that the erythema and hyperpigmentation over the ventral abdomen had markedly reduced and there was partial dorsal hair regrowth (Fig. 43.4). The greasy nature of the skin and hair coat had resolved. The patient was not longer pruritic and, interestingly, the owners reported that the dog was more alert and energetic. A 4- to 6-hour post-pill administration basal thyroxine concentration was 48 nmol/l, which indicated adequate thyroid supplementation.

After 6 months of therapy, there was complete regrowth of hair and resolution of the ventral hyperpigmentation (Figs 43.5 and 43.6). The dosage of sodium levothyroxine was reduced to 0.02 mg/kg s.i.d. and the patient was maintained on this dosage over a 2-year period.

CUTANEOUS NODULES OR SWELLINGS WITH OR WITHOUT DRAINING SINUS TRACTS

44 Introduction to cutaneous nodules and swelling

A nodule is a solid, palpable, circumscribed elevation of more than 1 cm in diameter above the epidermis (Fig. 44.1), which may extend down into the dermis, subcutis and the underlying muscle. Most commonly they result from a massive accumulation of either inflammatory or neoplastic cells, or, uncommonly, due to accumulation of calcium or other deposits such as amyloid. A tumour is a large nodule or mass which is not necessarily neoplastic. A draining or sinus tract connects an area of inflammation in deeper tissue, such as the dermis and subcutis, to the skin surface. Drainage through the tract is a means of removing the by-products of inflammation and other debris. Single or multiple nodules may be present in the same animal.

According to the type of cellular infiltrate, they are generally divided into inflammatory or neoplastic nodules.

Inflammatory nodules:
- Infectious:
  - Bacterial
  - Fungal
  - Protozoal
  - Parasitic infections
- Non-infectious:
  - Allergic
  - Immune mediated
  - Sterile or metabolic processes.

Neoplastic nodules:
- Benign:
  - Single or multiple
- Malignant:
  - Single or multiple
  - With or without systemic involvement.

In small animal practice, solitary and multiple cutaneous neoplasms are common in dogs, especially over the age of 6 years, with the incidence increasing with age. Fight wound abscesses are more common in cats. Most cats with abscesses will respond to surgical drainage and systemic antibiotics. However, non-healing abscesses, nodules and draining tracts can present a diagnostic and therapeutic challenge in both dogs and cats.

Neoplastic nodules with or without draining tracts may be easier to diagnose on histology after either wedge or excisional biopsies. However, with certain neoplastic nodules, wide-margin surgical excision is essential and needs to be planned, depending on the site of the tumour.

When presented with such cases it is important to take a complete history, because the animal's management and environment may provide important clues of potential aetiologies. Certain infectious organisms are more prevalent in some geographical locations and are carried by some small mammals. A full physical and dermatological examination will provide clues of systemic involvement, if any. The diagnostic steps to confirm a diagnosis involve cytology either of fine-needle aspirates, smears from exudate or impression smears; depending on the findings, histopathological examination, culture of microorganisms, haematology and biochemistry, etc. can be prioritized. Once the diagnosis is confirmed the appropriate treatment is introduced.

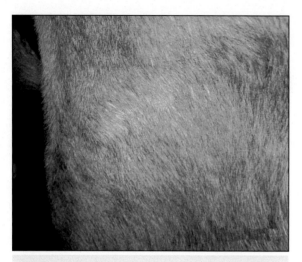

Figure 44.1 Nodule in the dermis and subcutis on the stifle of a dog.

The aetiologies of infectious organisms and types of neoplasms are numerous. It is beyond the scope of this book to review all cases; however, the few selected cases in this section demonstrate the steps to take to achieve a diagnosis and some aspects of treatment.

Acral lick dermatitis

Swelling with eroded surface on the distal forelimb.

INTRODUCTION

Canine acral lick dermatitis is a condition characterized by a firm, alopecic, frequently ulcerated plaque on a distal limb or limbs, caused by licking and usually complicated by a secondary bacterial infection. It used to be considered that the licking was purely the result of a psychogenic disorder, but it is now known that in many cases it is caused by a variety of pruritic or painful organic diseases, sometimes with a psychogenic component. This report describes a case of acral lick dermatitis in a Labrador.

CASE PRESENTING SIGNS

A 6-year-old, neutered male Labrador was presented with a swelling over the left forelimb.

CASE HISTORY

A detailed history and full physical and dermatological examinations should help the clinician in determining whether the licking is the result of underlying organic disease, a psychogenic disorder or a combination of the two. The history should ascertain whether the skin disease is confined to the limb or whether there is, or ever has been, evidence of a more generalized skin problem. It is also important to establish the presence or absence of lameness in the affected limb, or previous injury.

The relevant history in this case was:

- There was no history of other skin disease or more generalized pruritus.
- There was no history of systemic illness, pain, lameness or previous injury.
- Nine months previously, the dog had started to lick the left forelimb and, despite topical antibacterial and glucocorticoid therapy (sodium fusidate and beta-methasone), the licking had persisted, resulting in two eroded and exudative plaques.
- A similar lesion had developed 3 years previously that had resolved with the above therapy.
- The licking behaviour would not occur when the dog was being observed. It had become evident that licking occurred whenever the dog was left unattended.
- An Elizabethan collar was used at night to prevent further self-trauma.
- There was one other dog in the household, a male sibling that was unaffected.
- There was no evidence of zoonosis.
- Both owners worked full time. They had moved house two and a half years previously. Prior to that, one or other of them had been able to return home during the day to exercise the dogs, but this had not been possible since the move. The dogs were in a kennel with a dog flap and a large outside run from 7.30 a.m. until 6.00.p.m. 5 days a week.
- Routine flea control consisted of monthly applications of fipronil spot-on during the summer and every 6–8 weeks during the winter.
- The diet consisted of a proprietary tinned and dried food, occasional bones and just water to drink.

CLINICAL EXAMINATION

Acral lick dermatitis usually develops on the limbs at the level of, or distal to, the mid radius or tibia. The anterior aspect of the carpus is commonly affected. Lesions may be single or multiple. The typical lesion is a raised, alopecic plaque with an eroded or ulcerated area at the centre of the lesion and a hyperpigmented margin. Some lesions may have draining sinus tracts and this should alert the clinician to the possibility of deep bacterial or fungal infection. There may be evidence of more generalized skin disease, such as otitis externa or pyoderma.

The examination should include manipulation of local joints and the neck (to assess for cervical pain), and palpation of underlying bone. If there is evidence of orthopaedic or generalized skin disease, these symptoms should be investigated and treated accordingly.

- No abnormalities were detected on full physical examination.
- There was no lameness and no pain on manipulation of the carpal joint.
- There were two eroded and slightly exudative plaques over the lateral aspect of the left carpus (Fig. 45.1).
- Apart from moderate erythema of both external ear canals, there were no other skin lesions.

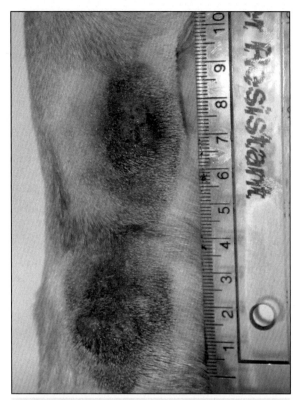

Figure 45.1 Case of acral lick dermatitis at initial presentation. Two eroded and slightly exudative plaques over the lateral aspect of the left carpus.

DIFFERENTIAL DIAGNOSES

There are focal inflammatory, or neoplastic, disorders which may resemble acral lick dermatitis and that result in licking. In this case, there was evidence of aural erythema, which might have been evidence of a hypersensitivity disorder. The differential diagnoses included:

- Acral lick dermatitis
- Deep bacterial or fungal granuloma
- Demodicosis
- Histiocytoma
- Mast cell tumour
- Other cutaneous neoplastic disease
- Underlying allergic dermatitis (atopy or adverse food reaction)
- Underlying hypothyroidism.

CASE WORK-UP

A range of diagnostic tests, including therapeutic and diet trials, are required to rule out the involvement of ectoparasitism, infection, hypersensitivity disorders, neoplasia and systemic disease. Histopathological examination is helpful to confirm the diagnosis.

The findings from the diagnostic tests undertaken in this case were:

- No *Demodex* mites were evident on skin scrapes from the lesions.
- A pyogranulomatous inflammation without evidence of bacteria was evident on examination of a fine-needle aspirate from the mass (Fig. 45.2).
- Material was taken for routine fungal culture using a toothbrush technique, which was negative.
- Two skin samples taken using a 6-mm punch biopsy were submitted for histopathological examination, which showed parakeratotic hyperkeratosis, acanthosis, surface erosions, marked fibrosis with vertical

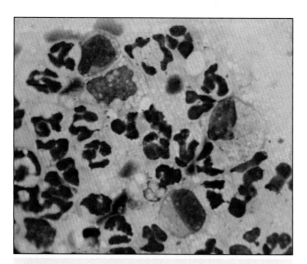

Figure 45.2 Cytological examination of a fine-needle aspirate from the plaques shown in Fig. 45.1. Pyogranulomatous inflammation without evidence of bacteria (×1000 original magnification).

orientation of collagen fibres within the dermis, and sebaceous gland hyperplasia signs consistent with a lick-induced lesion. Special stains failed to reveal the presence of fungal elements.
* A blood sample was taken for basal thyroxine and TSH. Basal thyroxine was 21 nmol/l (15–45 nmol/l) and TSH 0.12 ng/ml (<0.6 ng/ml), indicating normal thyroid function at that time.

DIAGNOSIS

The history, clinical signs and histopathology were consistent with a diagnosis of acral lick dermatitis.

PROGNOSIS

The prognosis for acral lick dermatitis is guarded for a complete and permanent resolution of lesions. In cases where there is significant secondary bacterial infection, the appearance of the lesion will improve with prolonged antibacterial therapy. Prevention of licking depends on whether the primary cause or causes can be identified and corrected.

AETIOPATHOGENESIS OF ACRAL LICK DERMATITIS

Organic disease plays a significant and sometimes major role in the formation of canine acral lick dermatitis.

Localized pruritogenic stimuli, such as wounds, may initiate the licking behaviour. Similarly, generalized pruritic conditions, including atopic dermatitis or an adverse cutaneous food reaction, may also play a role, although in the latter diseases there will usually be evidence of generalized skin disease or pruritus, and acral lick lesions are frequently multiple. Osteoarthritis, or referred pain, may stimulate licking. Secondary bacterial infection, most commonly with *Staphylococcus intermedius*, but also at times with Gram-negative organisms, is a frequent complication whatever the underlying aetiology. The infection further exacerbates the clinical signs.

Canine acral lick dermatitis of psychogenic origin is usually seen in large breeds of dog and is considered to be a form of compulsive disorder. Triggering factors include frustration and anxiety as a result of being left alone for long periods of time, or otherwise being kept in a restrictive or stressful environment. To relieve this conflict, the dog adopts the habit of licking at a limb, resulting in the stimulation of nerve endings and, ultimately, it is thought, the release of endogenous opioids such as endorphins, which induce a euphoric and addictive state. Other neurotransmitters, especially serotonin, are thought to be involved in compulsive disorders in animals as well as in humans. Persistent licking results in the formation of the alopecic eroded plaque.

EPIDEMIOLOGY

Predisposed breeds include the Great Dane, Labrador, German shepherd, Dobermann pinscher, golden retriever and Irish setter. Males are predisposed and outnumber females by 2 : 1.

MEDICAL TREATMENT OPTIONS

Clinical management

Clinical management falls into three main categories – treatment of the lesion itself, resolution of any underlying painful or pruritic disease, and identification and correction of psychogenic factors. Canine acral lick dermatitis is often refractory to treatment and the most successful approach will involve one that attempts to address all the causative factors.

Antibacterial therapy: As secondary bacterial infection is common, antibacterial therapy is indicated as the first line of treatment. The treatment may be combined with physical measures to prevent further self-trauma, such as dressings or an Elizabethan collar, but glucocorticoids should not be used at this stage. The antibacterial used should be effective in deep pyoderma lesions and active against *Staphylococcus intermedius*. Treatment should be administered for at least 6 weeks and at least 2 weeks past any clinical cure. Antibacterial therapy may result in partial or complete resolution of symptoms. If there is only a partial response to treatment, *and there is no other evidence of the involvement of organic disease*, further measures will be required to address psychogenic disorders and prevent further self-trauma. Although not done in this case, the clinician should consider submission of swabs or tissue samples for culture, prior to starting antibacterial therapy.

Treatment of psychogenic disorders: Relieve any environmental stressors by avoiding leaving the dog alone for long periods, increasing the frequency and duration of exercise, avoid confinement in a crate and consider the introduction of a companion animal, although the latter can have a detrimental rather than beneficial effect. Referral to a behaviourist should be considered if the underlying cause cannot be identified or easily corrected.

In the short term, it may be necessary to use drug therapy to break the cycle of obsessive behaviour, that can subsequently be discontinued if the underlying causes are addressed. Treatment may need to be continued if the underlying causative factors are not removed. Tricyclic antidepressants and selective serotonin reuptake inhibitors (SSRIs) are reported to be of benefit in the treatment of canine acral lick dermatitis. Drugs and dosages are shown in Table 45.1. Clomipramine is the only such treatment currently available in the UK that is licensed for use in dogs. The narcotic antagonist naltrexone has also been used successfully to manage acral lick dermatitis by antagonizing the effect of endogenous opioids and thereby increasing the perception of pain, although its use is controversial.

Other available treatment measures

The following treatments may also be of value in individual cases. Whilst these measures may help to break the itch–lick cycle, or in the case of surgery actually result in lesion removal, they are unlikely to result in permanent resolution without addressing contributory psychogenic and organic disease factors.

Prevention of licking: Elizabethan collars and/or the use of dressings may help to break a continuing itch–lick cycle.

Glucocorticoids: Glucocorticoids used topically, systemically and by intralesional injection are widely used and may be beneficial in reducing pruritus. However, care should be taken because glucocorticoids are contraindicated if pyoderma is present.

Acupuncture: Acupuncture has been reported to be beneficial in the management of acral lick dermatitis, but further documentation of efficacy is required.

Surgical removal: Surgical removal of single small lesions may be beneficial provided the wound can be sutured without undue skin tension and further self-trauma can be prevented. However, there is a significant risk of self-trauma and wound dehiscence with the end result being a large, non-healing skin defect. Surgical removal should not be contemplated without addressing underlying organic and/or psychogenic contributory factors.

Cryosurgery: Cryosurgery may be used for large lesions which are not amenable to surgical excision and are refractory to other treatments. One potential advantage of cryosurgery is desensitization of peripheral nerve endings, helping to block the itch–lick cycle.

Treatment administered and further case work-up

The first step was to rule out bacterial involvement using a prolonged course of systemic antibacterial therapy. In addition, although there was no generalized pruritus, there was aural erythema, tentative evidence of a possible hypersensitivity disorder, and the decision was made to run a diet trial concurrently with antibacterial therapy.

Table 45.1 Drug treatment for psychogenic disorders

Tricyclic antidepressants	
Clomipramine	1–3 mg/kg p.o., q12 h
Amitriptyline	1–3 mg/kg p.o., q24 h
Doxepin	3–5 mg/kg p.o., q12 h
SSRI	
Fluoxetine	1 mg/kg p.o., q24 h
Narcotic antagonist	
Naltrexone	2 mg/kg p.o., q24 h

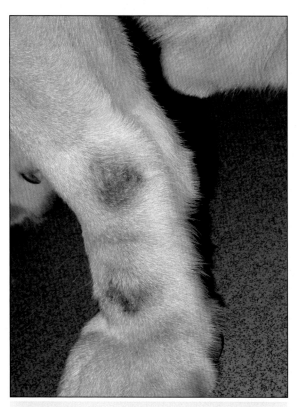

Figure 45.3 The same dog as in Fig. 45.1 after 6 weeks of antibacterial therapy. Decreased swelling and lesion surface area.

Re-examination 8 weeks later showed an improvement in the appearance of the lesions with decreased swelling, but there was no discernible reduction in licking (Fig. 45.3).

Further treatment options were discussed with the owner. They were interested in trying acupuncture and the dog was referred for acupuncture therapy as part of a clinical trial. Antibiotic treatment was continued and the dog received a weekly acupuncture treatment for 6 weeks. This made no significant difference to the level of licking behaviour.

> **CLINICAL TIPS**
>
> Bacteria are frequently scarce or not seen at all on cytology from deep pyoderma lesions, but this does not mean that bacterial infection is not involved. In this case, cytological examination of a fine-needle aspirate from the lesion showed a pyogranulomatous inflammation, referring to the presence of both neutrophils and macrophages, but no bacteria.

FOLLOW-UP

Follow-up after 2 years revealed that the dog had continued to lick the lesion. One family member had been at home for a 6-month period (maternity leave) and, during this period, there had been a noticeable improvement, with decreased licking and healing of the lesion. However, there had been recrudescence of licking behaviour when the owner went back to full-time employment. An Elizabethan collar was used on occasions during the night to prevent licking. The owners hadn't considered it necessary to seek further veterinary attention for the lesion.

A challenge with the original food would be conducted if there was an obvious response to ascertain whether the change of diet had been responsible for the improvement.

- The patient was started on a proprietary fish and corn, limited antigen restricted diet trial.
- Systemic antibacterial therapy was administered using cefalexin at a dosage of 23 mg/kg b.i.d.

46 Sterile pyogranulomatous nodular dermatitis

INITIAL PRESENTATION

Nodules, alopecia and draining tract in an 18-month-old Labrador.

INTRODUCTION

Nodules are raised elevations of the skin, of 1 cm or more in diameter. Nodular or diffuse dermatitis and panniculitis are essentially histological diagnoses, characterized by the accumulation of inflammatory cells in the dermis or the subcutaneous tissue. The types of inflammatory cells include neutrophils, macrophages, eosinophils and lymphocytes. This accumulation may result from infectious or non-infectious causes, such as neoplasia, immune-mediated conditions, nutritional causes, blunt trauma or a sterile idiopathic process. A diagnosis of a sterile idiopathic process is made only when all other causes have been ruled out.

CASE PRESENTING SIGNS

An 18-month-old, neutered male Labrador was presented with a history of multiple nodules, draining tracts and erythema on the dorsum.

CASE HISTORY

Sterile nodular pyogranulomatous dermatitis in dogs usually has a spontaneous onset, with no history of trauma. Pain and pruritus are variable and, depending on the underlying trigger, systemic signs such as vomiting, abdominal pain and lethargy may be reported. Some dogs may be anorexic or have a depressed appetite.

The history in this case was:
- The nodules had a rapid onset, with history of pruritus at the site.
- There was no reported history of any previous dermatological disease.
- There was no contact with other animals and no history of trauma.
- A high-fibre diet (canine Hills r/d) was being fed because the dog was overweight.
- The dog was otherwise in good health.

CLINICAL EXAMINATION

Pyrexia, pain and a reluctance to move may be evident on physical examination. Single or multiple nodules are normally located on the trunk or on the neck. Nodules present deep within the subcutis would suggest a panniculitis. They may vary in size, ranging from a few millimetres to several centimetres in diameter. The nodules may be well demarcated or ill defined, and on palpation they may appear either soft and/or fluctuant, or hard. Some cases may have draining tracts that release a purulent or even oily exudate (in the case of panniculitis) of variable colour.

In this case:
- Physical examination was within normal limits.
- Multiple ill-defined nodules were present on the dorsal lumbar area. There was no evidence of pain on nodule palpation.
- Erythema, scarring and sinus tracts were evident when the fur was clipped (Fig. 46.1) over affected areas.
- There was a yellowish to red coloured exudate discharging from sinus tracts.

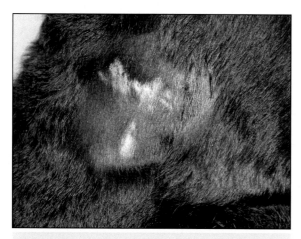

Figure 46.1 Raised swelling with erythema, scarring and depigmentation is evident when the fur was clipped. Note a pinpoint draining tract.

DIFFERENTIAL DIAGNOSES

Ill-defined nodules with discharging sinus tracts can occur due to a number of conditions, and the differential diagnoses in this case included:
- Deep folliculitis and furunculosis
- Bacterial or fungal pseudomycetoma
- Opportunistic mycobacterial infection
- Subcutaneous mycoses
- Cutaneous cysts
- Sterile pyogranulomatous nodular dermatitis and/or panniculitis
- Xanthomatosis
- Cutaneous histiocytosis
- Multiple cutaneous histiocytomas.

Other causes of nodular disease which were unlikely differentials in view of the signalment and clinical lesions included injection site reaction, foreign body reactions, abscess formation and cutaneous neoplasia including epitheliotropic lymphoma and mast cell tumour.

CASE WORK-UP

It is essential to systematically and carefully rule out all the other differential diagnoses in order to make a diagnosis of idiopathic sterile pyogranulomatous dermatitis. In any nodular disease, cytological examination of fine-needle aspirates and/or impression smears of exudate is indicated. A pyogranulomatous inflammation (neutro-phils and macrophages) and an absence of microorganisms will be seen in cases of sterile pyogranulomatous disease. Biopsied specimens are essential for bacterial and fungal cultures, and also for histology. Either an excision biopsy of a nodule or a wedge biopsy of a larger lesion should be taken for this purpose. Special staining techniques of histological sections can help to rule out the presence of bacterial and fungal organisms. Ziehl–Neelsen (ZN) stain may reveal acid-fast bacteria such as *Mycobacteria* and *Nocardia*. Other bacteria may be identified by their Gram-staining properties. Periodic acid–Schiff (PAS) stain and Gomori's silver stain are used to identify the presence of fungal elements.

As nodular skin disease is sometimes associated with systemic conditions, haematology and biochemistry, including serum amylase and pancreatic-specific lipase, are indicated, especially if gastrointestinal signs or abdominal signs are present. If pancreatic disease is suspected, abdominal ultrasonography and radiography, followed by exploratory surgery, may be necessary.

In this case the following tests were performed:
- Cytological examination of smears of the exudate, stained with modified Wright's stain, revealed pyogranulomatous inflammation with fat necrosis (Fig. 46.2a, b).
- Haematology revealed mild eosinophilia (1.2×10^9/l; normal range $<1.0 \times 10^9$/l) and monocytosis (1.2×10^9/l; normal range $<0.8 \times 10^9$/l). All biochemical parameters, including amylase, pancreatic-specific lipase and trypsin-like immunoreactivity (TLI), were within normal reference ranges.
- A large wedge biopsy specimen was obtained under general anaesthesia, which was divided into three sections (one for histology, one for bacterial culture and one for fungal culture). Additional biopsy specimens were taken and kept in the freezer in case further tests became necessary. The biopsy specimens submitted for bacterial and fungal culture failed to grow any organisms. Given the negative result from the PAS staining and ZN staining (see below), further culture for mycobacteria and saprophytic fungi was not pursued.
- Histopathological examination showed focal subcutaneous fat necrosis and pyogranulomatous inflammation of the dermis and panniculus. Macrophages forming granulomas interspersed with neutrophils and lymphocytes were present around the follicles and the subcutaneous fat. The sections, stained with Geimsa, Ziehl–Neelsen, PAS and Gram stains, failed to reveal any bacteria, protozoa or fungi.

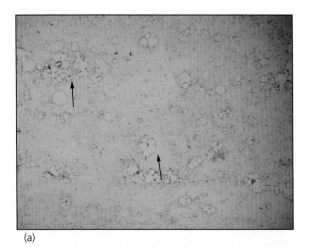

(a)

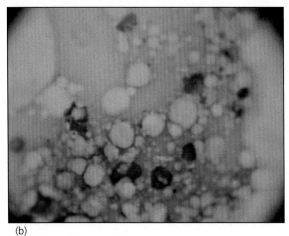

(b)

Figure 46.2
(a) Fatty necrosis showing large vacuoles and inflammatory cells under low power.
(b) Fat necrosis and neutrophils under high power (×1000, oil immersion).

Given that the dog in this case report did not show any systemic signs, further investigation by ultrasound examination and radiography was not carried out.

DIAGNOSIS

A diagnosis of sterile idiopathic nodular dermatitis and panniculitis was finally made after all the other differential diagnoses had been ruled out.

PROGNOSIS

The prognosis in this case was good and most dogs respond favourably to treatment, although long-term therapy may be required to maintain remission. Cases associated with pancreatic disease or immunological conditions such as systemic lupus erythematosus tend to have a poor to guarded prognosis.

AETIOPATHOGENESIS

Nodular dermatitis

Nodular dermatitis is an accumulation of inflammatory cells in discrete nodules in the dermis but in some cases the inflammation may involve the subcutaneous fat, resulting in panniculitis (see below). In some advanced cases the nodules coalesce together to form a diffuse pattern of inflammation on histopathological examination. Nodular dermatitis is usually classified according to the type of inflammatory cells involved. Pyogranulomatous dermatitis is characterized by an accumulation of neutrophils and macrophages, whereas granulomatous dermatitis is characterized by a predominance of macrophages and, in chronic cases, by the presence of giant cells. Macrophages are derived from the bone marrow as promonocytes. They enter the circulation as monocytes, from where they migrate to different tissues (skin, lung, etc.) and then differentiate into macrophages. Macrophages (also referred to as histiocytes when in the skin and connective tissue) are found in small numbers in normal skin. They form part of the innate immune system and they respond non-specifically to antigens by phagocytosis. They are involved in antigen processing and presentation to T cells. In chronically inflamed tissue, activated macrophages produce cytokines and other factors that promote continued inflammation.

Panniculitis

Panniculitis is an inflammation of subcutaneous tissue involving damage to lipocytes, which release free lipid into the extracellular space. There are a number of recognized trigger factors. It has been suggested that pancreatic enzymes, released into the circulation during episodes of pancreatitis, can be responsible for the damage to the fat. Hydrolysis of the lipids into free fatty acids and glycerol induces an inflammatory process that leads to the accumulation of inflammatory cells. Other triggers, including microbial, parasitic or self-antigens, can lead to recruitment of cells of the innate immune system.

EPIDEMIOLOGY

This condition is uncommon and is associated with a variety of triggers, but many canine cases are idiopathic. There have been no age or sex predispositions reported;

however, there is an increased incidence in dachshunds and poodles. The condition has been associated with pancreatic disease and, more recently, it has been reported in unrelated Weimaraners with a suspected immune-mediated disorder.

In humans the condition has been associated with systemic lupus erythematosus, rheumatoid arthritis and pancreatic disorders. It has been suggested that a deficiency of α-antitrypsin predisposes individuals to panniculitis, but in a canine study no link between the two was demonstrated.

TREATMENT OPTIONS

Every attempt should be made to identify and correct any underlying trigger factors for the pyogranulomatous disease.

In idiopathic conditions, the following treatments may be of benefit.

Glucocorticoids

Glucocorticoids are commonly the initial treatment of choice for most cases of sterile idiopathic nodular panniculitis. Methylprednisolone (0.8–1.6 mg/kg s.i.d.) or prednisolone (1–2 mg/kg s.i.d.) are the drugs of choice and most dogs will respond after 2–6 weeks of treatment. The dosage frequency is reduced to alternate days as soon as the condition is in remission and then the dose is tapered off to the lowest dosage that will prevent recurrence. Depending on the trigger, some animals may go into remission for a prolonged period or even be completely cured.

Ciclosporin

Recently, anecdotal reports have suggested that ciclosporin may be of benefit in the management of idiopathic sterile nodular dermatitis/panniculitis at a dosage of 5 mg/kg s.i.d.

Oxytetracycline/nicotinamide

The combination of oxytetracycline and nicotinamide is effective in the management of idiopathic, pyogranulomatous dermatitis in some dogs. Initial dosages were 250 mg of each t.i.d. for dogs <10 kg and 500 mg of each t.i.d. for dogs >10 kg body weight (for further information on this drug combination see Chapter 53).

Vitamin E

Vitamin E has antioxidant and anti-inflammatory properties, and is useful in some cases as a glucocorticoid-sparing agent. The recommended dosage is 400 IU b.i.d.

Surgical excision may be curative in cases where there is a solitary mass.

Treatment in this case

The dog in this case was treated with prednisolone at 2 mg/kg s.i.d. for 3 weeks and vitamin E at 400 IU b.i.d. After 3 weeks the surface lesions had almost resolved, but there was scarring of the subcutaneous tissue. The dosage frequency of prednisolone was then reduced to 2 mg/kg on alternate days for a further 2 weeks, after which the dog was showing signs of polydipsia, polyuria and polyphagia. At the 5-week examination, there were no cutaneous signs present, so the prednisolone dosage was reduced to 1 mg/kg every other day for a further 2 weeks and then down to 0.5 mg/kg every other day. Prednisolone was finally withdrawn after a total of 16 weeks of therapy. Vitamin E was continued indefinitely.

Systemic antibiotic treatment may be required if, during treatment, there is cytological or other evidence of secondary bacterial infection of ulcerated lesions.

NURSING ASPECTS

There are no specific nursing aspects, unless there are systemic signs of pancreatitis. In these cases, intravenous fluid therapy and dietary management are required.

CLINICAL TIPS

- Culture from a biopsy specimen and special staining procedures are essential to confirm that the inflammatory process is sterile.
- It is best to take an excision biopsy of a nodule, divide it into three or four sections for the different procedures and freeze excess tissue in case histopathological examination indicates a possible mycobacterial infection and culture is required, thus avoiding the need to repeat the biopsy and incurring unnecessary costs.
- Dogs with systemic signs should be investigated for internal diseases, especially those affecting the pancreas.

FOLLOW-UP

The dog remained in remission over a follow-up period of 12 months.

47 Feline mycobacterial disease

INITIAL PRESENTATION

Non-healing draining nodules, ulcers and cellulitis in a cat.

INTRODUCTION

Most cutaneous and subcutaneous abscesses, cellulitis and wounds seen in cats are due to fights, and are infected by both aerobic and anaerobic bacteria. *Pasteurella multocida*, B-haemolytic streptococci, *Actinomyces* spp., *Bacteroides* spp. and *Fusobacterium* spp. are commonly isolated from abscesses. In most cases, surgical drainage and routine antibacterial therapy resolves the infection.

Non-healing draining wounds and nodules, however, although uncommon, can be a diagnostic and therapeutic challenge. They can be caused by infectious organisms (bacterial, fungal, viral and protozoal organisms), foreign body reactions, sterile panniculitis and neoplasia (Table 47.1). Concurrent infections with FIV, FeLV or corona virus and the use of immunosuppressive drugs may be underlying causes of infection. Identification of the infectious organism is important, as some may have zoonotic implications and others may be life threatening. Cats presented with non-healing abscesses, non-healing wounds, nodules, draining tracts and cellulitis require extensive investigation and treatment.

One of the causes of persistent non-healing wounds, nodules and draining sinus tracts in cats is infection with rapidly growing mycobacteria (previously known as opportunistic or atypical mycobacteria). The report describes the investigation and treatment of such a case in which there was also a concurrent *Nocardia* infection.

CASE PRESENTING SIGNS

A 10-year-old, neutered female domestic long-haired cat was presented with a long-standing history of draining tracts with seropurulent exudate, nodules, ulceration and alopecia on the trunk.

CASE HISTORY

The various forms of feline mycobacterial disease are poorly responsive to short courses of antibiosis used for the treatment of routine cat-bite abscesses. There may be a history of a fight or the individual may have a history of hunting small rodents. Some individuals may have had surgery in an attempt to remove the diseased tissue, and this sometimes results in wound breakdown and subsequent failure to heal. The cat may have a history of anorexia, weight loss and pain.

In this case the relevant history was:
- Lesions had first appeared 1 year previously, consisting of a small patch of alopecia with draining tracts over the trunk.
- There had initially been some response to short courses of potentiated amoxicillin and clindamycin, but the lesions recurred within 3–4 weeks of treatment withdrawal.
- The lesions recurred within 3 weeks of attempted surgical excision.

Table 47.1 Causes for cutaneous nodules and draining tracts in cats

Bacteria	Non-acid-fast organisms	*Actinobacillus* spp., *Arcanobacterium pyogenes* (previously known as *Actinomyces pyogenes*), *Rhodococcus equi*, *Staphylococcus* spp., *Streptococcus* spp., *Pseudomonas* spp., *Proteus* spp.
	Acid-fast organisms	*Norcardia asteroides, Mycobacterium lepraemurium, M. tuberculosis, M. microti, M. chelonei, M. fortuitum, M. phlei, M. thermoresistible, M. smegmatis*
Fungi	Subcutaneous mycoses	*M. canis, Rhizomucor, Mortierella, Fusarium, Paecilomyces, Alternaria, Cladosporium, Exophiala, Moniliella, Curvularia, Madurella, Pythium insidiosum, Sporothrix schenckii*
	Systemic mycoses	*Cryptococcus neoformans, Sporothrix schenckii, Histoplasma capsulatum, Blastomyces dermatidis, Coccidioides immitis*
Parasitic or protozoal		*Leishmania* spp., cutaneous habronemiasis
Viral		Cowpox virus, calcivirus, herpes virus
Non-infectious causes		Foreign body reactions, eosinophilic granulomas, sterile nodular panniculitis, xanthamatosis, cutaneous histiocytosis and neoplasia

After Patel A (2002): Pyogranulomatous skin disease and cellulitis in a cat caused by *Rhodococcus equi*. J Small Anim Pract 43, 129–132, with permission of Blackwell Publishing.

- Histology of excised tissue revealed a severe granulomatous dermatitis, with furunculosis and foreign material.
- No organisms were cultured from swab samples of exudate submitted on two separate occasions.
- None of the other four cats in the house were affected.
- No zoonosis was reported.
- The cat had occasional bouts of gastritis and vomited fur.
- The cat licked the affected area.
- In general, the cats in the house did not fight with one another, but they were allowed to roam freely through a cat flap and there were other cats in the neighbourhood so fight wounds were a possibility.
- The owner did not know whether this cat hunted or not.
- The cat's appetite was unaffected.
- There were no other signs of systemic illness.

CLINICAL EXAMINATION

In general, cats with infections caused by the rapidly growing mycobacteria (RGM) have few signs of systemic illness, although more extensive disease may result in pyrexia, reluctance to move, peripheral lymphadenopathy and other constitutional signs. Typically, fight wounds are the cause of RGM infections and lesions tend to start in areas subject to biting and scratching such as the dorsum, flanks and inguinal fat pad. Early on in the clinical course, the lesions resemble catfight abscesses, but they generally do not have the putrid malodour associated with them. As lesions progress, the affected areas become alopecic with numerous discharging punctuate sinus tracts. The surrounding subcutis may be thickened and the overlying skin may become adherent to the underlying tissue. Some areas may have ulcers of varying sizes and necrotic skin. Hypercalcaemia has been reported in some cats.

A clinical examination revealed:

- The cat was in poor body condition and weighed 3.35 kg.
- The skin lesions were confined to the dorsal and lateral aspects of the thoracolumbar region.
- Ulcers of varying sizes, a thickened subcutis due to scarring and nodules, and alopecia were also evident (Fig. 47.1).
- Multiple draining tracts from the subcutaneous fat to the skin surface were discharging a seropurulent exudate (Fig. 47.2).
- The nodules were not painful on palpation.
- General physical examination was unremarkable.

CASE WORK-UP

The history and the clinical signs were suggestive of an atypical bacterial infection, possibly due to one of the rapidly growing mycobacterial organisms. Meticulous

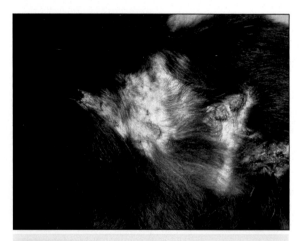

Figure 47.1 Ulcers, draining sinuses, scarring and alopecia on the lateral thorax and flank.

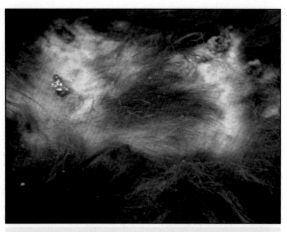

Figure 47.2 Seropurulent exudate from draining sinuses and ulcers.

investigation is required to identify the causative organism. A tentative diagnosis may be based on finding organisms within macrophages, giant cells or lipid vacuoles on cytological preparations stained with modified Wright or Gram stains. However, in cases with this sort of presentation, tissue samples should ideally be obtained both for histopathology, and also bacterial and fungal culture, to confirm the diagnosis.

Samples for both culture and histopathology should be obtained by surgical excision rather than biopsy punch in order to include the subcutis. Depending on the type of lesions present, an excision biopsy of a nodule, a deep wedge biopsy from a large lesion or sequential biopsies can be obtained. For histology, wedge or elliptical biopsies should have healthy tissue at the margins and on the depth of the tissue. If submitting tissue for initial histopathological examination it can be helpful to retain and freeze half the excised tissue for later mycobacterial culture if indicated by the histopathology results.

Tissue samples for culture should be submitted in a sterile container with a small amount of sterile saline or wrapped in a sterile guaze swab moistened with sterile saline. Exudate or needle aspirates of fluid and cellular material may also be submitted for culture.

Histology: When bacterial or deep fungal infections are involved, histology reveals nodular to diffuse granulomatous and/or pyogranulomatous dermatitis and panniculitis. In some cases, organisms may be visible on H&E sections. Special staining of histological sections can aid detection of specific organisms:
- Periodic acid–Schiff (PAS) stain for fungi
- Ziehl–Neelsen staining (ZN) for *Mycobacterium* or *Nocardia* spp.
- Gram staining for other bacterial infections (including *Nocardia* spp.).

Culture: Ultimately, identification of the exact aetiological agent in most cases of granulomatous or pyogranulomatous disease is based on culture. As the different agents each have specific growth requirements, the laboratory ought to be notified as to what organisms might be involved. In general, the clinician should ask for aerobic and anaerobic bacterial cultures and fungal culture. A specialist mycobacterial reference laboratory is recommended for the isolation of *Mycobacterium* spp., because of the particular requirements for growth.

Further investigations: Haematology, biochemistry, viral serology, urinalysis and diagnostic imaging may be

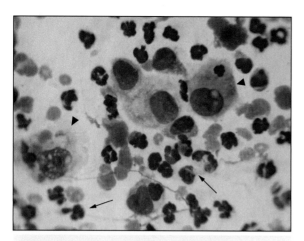

Figure 47.3 Neutrophils (arrows), macrophages (arrowheads) and red blood cells on an impression smear. Note the formation of a multinucleated giant cell.

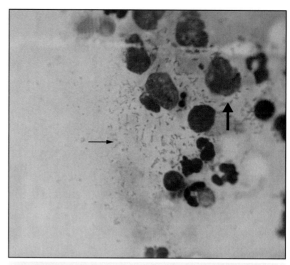

Figure 47.4 Intra- (bold arrow) and extracellular (arrow) rod-shaped organisms.

indicated if there is any evidence of systemic involvement or underlying immunosuppressive disease.

The following diagnostic tests were performed:

- In-house cytology of smears made from the exudate revealed pyogranulomatous inflammation, with mainly neutrophils, macrophages, giant cells and few lymphocytes (Fig. 47.3). Furthermore, extracellular pleomorphic rod-shaped organisms were present (Fig. 47.4) and, on others, filamentous organisms were present within a vacuole (Fig. 47.5).

- A swab sample of the seropurulent exudate did not produce any growth on either aerobic or anaerobic culture after 48 hours.

- Multiple deep biopsy samples, including skin and subcutaneous fat, were obtained under general anaesthesia. One was submitted for aerobic and anaerobic bacterial and fungal cultures, and one was submitted to a mycobacterial reference laboratory for mycobacterial culture. A *Nocardia* sp. and *Staphylococcus intermedius* were isolated from the aerobic culture of biopsy tissue. The exact species of *Nocardia* was not identified. The *Norcardia* sp. was sensitive to enrofloxacin, amoxicillin/clavulanate, ampicillin, cefalexin, oxytetracycline, penicillin and sulphonamide/trimethoprim. *Staphylococcus intermedius* was sensitive to enrofloxacin, cefalexin, oxytetracycline and sulphonamide/trimethoprim. Acid-fast bacilli were identified on cytological examination of impression smears of submitted tissue and *Mycobacterium fortuitum* was cultured from the tissue submitted to the TB reference laboratory.

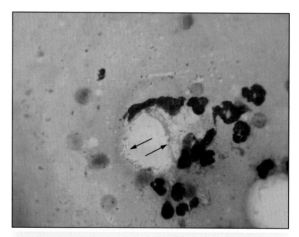

Figure 47.5 Filamentous bacteria (arrows) in vacuoles on an impression smear made from the exudates.

- Some tissue was fixed in formal saline and submitted for histology, which revealed pyogranulomatous dermatitis and panniculitis. In this case, microorganisms were not demonstrated, even with special stains. This is not unusual because acid-fast bacilli may be very difficult or impossible to find on ZN-stained tissue sections.

- Routine haematology, biochemistry and serology for FIV and FeLV were performed in an attempt to identify any potential underlying immunosuppressive conditions. The results of these tests were all within normal limits.

- Thoracic radiography failed to reveal any abnormalities in the lung tissue.

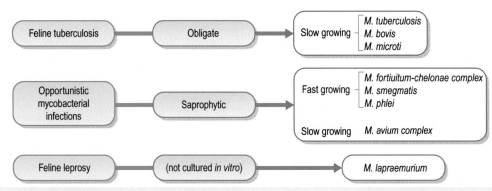

Figure 47.6 Feline mycobacterial syndromes and causative agents.

DIAGNOSIS

Pyogranulomatous dermatitis and panniculitis caused by concurrent infections with *Nocardia* and *Mycobacterium fortuitum*, which were confirmed on culture. It is likely that the *Staphylococcus intermedius* was a secondary invader or a contaminant in this case. How the organisms were introduced into the skin was not known, but a bite wound was suspected. No underlying cause of immunosuppression could be identified in this case.

PROGNOSIS

The prognosis depends on the causative organism, and the owner has to be made aware of the long duration of treatment required to cure pyogranulomatous or granulomatous dermatitis and panniculitis caused by RGM and other saprophytic bacteria. Owner compliance and willingness to treat for a long time are paramount for a successful outcome. The limiting factor in many cases is the ability of the client to administer the medication.

If investigations reveal an infection caused by *Mycobacterium tuberculosis* or *M. bovis*, public health issues should be considered and euthanasia should be advised.

AETIOPATHOGENESIS

In cats, there are numerous potential causes of nodules and draining tracts (Table 47.1), the most common route for the infection being a deep penetrating wound during a fight. In this case, two potentially causative organisms were isolated.

Mycobacterium spp. comprise a variable group of non-motile, non-spore-forming bacteria with different host specificities and pathogenic potential. The mycobacteria reported to cause cutaneous disease in cats are generally divided into obligate, facultative and saprophytic organisms (Fig. 47.6). This large genus may also be classified according to their cultural characteristics with slow-growing organisms that do (*M. tuberculosis*, *M. bovis* and *M. microti*) or do not (*M. avium* complex) produce tubercles, leproid granuloma-producing organisms (*M. lepraemurium*) and the rapidly growing mycobacteria that were previously termed opportunistic or atypical mycobacteria. The latter are a large group of organisms that are ubiquitous in soil and water. This group of organisms includes *M. fortuitum*, *M. chelonei*, *M. smegmatis* and *M. phlei*. Three different syndromes – panniculitis, pyogranulomatous pneumonia and disseminated systemic disease – are recognized as resulting from these rapidly growing mycobacteria.

Rapidly growing mycobacteria are not particularly virulent organisms. They gain entry via a penetrating wound, either a bite or foreign body. These organisms are lipophilic and there is a tendency for the disease to occur in obese cats, where it tends to affect the inguinal fat pad resulting in panniculitis. The organism tends to elicit a strong immune response that may or may not eliminate the organism. Unless the host is markedly immunosupressed, the organism is unlikely to produce disseminated disease.

Nocardia spp. are aerobic, Gram-positive, filamentous organisms that can cause a pyogranulomatous to granulomatous localized or generalized bacterial infection. The most commonly isolated species is *Nocardia asteroides*, but several other species are reported to affect the cat and dog. As with the RGM species, these are ubiquitous environmental organisms that are found in soil and water and gain entry either via inhalation or puncture wounds to the skin or mucosae. Although nocardiosis can result in pneumonia, cutaneous involvement is the most common presentation in cats with abscesses and pyogranulomatous lesions predominating. Some lesions may discharge sulphur granules. The severity of disease depends partly on the strain of organism and also on the susceptibility of the host. Immunosuppressed animals are predisposed to more severe disease manifestations.

Table 47.2 Antibiotics of choice for opportunistic mycobacterial infections

Drug	Dose and frequency
Enrofloxacin	5–15 mg/kg once daily
Marbofloxacin	2 mg/kg once daily
Doxycycline	5–10 mg/kg once daily
Clarithromycin	10–15 mg/kg twice daily

EPIDEMIOLOGY

Infections by rapidly growing mycobacteria and saprophytic bacteria are uncommon to rare, and are associated with wound contamination by organisms found in the environment. Some reports have suggested that RGM infections are more common in warm, humid climates but the disease is seen in cats from temperate climates and the organisms may be isolated from the soil of many temperate countries. In one study of feline RGM infections, there was no age predilection but females were markedly over-represented. Interestingly, males are reportedly predisposed to develop feline nocardiosis, presumably a reflection of their territorial behaviour. There was no age predisposition.

Feline tuberculosis is caused by slow-growing obligate mycobacteria (Fig. 47.6), such as *Mycobacterium bovis*, which is associated with cattle, and *Mycobacterium microti*, which are associated with voles and wild mice. Infections by *Mycobacterium tuberculosis* are very rare in cats.

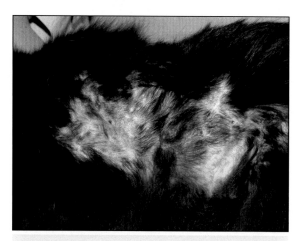

Figure 47.7 The cat 12 weeks post-treatment – there are still small draining lesions.

TREATMENT

Treatment for *Nocardia* and RGM infections should ideally be based on culture and sensitivity testing.

In most cases, the initial treatment of choice for nocardiosis is sulphonamide therapy, although a range of other antibacterials including ampicillin, cephalosporins, clarithromycin, doxycycline, erythromycin and ofloxacin have reportedly been effective.

Fluoroquinolones, doxycycline or clarithromycin are the treatments of choice for RGM infections (Table 47.2). Enrofloxacin is recommended in the interim period while waiting for the results of the tests. Doxycycline is the second line treatment for such infections. In some cases, combination therapy may be indicated. Doxycycline was the choice in this case because of the long-standing history and because the other two pathogenic microorganisms involved had shown in vitro susceptibility to it. It is a lipid-soluble tetracycline, which gives it good intracellular pen-

etration. As already stated, many months of treatment may be required to achieve a cure in these cases.

In some cases of severe disease, planned surgical debulking of infected tissue and reconstructive surgery for the wound closure is indicated. Extreme care is needed during surgery to prevent seeding organisms on to other sites and to prevent wound breakdown. It is best to refer these cases to an experienced soft-tissue surgeon. The residual infection is treated with post-surgical antibiosis.

Treatment in this case

The cat in this case was treated with enrofloxacin (5 mg/kg) for 14 days followed by doxycycline at the dose of 5 mg/kg every 12 hours before feeding, for 10 months (see 'Clinical tips'). The treatment was continued for 4 weeks beyond clinical cure (Figs 47.7 and 47.8).

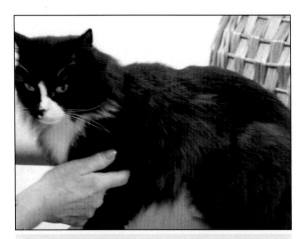

Figure 47.8 Complete hair regrowth after 10 months of treatment.

then forward it on if they are unable to do it themselves. It is best not to rely on a single test such as histology to rule out infectious causes.

The owner's ability to medicate the cat for prolonged periods should be taken into consideration when choosing the drug. Often, treatments fail because they are not administered for the extended periods necessary to effect a cure.

Some of these drugs are not licensed for veterinary use and written informed consent should be obtained from the client for their use. The patient should always be monitored for any adverse effects of the medication – e.g. oesophagitis, oesophageal ulceration and gastritis are reported with doxycycline – and it is therefore best to administer the medication prior to feeding, or followed by a drink.

The most common reason why surgery fails is wound breakdown, resulting from tension across the wound. This can be overcome by proper planning of the procedure and with adequate reconstruction for wound closure. It is possible that, even with well-planned surgery, not all the infected tissue will be removed and another reason for surgery to fail is too short a course of, or inappropriate choice of, postoperative antibiotic treatment.

FOLLOW-UP

This cat has been followed for 3 years and, up to the time of writing, there had been no recurrence of disease.

48 Multiple canine mast cell tumours

INITIAL PRESENTATION

Multiple cutaneous nodules in a Weimaraner.

INTRODUCTION

Mast cell tumours are the most common canine cutaneous neoplasm. They are challenging tumours to deal with in a clinical situation, because of their variable clinical appearance, variable behaviour and potential for malignancy. This report describes a case of multiple mast cell tumours in a Weimaraner.

CASE PRESENTING SIGNS

A 6-year-old, spayed female Weimaraner was presented with multiple cutaneous nodules.

CASE HISTORY

The history in cases of mast cell tumour (MCT) is variable. Tumours may have developed recently, or can have been present for months or even years and then suddenly start to behave in a malignant manner. Mast cell tumours are variably pruritic. There may be a history of sudden increases and decreases in tumour size over a period of hours to days. Alternatively, some dogs with MCT have a history of repeated episodes of erythema and urticaria or angioedema ('Dariers sign'). Both these scenarios are the result of a massive release of vasoactive mediators from the mast cells. Systemic signs, including vomiting, delayed wound healing and coagulopathies, may be evident.

This dog presented with the following history:

- A 12-month history of intermittent episodes of widespread urticaria, and angioedema involving the pinnae and eyelids.
- A 5-month history of multiple dermal nodules. According to the owner, some nodules appeared to be spontaneously resolving whilst others were increasing and decreasing in size.
- Over the past 3 months there had been a more rapid increase in the number of nodules and some lesions had ulcerated.
- Some of the nodular lesions had been mildly pruritic.
- Apart from occasional vomiting, there were no other signs suggestive of systemic involvement.
- There was no zoonosis.
- Recent treatment had consisted of chlorphenamine at a dosage of 0.4 mg/kg b.i.d. to treat any episodes of urticaria or angioedema, and systemic antibacterial therapy to treat secondary infection of ulcerated lesions. The use of chlorphenamine had, to a large extent, prevented the urticarial episodes.

CLINICAL EXAMINATION

Mast cell tumours most commonly present as raised or ulcerated cutaneous masses. They may be haired or hairless, single or multiple, dermal or subcutaneous. MCTs are often reported to resemble lipomas, but they can look and feel like many different skin diseases. They are seen most commonly on the skin of the trunk and hindquarters, and on the extremities. In most cases MCTs are solitary lesions, but around 10% of dogs present with multiple tumours.

In this case the findings were:
- A general physical examination was within normal limits.
- There were numerous subcutaneous nodules ranging from a few millimetres to 1–2 cm in diameter over the entire integument. Some of these nodules had an ulcerated surface, particularly those over the left hindlimb and one over the left pinna (Figs 48.1, 48.2 and 48.3).

DIFFERENTIAL DIAGNOSES

The differential diagnoses for multiple nodular lesions included:
- Neoplasia, including:
  - Mast cell tumour
  - Cutaneous lymphoma
  - Lipoma
  - Histiocytoma
- Sterile granulomatous/pyogranulomatous disease
- Bacterial or fungal granuloma.

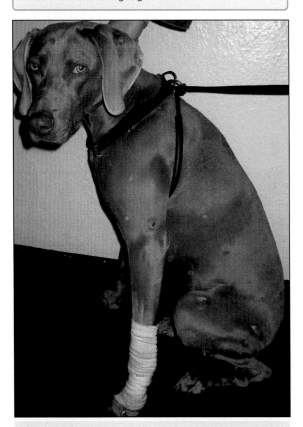

Figure 48.1 Generalized subcutaneous nodules on the entire body.

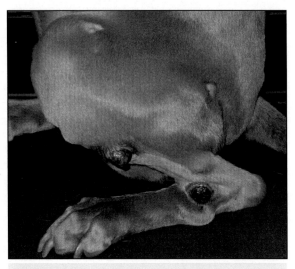

Figure 48.2 Ulcerated nodules on a hind limb.

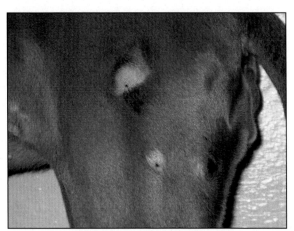

Figure 48.3 Close-up view of nodules on the left thigh.

CASE WORK-UP

The first step with any nodular disease is to perform fine-needle aspiration. Except in the case of poorly differentiated tumours, the diagnosis of MCTs is usually easily made on cytological examination of fine-needle aspirates. Diff Quik® or Rapi-Diff® are appropriate stains for cytological examination. Mast cells appear as small to medium-sized round cells, the nuclei are centrally placed within the cell, giving a 'fried egg' appearance, and the cytoplasm usually contains abundant dark staining granules (see Chapter 2). Eosinophils are frequently encountered. NB: Mast cell granules may be difficult to visualize in poorly differentiated MCTs.

The advantages of fine-needle aspiration over excisional biopsy are that it is inexpensive, it can be performed with the animal conscious and, in the case of mast cell tumour, is usually diagnostic. Additionally, an effective first surgery is most likely to result in a cure and prior fine-needle aspirates allow for effective surgical planning. The major limitation of fine-needle aspiration is that it is not possible to predict the behaviour of the tumour; histology is much more useful in this respect.

- Fine-needle aspirates were taken of several non-ulcerated nodules. Cytological examination of the aspirates showed large numbers of mast cells and occasional eosinophils (Fig. 48.4).

The cytology was consistent with a diagnosis of mast cell tumour. All mast cell tumours have metastatic potential, and the next stage was to clinically stage the case and establish the likelihood of metastasis prior to deciding on a treatment strategy.

Staging the tumour: Traditionally, a range of tests have been used to try and establish the presence or absence of metastatic disease. The tests include analysis of buffy coat smears, bone marrow aspiration, splenic and hepatic ultrasound-guided biopsies, radiographs and ultrasonography. Recent evidence has shown that some of these tests are of low specificity or sensitivity. For example, buffy coat smears were only positive in 30% of dogs with poorly differentiated tumours and were positive in dogs with 85 other diseases. Lymph node aspirates are of value, but mast cells may be seen in aspirates from dogs that do not have MCTs. Note that mast cell tumours tend to metastasize diffusely to visceral organs, and thoracic radiography is usually negative for the classic 'cannon-ball' metastases.

Bearing in mind these limitations, the following tests were carried out:
- Routine haematological and biochemical examinations showed a moderate basophilia (0.2×10^9/l).
- Urinalysis was unremarkable.
- No mast cells were seen on examination of fine-needle aspirates from the superficial lymph nodes.
- Abdominal ultrasound examination revealed splenomegaly, hyperechoic areas within the liver and an enlarged mesenteric lymph node. There was no evidence of systemic mastocytosis on cytological examination of fine-needle aspirates from these organs.
- Submission of four masses for histopathological examination confirmed that these were grade 1 mast cell tumours consisting of well-differentiated mast cells (see Table 48.2).

A clinical staging system has been developed (Table 48.1) that is of some value in predicting the behaviour of canine mast cell tumours. It can be seen from the table that this case fitted the criteria for stage 3B, on the basis of the clinical signs and diagnostic tests.

DIAGNOSIS

A diagnosis of multiple grade 1 mast cell tumours was made in this case.

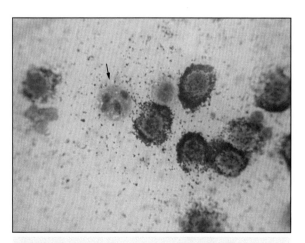

Figure 48.4 Mast cells with both intracellular and extracellular granules. Also shows an eosinophil (arrow).

Table 48.1 The World Health Organization staging for mast cell tumours

Clinical stage	Description
1	Solitary tumour confined to the dermis; no regional lymph node involvement
2	Solitary tumour confined to the dermis; regional lymph node involvement
3	Multiple dermal tumours or large infiltrative tumour; with or without regional lymph node involvement
4	Any tumour in which distal metastasis or recurrence with metastasis occurs; also includes blood or bone marrow involvement
A	Without systemic signs
B	With systemic signs

PROGNOSIS

No accurate estimate of malignancy or prediction of prognosis can be made on the clinical appearance of a mast cell tumour. The most important prognostic factor is the histological grade of the tumour. Tumours are classically categorized as well, intermediately or poorly differentiated. The grade is dependent on several factors relating to the cells, invasiveness and heterogeneity of the tumour (Table 48.2). The success of treatment correlates closely with the histological grade.

Well-differentiated mast cell tumours generally behave clinically as locally invasive tumours with a metastatic rate of less than 10%. Poorly differentiated tumours are more deeply infiltrative and metastasize in around 80% of cases to local lymph nodes, liver and spleen. Metastatic rates in intermediately differentiated tumours vary between 5% and 22%, and clinical behaviour of these tumours is difficult to predict.

In addition to the histological grade, various other prognostic indicators have been established and they are summarized in Table 48.3.

There were variable prognostic indicators in this case. Although histologically this was a well-differentiated tumour, it was at clinical stage 3B with evidence of vomiting and the tumours were rapidly growing, which potentially indicated a poor prognosis.

AETIOPATHOGENESIS OF MAST CELL TUMOUR

Mast cells are found in many tissues and play an important role as effecter cells in IgE-mediated allergic reactions and responses to parasitic disease. They are also important in non-IgE-mediated disease as 'orchestrators' of immunological reactions, via the production of many preformed and newly formed inflammatory mediators, including histamine, heparin, various enzymes and a vast array of cytokines. Some of the effects of these molecules are recognized in animals with mast cell tumours when degranulation occurs in response to mechanical trauma of the tumour mass. Histamine release can cause vomiting, gastric or duodenal ulceration and hypotensive episodes. Coagulopathies are associated with heparin release. Thus, these tumours should be handled gently.

The aetiopathogenesis of mast cell tumours is unknown, but a relationship to chronic inflammatory disease and in particular atopic dermatitis has been speculated, but remains unproven. Links between tumour grade and various genetic mutations, including the tumour suppressor gene p53 and the c-kit mast cell receptor, have been identified that may play a role in mast cell tumour development. The production of certain matrix metalloproteinases has been linked to the malignancy of mast cell tumours.

EPIDEMIOLOGY

Canine mast cell tumours are seen most commonly in middle-aged dogs, but have been reported in a wide age range from a few months to 20 years of age. Boxers, Boston terriers, golden retrievers, Staffordshire bull terriers, Weimaraners, Labradors, beagles and Shar Peis are reported to be predisposed. Interestingly, they are almost never encountered in hound breeds.

SURGICAL TREATMENT OPTIONS

Surgical excision is the most successful treatment for the management of canine mast cell tumour. For well-differentiated and for many intermediately differentiated

Grade	Histological criteria
1 (well differentiated)	Compact groups or rows of neoplastic cells confined to dermis separated by collagen fibres. Cells round, monomorphic, distinct cytoplasm, medium-sized intracytoplasmic granules, no mitotic figures, minimum oedema, no ulceration.
2 (intermediately differentiated)	More cellular tumour infiltrating lower dermis/subcutaneous tissue. Round to ovoid cells, some pleomorphic. Some cells have less distinct cytoplasm with large and hyperchromatic intracytoplasmic granules. Most have distinct cytoplasm with fine granules. Mitotic figures are 0–2 per high-power field. Areas of diffuse oedema or necrosis.
3 (poorly differentiated)	Dense sheets of pleomorphic cells. Indistinct cytoplasm with fine or not obvious intracytoplasmic granules. Binucleated cells common. Mitotic figures 3–6 per high-power field. Oedema, haemorrhage, necrosis common.

Table 48.2 Histological criteria used in determining grade of mast cell tumours

Table 48.3 Prognostic indicators in canine mast cell tumour

Prognostic factor	Description
Breed	Boxers are prone to developing mast cell tumours but they tend to be well differentiated and carry a better prognosis. Shar Peis may have more aggressive tumours.
Clinical stage	Higher stage disease carries a poorer prognosis.
Histological grade	Anaplastic tumours carry a poor prognosis – most dogs dead within 6 months. The majority of dogs with well-differentiated tumours should be cured with good surgical treatment.
Location	1. Tumours of the perianal, preputial, inguinal or subungual areas, or at mucocutaneous junctions, seem to have the poorer prognosis in some studies. 2. Tumours located at peripheral locations may carry a poorer prognosis because of failure of inexperienced surgeons to apply adequate surgical margins.
Rate of growth	Mast cell tumours that remain localized and are present for prolonged periods prior to presentation are usually well differentiated and behaviourally benign.
Number of tumours	It was thought that dogs presenting with multiple tumours had a poorer prognosis, but recent evidence has shown no difference in prognosis between dogs with single or multiple tumours.
Recurrence	Recurrence following surgical excision may make subsequent curative surgery difficult to attain.
Systemic signs	The presence of systemic signs (anoriexia, vomiting, melaena) is often indicative of more aggressive forms of mast cell tumour.
Argyrophilic nucleolar organizer regions (AgNORs)	This test is commercially available. The presence of these areas is said to relate to the proliferative ability of the tumour, with the higher grade mast cell tumours having a higher number AgNOR count.

tumours, surgical excision is likely to result in clinical cure. Because of the infiltrative nature of mast cell tumours, wide surgical margins of 3 cm and the removal of one fascial plane below the tumour is recommended, to ensure complete excision of the tumour cells. However, there is evidence that wide surgical excision may not necessarily affect outcome in dogs with well-differentiated tumours and that 'clean' margins are not a prerequisite for a good prognosis for these tumour grades.

Despite this, it should be borne in mind that the first surgery performed on a mast cell tumour provides the greatest opportunity for cure and, wherever possible, wide margins should be obtained. In some cases, referral should be considered if the surgeon is inexperienced and the site or tumour size precludes simple closure. In the case of well, or intermediately, differentiated tumours, a decision on appropriate margins may be made where aggressive surgical resection will potentially affect the function or quality of life. Clearly, prior histological evaluation of the mass is required in this situation.

In this case, after discussion with the owner, surgical excision of every tumour was not considered an appropriate therapy, because of the number of tumours and the likelihood of additional tumours developing following surgical excision of the current crop.

MEDICAL TREATMENT OPTIONS

Radiotherapy: Mast cell tumours are sensitive to the effects of moderate doses of radiation and good results have been reported in cases where there has been an incomplete excision of tumour.

Chemotherapy: Glucocorticoids are cytotoxic to mast cells and are the most frequently recommended therapy for the management of canine mast cell tumours, where there has been metastasis, or local recurrence and surgical excision or radiotherapy are no longer options. Treatment is considered to be palliative, but longer-term responses can occur. Prednisolone has been recommended at a dosage of 2 mg/kg s.i.d., p.o., for 2 weeks, then 1 mg/kg s.i.d., p.o., for 2 weeks then 1 mg/kg p.o., e.o.d., for 6 months. Uncontrolled studies have reported prednisolone to be very helpful in the management of canine mast cell tumour and to prevent tumour proliferation, but one controlled study demonstrated only a 24% response rate.

Other chemotherapeutic protocols described include CCNU (lomustine – 90 mg/m^2 every 4 weeks, p.o.), and a combination of prednisolone and vinblastine with response rates of 42% and 47% respectively. No single chemotherapeutic protocol has shown consistently reliable results. Vinblastine is myelosuppressive and a weekly CBC should be performed. If using CCNU, monitor CBC and liver enzymes prior to each administration and discontinue therapy if thrombocytopaenia or increased liver enzymes are seen.

The use of H2 receptor antagonists such as cimetidine or ranitidine should be considered to protect the gut against ulceration caused by histamine stimulation of gastric parietal cells. Gastric ulceration is most likely to occur in dogs with larger, bulky tumours, with recurrence of cutaneous disease or with systemic spread of MCTs. Animals undergoing surgery should be given H1 blocker premedication to prevent the risk of anaphylaxis due to massive histamine release.

Deionized water: The use of localized injections of deionized water around tumour excision sites has been proposed as an adjunct to surgical therapy for mast cell tumours. The presence of water has been shown to result in mast cell lysis. The proposed protocol was a minimum of four injections at 7- to 21-day intervals. Sufficient volume of water should be injected along the length of both edges of the skin incision to cause raised turgidity of the wound surface. General anaesthesia or sedation may be required as the injections can be painful.

If effective, this technique would be a useful alternative to radiation therapy for the management of cases where wide surgical excision was not possible, perhaps due to financial constraints. However, there have been conflicting reports on efficacy and larger-scale studies are required.

Treatment in this case:
- Radiation therapy was neither readily available nor appropriate because of the large numbers of tumours.

- After discussion with the owner, it was decided to excise the remaining ulcerated tumours and to treat palliatively with prednisolone at an initial dosage of 1 mg/kg.
- Treatment with ranitidine was also started at a dosage of 2.5 mg/kg b.i.d.

CLINICAL TIPS

Fine-needle aspiration is a very useful technique in nodular skin disease. In this case it would have been tempting to take impression smears from the surface of ulcerated tumours, avoiding the necessity of inserting a needle. This might have revealed the presence of large numbers of mast cells, but as the surface of such lesions is likely to have a granulating surface colonized by bacteria, the danger of this approach is that a misdiagnosis may be made. A far better technique is to sample intact, non-ulcerated lesions by fine-needle aspiration. If only ulcerated lesions are present, then the needle should be inserted through normal skin adjacent to the lesion deep into the nodule.

In any case, where multiple nodular lesions are present, it is good practice to sample all the lesions present. This is because mast cell tumours can resemble many different lesions and a single mast cell tumour may be missed if only one of the multiple lesions is sampled.

FOLLOW-UP

After around 6 weeks of this therapy there had been no significant beneficial response and prednisolone was discontinued due to unacceptable side-effects. Ranitidine was continued. Over the course of the next 3 years, further tumours appeared; occasionally, they ulcerated and were excised. The dog remained well with no evidence of systemic disease. Three years after initial diagnosis the dog was re-presented with multiple ulcerated tumours and was euthanized at the owner's request.

49 Histiocytoma

INITIAL PRESENTATION

A circumscribed nodule with haemorrhagic exudate and crusting in a dog.

INTRODUCTION

Canine cutaneous histiocytoma is a common benign solitary tumour that usually undergoes spontaneous regression. They tend to occur in younger dogs, on the pinnae, face or distal extremities. Histiocytoma can be difficult to differentiate from other tumours, such as plasmacytoma or mast cell tumour, and from localized granulomatous infections, just on clinical presentation alone. A systematic approach is required to make a diagnosis and then to taking the appropriate action, which will depend on the individual assessment.

CASE PRESENTING SIGNS

An 18-month-old female boxer was presented with a cutaneous nodule on the distal limb.

CASE HISTORY

The tumour has usually been noticed by the owner prior to presentation, although it may be detected on veterinary examination of the dog for other reasons. Dogs may draw their owner's attention to the tumour by obsessive licking. There are no systemic signs associated with histiocytoma.

In this case a small mass on the dog's left forelimb was noticed by the owner about 10 days prior to presentation. The dog had started to lick it and its size had increased. The dog's general health was unaffected.

CLINICAL EXAMINATION

Histiocytoma appears as a small (1–3 cm), solitary circumscribed dome or button and may, by the time of presentation, have an ulcerated surface with haemorrhagic crusts. The tumour is most commonly located on the face, pinnae or limbs and some dogs may have lymphadenopathy of the draining lymph node.

In this case a small, dome-shaped tumour with haemorrhagic surface crust was present on the lateral aspect of digit 5 of the left forefoot (Fig. 49.1). The draining lymph node was not palpable.

DIFFERENTIAL DIAGNOSES

The differential diagnoses in this case were:
- Cutaneous histiocytoma
- Plasmacytoma
- Mast cell tumour
- Sebaceous adenoma
- Melanoma
- Bacterial granuloma
- Fungal granuloma.

CASE WORK-UP

The history (age, breed and duration of onset) and clinical examination were suggestive of a cutaneous histiocytoma; however, the other differentials could not be ruled out on clinical examination alone. Boxers in particular are predisposed to mast cell tumour, so confirmation of the diagnosis of histiocytoma was essential, before deciding on the best course of treatment.

A fine-needle aspirate sample was obtained aseptically with a 23-gauge needle. The author's technique is to insert the needle into the lump and redirect it in and out in several directions and then remove it. A 10-ml

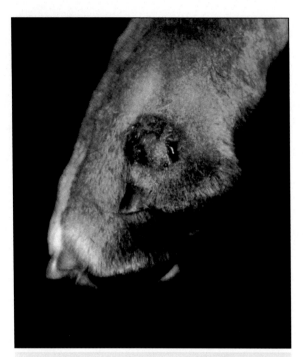

Figure 49.1 Small, button-shaped tumour with haemorrhagic crusts on the surface on the foot.

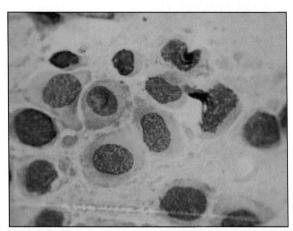

Figure 49.2 Round cells with round or indented nucleus and pale blue staining cytoplasm (note lack of granules).

syringe *containing air* is attached to the needle and the contents expressed onto a clean microscope slide by pushing in the plunger. Usually, this method produces a good harvest of cells. The slide is stained with modified Wright's stain or sent to a cytopathologist. A correct interpretation of the sample is essential to avoid a misdiagnosis, which could lead to major surgery or to other life-threatening treatments.

In this case, the fine-needle aspirate revealed a population of mononuclear cells with oval to round nuclei (some with indented nuclear membranes) and pale blue cytoplasm (Fig. 49.2). The cells lacked the granules that one would expect to see with mast cells, thus ruling out a mast cell tumour. Plasmacytomas have a smooth surface that is rarely ulcerated. Cells from a plasmacytoma generally have a more basophilic staining cytoplasm, and the cells show increased anisocytosis (variation in cell size) and anisokaryosis (variation in the size of the nucleus). Sebaceous gland adenomas and hyperplasia yield epithelial cells containing lipid vacuoles, which were not seen in this case, and infectious granulomas would yield large numbers of inflammatory cells such as neutrophils and macrophages that also were not present in this case.

However, with any fine-needle biopsies the quality of samples varies considerably. It may bleed, which results in a poor cell harvest, or it may just not be a representative sample of the cells. In these cases, the next best option is to take a wedge biopsy, or an excision biopsy if the site is in an area where a good margin of excision and wound closure can be guaranteed.

On this occasion, in addition to cytological examination, a wedge biopsy was also performed. Histology revealed a dense infiltration of large epitheloid cells in the epidermis and in the dermis (Fig. 49.3). The tumour cells had clear or lightly staining eosinophilic cytoplasm; and had the tumour been in a regression phase, lymphocytes and neutrophils would also have been seen. The epitheloid cells in the superficial dermis appear as loose cords arranged at right angles to the epidermis and the cells in the deep dermis appear as dense cords or nodules.

DIAGNOSIS

The tentative diagnosis of a histiocytoma was confirmed on histology.

PROGNOSIS

The prognosis for histiocytoma is good. The majority of tumours undergo spontaneous resolution without requiring treatment.

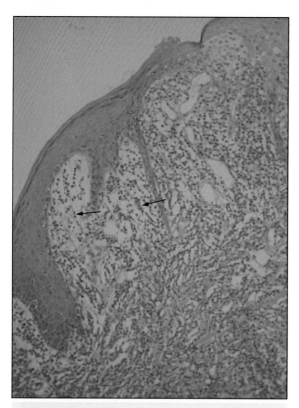

Figure 49.3 Histological section showing vertically orientated loose cords of epitheloid cells (arrows) with a denser infiltrate in the deeper portion of the dermis.

especially common in boxers, dachshunds, terriers, Labradors, cocker and English spaniels. There is no sex predilection. Although histiocytomas are benign, they have a tendency both to grow fast and to undergo spontaneous regression.

TREATMENT OPTIONS

Treatment options include wide-margin surgery or monitoring the tumours while waiting for them to regress spontaneously. Surgery has to be well planned, especially on the distal limb, to ensure that there is sufficient skin to close the wound. If there is increased tension in the wound, it invariably breaks down.

After a discussion of the options, because of the site involved in this case (distal limb) and given that spontaneous regression occurs in most cases, a decision to monitor the lesion was taken.

NURSING ASPECTS

An Elizabethan collar is used to prevent self-trauma during the regression phase. If surgical excision or biopsies are taken, appropriate postoperative advice and wound management are required.

IMMUNOPATHOGENESIS

Canine histiocytoma is a Langerhans' cell tumour. Langerhans' cells are antigen-presenting cells, capable of phagocytosing and presenting processed antigen to naive T lymphocytes that then mount a primary immune response, and also to memory T cells. They therefore play a major role in the induction of an immune response and in immune surveillance. They express CD1, CD11/18, CD45, MHC class II and E-cadherin. CD8+ lymphocytes often infiltrate the tumour and it is thought they are involved in the regression of the tumour. The cause of the proliferation of the Langerhans cells is not known.

EPIDEMIOLOGY

This tumour is most commonly found in young dogs under the age of 2 years, although it has been seen in older animals. There is a breed predisposition, and it is

CLINICAL TIPS

- Most cases resolve spontaneously and therefore a diagnosis based on cytology can be very useful.
- Surgery should be planned to allow proper wound closure and to avoid tension, which leads to wound breakdown.
- Regressing tumours have been known to develop secondary infections, so topical or possibly systemic antibacterial therapy may be required.

FOLLOW-UP

The lesion regressed completely within 4 weeks and no further treatment was required.

SECTION 7

DERMATOSES AFFECTING SPECIFIC SITES

50 Dermatoses of specific sites

INTRODUCTION

There are areas of skin that, by virtue of their anatomical location or specialized structure and function, deserve special attention when it comes to consideration of diseases affecting these sites. These areas include the face, eyelids, nasal planum, ears, pinnae, claws and claw beds, footpads and anal sacs. It is beyond the scope of this brief introduction to review all these sites in detail, but some consideration of the effect of the specialized structure or anatomical site may be of help.

SITES OF SPECIALIZED STRUCTURE AND FUNCTION

Footpads and nasal planum: The footpads and nasal planum are specially adapted to the function they perform. The footpads have a thick epidermis and an underlying fat pad that protect against mechanical trauma. The nasal planum also has a thick, protective epidermis and, grossly, has a cobblestone appearance. Perhaps in part due to the very thick epidermis, diseases affecting the keratinization process tend to be exaggerated in these sites (Fig. 50.1). The footpads, particularly, are sites of mechanical stress and are susceptible to trauma-exacerbated blistering diseases affecting the basement membrane zone. On the other hand, demodicosis does not occur and dermatophytosis is very rare in these sites, due to the absence of hair follicles.

Claws: Claw anatomy is covered in Chapter 56. There are a wide range of cutaneous and systemic diseases that may directly or indirectly result in claw involvement,

in both dogs and cats. The nail folds are a site of bacterial and yeast colonization, and secondary bacterial or yeast paronychia is a frequent finding in many generalized skin diseases (Fig. 50.2). Onychodystrophy is also a feature of many metabolic diseases, including hyperthyroidism in cats and hepatocutaneous syndrome and zinc-responsive dermatosis in dogs. Onychomadesis (loss of nails) may be a manifestation of autoimmune diseases that target the basement membrane. Claw disease, as a sole entity, is relatively uncommon, with a reported incidence of only 1–2% of referral dermatology cases.

Ears: The ears are highly specialized structures and this specialization has given them particular disease susceptibility. The ear canal is a cartilaginous structure lined by modified skin with hair follicles, and ceruminous and apocrine glands. Humidity within the ear canal naturally predisposes it to colonization by commensal organisms. Any alteration in the microclimate or local immune response within the ear canal can alter and/or increase glandular secretion, increase humidity and predispose it to overgrowth of potential pathogens.

Eyelids: The eyelids are complicated skin folds containing meibomian and Zeis glands that are modified sebaceous glands and the modified sweat glands known as Moll's glands. Diseases that affect the eyelids can affect tear film production and result in eye involvement. The eyelids are mucocutaneous junctions and the skin is thin and easily damaged by self-trauma. There are a number of generalized skin diseases, including demodicosis, *Malassezia* dermatitis and pyoderma (Fig. 50.3), and hypersensitivity disorders that produce an exagger-

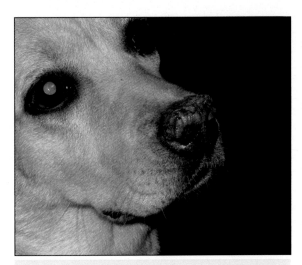

Figure 50.1 Hereditary nasal parakeratosis of Labradors, a disease confined to the nasal planum resulting in excessive thick adherent scale.

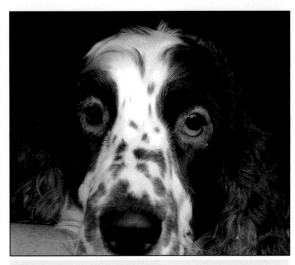

Figure 50.3 Deep pyoderma affecting the eyelids in a cocker spaniel. The underlying cause for the pyoderma was atopic dermatitis.

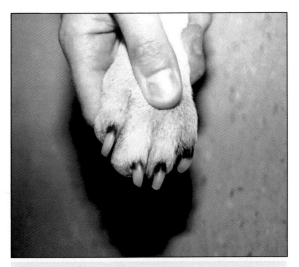

Figure 50.2 *Malassezia* paronychia. Brown staining over the proximal nails is a prominent feature of this disease.

ated response in the eyelids and periocular skin. Diseases such as hordeolum, a pyogenic infection of sebaceous glands of the eyelids, and chalazion, a chronic inflammation of meibomian glands, are examples of diseases confined to the eyelids.

Anal sacs: The anal sacs are hemispherical skin invaginations, lined by a squamous cornifying epithelium, with numerous apocrine and sebaceous glands that are located bilaterally to the anus and surrounded caudally

and laterally by the sphincter muscles. The anal sac duct opens at the mucocutaneous junction of the anus. Anal sac contents consist of products of apocrine and sebaceous glands, epidermal exfoliation, and local bacterial and yeast metabolism. Anal sac disease is a common but still poorly understood presentation in small animal practice. Disease may present as impaction, infection, abscessation and neoplasia. Anal sac disease may be a manifestation of a generalized skin problem and apparent repeated anal sac impactions may be a manifestation of a hypersensitivity disorder, although whether the irritation is due to perineal pruritus rather than the anal sac impaction is not always clear. Some work has been done in recent years on characterizing the nature and microbial content of anal sac secretions, and cytological examination of anal sac contents should be standard practice.

Effect of anatomical location: The anatomical site of some of the specialized areas of skin has a bearing on disease predisposition. The nails, footpads, nasal planum and pinnae are situated on the extremities. These are sites that are exposed to a variety of different sorts of trauma and environmental factors. Traumas include fight wounds and penetrating foreign bodies. Sites such as the face and pinnae are highly exposed to ultraviolet light, and this is a major factor in the development of actinic keratoses and squamous cell carcinoma, particularly in non-pigmented animals. The extremities tend to

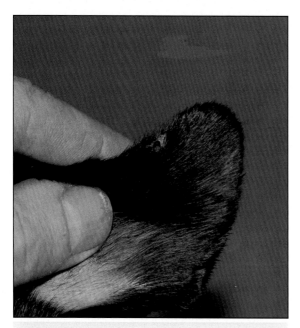

Figure 50.4 Ulceration and scarring of the pinnal margin in a cross-bred dog: cold-induced vasculopathy.

have poorer vascular perfusion and are thus predisposed to the effects of vascular disease. On a similar note, these are sites that are also susceptible to cold-induced disease, where decreased temperature may precipitate agglutination of serum proteins, leading to infarction and tissue damage, as in cold agglutinin disease (Fig. 50.4).

CLINICAL APPROACH

A structured approach is required when investigating disease in these specialized areas of skin when such a diverse range of aetiologies can be involved. A detailed history and full physical and dermatological examinations are required to draw up a complete differential diagnosis list, and then a series of diagnostic tests are likely to be required in order to make a specific diagnosis. The general approach is therefore the same as for any skin disease but there may be special requirements in the technique and interpretation of diagnostic tests and the management of disease in these sites.

These are areas that may be difficult to sample for skin scraping and cytology, and some imagination may be required. Hair plucks are easily utilized for the investigation of demodicosis in sites such as the feet and eyelids (see Chapter 2), and cotton buds may be employed to obtain samples for cytology from sites where a direct impression would not be possible. The anatomical site may dictate the use of general anaesthesia for histopathological examination and in some cases complete amputation of a digit may be required.

Histopathological interpretation of skin biopsies from specialized sites can be challenging. The nasal planum and muzzle region are sites that are readily exposed to environmental microbes, contactants and allergens, and are highly involved in immune surveillance. This is reflected by the number of immunologically active cells (lymphocytes, plasma cells and histiocytes) found in the superficial dermis of healthy skin in these areas. It takes an experienced dermatohistopathologist to differentiate the normal from the abnormal on biopsy samples from these areas.

Lastly, the management of disease in these areas may pose special problems and require specific techniques. Disease affecting specialized areas is often focal and potentially amenable to topical therapy. Consideration must be given to the most effective method of applying medication and the use of an Elizabethan collar may be required to prevent licking. Ear flushing is an essential part of the effective management of otitis externa and is discussed in detail later in this section.

Feline cowpox virus infection

INITIAL PRESENTATION

Facial dermatitis and distal limb cellulitis in a cat.

INTRODUCTION

Cowpox virus infections in cats, although uncommon, have been increasingly recognized in certain parts of the UK and in Europe. They are referred to as feline cowpox or cat pox. Feline cowpox belongs to the genus *Orthopoxvirus* and is indistinguishable from cowpox virus. The infection is mainly seen in cats from rural areas that hunt and are bitten by small mammals. The first lesion appears at the site of inoculation (bite wound) and then spreads to other sites. The infection is of zoonotic importance, and is known to cause painful localized lesions and lymphadenopathy in people, particularly in those that are immunocompromised.

CASE PRESENTING SIGNS

A neutered male domestic short-haired cat, 4 years and 7 months of age, was presented with cellulitis and abscessation on the right forelimb, with an ulcerated lesion on the face.

CASE HISTORY

In most cases, the condition has a rapid onset and is of a short duration (a few days to a few weeks) at presentation, with no previous history of skin disease. In most cases, the owners are aware that the cat is a hunter because it brings prey into the house. Usually, at the time of presentation, there is no history of zoonosis and in-contact animals are usually unaffected. In some cases lethargy, inappetence and systemic signs may be reported.

The significant history in this case was:
- The cat was presented in late June.
- The owner had noticed a small crusted lesion on the foot a few days previously, which was now much larger, and developed further lesions on the face.
- The lesions were non-pruritic.
- The cat was not reported as being systemically ill.
- Cats were allowed to roam freely in a rural area.
- The in-contact cat and dog were unaffected and no zoonosis was reported.
- Flea control was only intermittently used; however, the cats were frequently wormed with proprietary wormer, because of their predisposition to tapeworm infestations.
- The cat was fed on a variety of commercial wet and dry foods.

CLINICAL EXAMINATION

Most cats present with multiple lesions but most cases start with a single lesion, either on the face or on the forelimbs. Usually, there is a secondary bacterial infection of the site resulting in an abscess, with necrosis and even sloughing by the time of examination. Some cases may present with a large ulcer where the necrotic skin has already sloughed off. Secondary lesions on distant sites are usually evident within 10 days, normally on the face, but sometimes on the trunk. Usually, they are single circumscribed raised papules, or nodules, which progressively become ulcerated and alopecic. Occasionally, larger areas become involved and then there will be marked ulceration and exudation. Unless the owner is very vigilant the very first lesion, the erythematous macule, is missed. In about 20% of cats, ulcerations in the oral cavity and the tongue are reported; systemic signs of pyrexia, lethargy, anorexia, conjunctivitis, respiratory and GIT involvement may also be reported. The lesions are self-limiting, unless the individual is immunosuppressed, due to concurrent conditions such as FIV, FeLV, or because of immunosuppressive therapy.

The relevant findings in this case were:

- Cellulitis, purulent exudate, erythema and skin necrosis involving an area of about 4 cm in length on the anterior right carpus (Fig. 51.1).
- Three single lesions at various stages were seen – a small erythematous macule (3 mm), a papule with surface crust (0.5 cm) and a larger lesion with ulcerated surface (1 cm) were present on the bridge of the nose and on the right medial canthus (Fig. 51.2).
- The peripheral lymph nodes were palpable.
- The results of the examination of other organ systems were within normal limits.

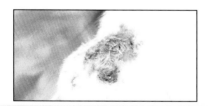

Figure 51.1 Large necrotic lesion on the distal foot.

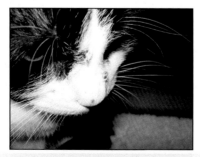

Figure 51.2 Facial lesions at different stages of the disease.

DIFFERENTIAL DIAGNOSES

The single lesion on its own could be easily diagnosed as a cat-bite abscess. However, when seen with the lesions at distant sites ranging from an erythematous macule to an ulcerated nodule, and when seen in a hunting cat, cowpox virus infection is high on the list of differentials. Other infectious diseases could also result in such lesions, but then the primary erythematous macule is not seen.

The differential diagnoses in this case were:
- Feline cowpox virus infection
- Mycobacterial or opportunistic mycobacterial infections
- Deep mycoses (sporotrichosis, cryptococcosis or phaeohyphomycosis)
- Cat-bite abscesses
- Eosinophilic granuloma complex and associated underlying conditions
- Dermatophytosis
- Bacterial granuloma (acid-fast or non-acid-fast organisms)
- Neoplasia.

CASE WORK-UP

In addition to the history and clinical examination, further investigations are needed to confirm the diagnosis of feline cowpox virus. The relevant tests include impression smears, histological examination of skin biopsies, virus isolation by culture, demonstration of rising pox virus-specific antibody titre in the serum, and demonstration of the virus by electron microscopy, or viral DNA by PCR.

In this case, impression smears from the ulcerated lesions on the face revealed mixed inflammatory cells, mainly neutrophils with few lymphocytes. There was no evidence of intracellular bacteria at this site; however, rod and coccoid bacteria were seen within neutrophils on a smear from the leg.

Under general anaesthesia, the crust from the main lesion was removed, placed in a sterile container and submitted for virus isolation. Pox virus was cultured from this material. Skin samples were taken at the same time, using a 6-mm biopsy punch, from the edge of the main lesion and an excision biopsy was taken from the lesion on the bridge of the nose. The histology revealed ballooning degeneration of keratinocytes, some with intracytoplasmic eosinophilic inclusion bodies.

DIAGNOSIS

Feline cowpox infection was confirmed by viral culture and histopathology in this case.

PROGNOSIS

The prognosis is good, as in most cases the infection is self-limiting; however, cats with concurrent immunosuppressive diseases, such as FIV and FeLV, can develop more serious lesions involving internal organs. The disease has a high zoonotic potential; care must be taken during the examination and appropriate advice on handling given to the owners (see 'Clinical tips').

AETIOPATHOGENESIS

Feline cowpox virus is closely related to other viruses in the family Poxviridae, which include the smallpox virus (now eradicated), vaccinia virus (smallpox vaccine) and infectious ectromelia virus. Although the name cowpox implies an infection in cattle, it is rarely reported in cattle and they are not the main source of infection for cats. The feline cowpox virus is very closely related to the cowpox virus and the two are indistinguishable; however, some of the European strains of cowpox virus differ from the traditional strains and they are referred to as 'cowpox virus-like strains'.

Feline cowpox virus infection is seen in hunting cats. The infection is through direct contact with an infected rodent, at a site where there is a bite wound or break in the skin. The virus multiplies at the site, causing a single primary lesion on the forelimb or the head. It then spreads to the local draining lymph node, resulting in viremia followed by spreading to other cutaneous sites and even internal organs. Infection can also occur oronasally, which tends to cause a less severe disease. Spread to in-contact cats sometimes occurs, but even if there is seroconversion, clinical lesions are not always seen.

EPIDEMIOLOGY

There is no age, sex or breed predilection, but the condition is more or less exclusively seen in cats that hunt. Infection has been reported in the UK and in European countries including the Netherlands, Germany, Belgium, France, Italy and Austria. The incidence of the disease is closely associated with the population dynamics of the small mammal reservoirs, such as bank voles (*Cletrionomys glareolus*), field voles (*Microtus agrestis*) and wood mice (*Apodemus sylvaticus*). Antibodies to cowpox virus have been detected in field voles and wood mice in the UK, supporting this theory of the source of infection. The cases peak in the autumn, although sporadic cases can occur at other times.

The incidence of cowpox virus infections in humans is not known, but less than a handful are reported each year. The infection in humans is mainly associated with infected pet cats, although in some cases the source cannot be traced.

Cowpox virus infections have been reported in other species, (cattle, dogs and foals) and in wild animals (cheetahs, elephants, rhinoceroses and okapi) in zoos.

TREATMENT

There is no specific treatment for the viral infection; however, cases with secondary bacterial involvement, as in this case, should be treated with a broad-spectrum bacteriocidal antibiotic. Cats with more severe systemic signs will require appropriate supportive care. The cat in this case was treated with 12.5 mg/kg, twice daily, of amoxicillin/clavulanate for 21 days.

Corticosteroids are contraindicated, even at anti-inflammatory doses, because their use can result in severe systemic infections.

NURSING ASPECTS

- The infection can potentially be transmitted to people and therefore barrier nursing should be practised when handling cats suspected to have feline cowpox virus infections.
- Some cats may need an Elizabethan collar to prevent self-mutilation.
- Severely affected cats may require supportive fluid therapy and additional nursing such as bandaging and wound cleansing with antiseptic solutions.
- The examination table, cat cage and baskets should be thoroughly cleaned out with a virucidal disinfectant or sodium hypochlorite (household bleach). The virus, like other pox viruses, can survive under dry conditions for several years.

CLINICAL TIPS

- Veterinary personal and owners should wear gloves when handling the animal, as this virus has zoonotic potential.
- Owners should keep handling of cats to a minimum while they still have lesions.
- Contact with immunosuppressed people, young children and the elderly should be avoided, as they are most at risk of infection.
- When presented with lesions, where an infectious organism (bacteria, virus or fungi) is suspected, *do not administer glucocorticoids* as a symptomatic treatment. Glucocorticoids invariably exacerbate the condition and may result in severe systemic involvement.

FOLLOW-UP

The cat recovered uneventfully within 4 weeks and there was no recurrence.

52 Eosinophilic folliculitis and furunculosis

INITIAL PRESENTATION

Sudden onset of nodules with ulceration, crusting and bleeding on the nose of a collie cross.

INTRODUCTION

Canine eosinophilic furunculosis is an uncommon condition with an acute onset. It is usually confined to the nose and the muzzle, although it can occur on the pinna and the trunk. The severity of the lesions varies and many dogs will exhibit signs of pruritus. In most cases, it is thought to result from an acute hypersensitivity reaction to arthropod antigens. The condition is similar to mosquito-bite hypersensitivity in cats.

CASE PRESENTING SIGNS

A 4-year-old, neutered female collie cross was presented with a sudden onset of pruritus, nodules, ulceration and crusting on the nose.

CASE HISTORY

Most dogs are presented with a history of a sudden onset of symptoms. Only when questioned is the owner likely to report a possible recent exposure to insects.

In this case the owner reported that:
- The dog had yelped during a walk on the previous day.
- The next day the dog was constantly rubbing its muzzle and haemorrhagic papules and plaques had appeared on the bridge of its nose.
- There was no previous history of dermatological disease.
- The dog's appetite and demeanour were unaffected.

- The dog was presented in December, when insect activity in the UK is assumed to be absent; however, this was in a year when mild autumn conditions extended into December.

CLINICAL EXAMINATION

A physical examination revealed enlarged submandibular lymph nodes, but all other parameters were within normal limits. Multiple nodules, some with an ulcerated surface and some with a haemorrhagic crust, were present on the bridge of the nose (Fig. 52.1). The dog resented examination of this site. None of the other sites were affected in this case.

DIFFERENTIAL DIAGNOSES

The most likely differential diagnoses based on the history were:
- Canine eosinophilic furunculosis of the face
- Bacterial folliculitis and furunculosis
- Sterile pyogranulomatous dermatitis
- Tick-bite hypersensitivity
- Contact irritant or allergic dermatitis.

An adverse drug reaction can also have a sudden onset, but the dog in this case had not been medicated for over 12 months. Other less likely diagnoses include:
- Dermatophyte kerions
- Pemphigus complex
- Neoplasia.

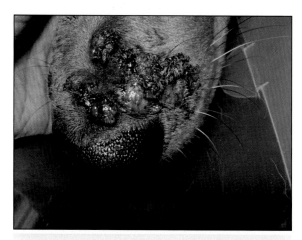

Figure 52.1 Large nodules with haemorrhagic crusts and oozing on the bridge of the nose.

However, the onset in these conditions is slow and the lesions progressively worsen. Furthermore, they usually involve multiple sites, so they can easily be ruled out during the case work-up.

CASE WORK-UP

The case work-up should include, or rule out, the differential diagnoses. In this case, the following tests were performed:

- Cytological examination of impression smears (obtained from the surface of the ulcerated lesions and stained with modified Wright's stain), which revealed numerous eosinophils and red blood cells, a few neutrophils and macrophages, but no bacteria.
- A swab sample was submitted for bacterial culture, which failed to produce any microbial growth after prolonged incubation.
- Gross and microscopic examination of coat brushings, which failed to reveal any evidence of ectoparasites.
- Hair plucks and skin scrapings taken from the edge of the lesions, which failed to reveal any *Demodex* mites.
- Routine haematology and biochemistry were within normal limits, although peripheral eosinophilia was reported.
- Three skin samples from the affected areas (one excision biopsy of a nodule and two 6-mm punch biopsies) were obtained under general anaesthetic for histopathological examination.

The excision biopsy and one punch biopsy were placed in pots containing 10% formal saline and submitted for histology.

A biopsy sample is required to culture certain bacterial organisms and fungi, so the second punch biopsy was placed in a sterile pot, in sterile saline to keep it moist, and was submitted for bacterial and fungal culture. In this case, there was no bacterial growth on aerobic and anaerobic culture after 72 hours, and no fungal growth after 3 weeks of incubation.

A tentative diagnosis of canine eosinophilic furunculosis was made, based on the history, clinical signs and the cytological findings before the results of bacteriology and histology were known. Treatment was started to provide relief to the dog, as this condition is intensely pruritic and in some cases painful.

Histological examination then revealed epidermal ulceration with moderate epidermal acanthosis, intense eosinophilic infiltrate around the intact and disrupted hair follicles, and fragments of keratin present in the dermis. Dermal oedema and haemorrhage were also present. These changes were consistent with eosinophilic furunculosis. Fungal elements were not demonstrated on Periodic acid–Schiff (PAS)-stained histological sections.

In recurring cases, further evaluation of the role of insects may be determined by intradermal testing using insect antigens. However, due to the limited availability of these allergens for intradermal testing and the wide range of insects that could have been involved, it was not undertaken in this case.

DIAGNOSIS

Canine eosinophilic furunculosis was confirmed on histology but the trigger for the condition was not determined, although an insect bite was implicated.

PROGNOSIS

The prognosis for this condition is good, although the owner has to be warned of possible recurrences if the dog is exposed to the allergens again. Rapid, appropriate glucocorticoid therapy is indicated in more severely affected cases because scarring may result if treatment is excessively delayed.

AETIOPATHOGENESIS

A hypersensitivity response to arthropod venom is the most likely cause of the symptoms in these cases, even though in most cases the actual exposure is not seen by the owner. Wasps, bees, mosquitoes, spiders, hornets, black flies, stable flies and other stinging insects have all been implicated.

In dogs, Type I and IV hypersensitivity mechanisms are thought to be involved, although in humans Type III and Type IV mechanisms have been proposed for arthropod-bite reactions. Type III and Type IV reactions are implicated for tick-bite reactions in dogs.

Exposure to insect venom in sensitized individuals leads to mast cell degranulation and the consequent release of inflammatory mediators. These mediators are involved in further recruitment of inflammatory cells, in particular eosinophils, to the site. The eosinophils in turn produce toxins, enzymes and cytokines, all of which lead to extensive tissue damage and help to perpetuate the lesions (see Chapter 36).

EPIDEMIOLOGY

Eosinophilic furunculosis is an uncommon condition that is seen in dogs of any age, although more than half the reported cases are in dogs less than 2 years old. This age distribution may arise because it is the younger, less experienced, dogs that are more likely to disturb insect nests.

There is no reported sex or breed predisposition, but it is thought that larger breeds, living outdoors, may be more prone to it than smaller, indoor, dogs. A higher incidence has been observed in the warmer months, when insect activity is at its highest; however, it is reported in winter months and in dogs living indoors.

TREATMENT

Systemic glucocorticoids are indicated in all cases for rapid response, although resolution without treatment has been reported. The treatment of choice is prednisolone administered at 1 mg/kg daily, ideally until resolution of lesions, then reduced to alternate days, and gradually tapered off and withdrawn. Most cases respond within 48 hours and resolve within 3 weeks.

Topical ointments or gels containing corticosteroids can be applied to the lesions; however, topical treatment alone is not sufficient to provide complete and quick relief to the dog.

Sedatives such as acetylpromazine may be prescribed for the first few days to stop self-trauma, if one is unable to make a tentative diagnosis based on surface cytology and needs to wait for results before starting glucocorticoids.

Treatment in this case

Treatment was started with prednisolone at 1 mg/kg for 10 days which was then reduced to 0.5 mg/kg every alternate day for 2 weeks until resolution of lesions when glucocorticoid therapy was withdrawn.

Cases should be monitored for evidence of secondary bacterial infection and antibacterial treatment started if required.

NURSING ASPECTS

A Buster collar should be used in most cases to prevent self-trauma.

CLINICAL TIPS

This is one of the few conditions that have both a sudden onset of severe lesions and pruritus. In most cases the history and clinical signs are suggestive of the condition, and in most cases a tentative diagnosis can be made by simple in-house cytology. Treatment should be started immediately, after obtaining the appropriate biopsy samples necessary to confirm the diagnosis.

FOLLOW-UP

There has been no recurrent episode of the condition up to the time of writing (2 years later).

53 Cutaneous lupus erythematosus

INITIAL PRESENTATION

Ulceration, crusting and leucoderma on the nasal planum in a dog.

INTRODUCTION

Although discoid (cutaneous) lupus erythematosus is uncommon, it is still the most frequently encountered immune-mediated disease in general practice. Generally, the lesions are confined to the bridge of the nose and the nasal planum; however, they can occur on feet and other mucocutaneous sites, such as the genitalia and anal mucosa. The condition is aggravated by sunlight. There has been some discussion on the use of the term 'discoid lupus erythematosus', as the clinical presentation is different from that seen in humans and the histology of the condition is not lupus specific (it is also commonly seen in mucocutaneous pyoderma). It has been suggested that the term cutaneous lupus erythematosus may be more appropriate. This case report describes the condition on the nasal planum and the feet of a dog and is referred to as cutaneous lupus erythematosus.

CASE PRESENTING SIGNS

An 8-year-old, neutered male boxer was presented with a crusting and ulcerative dermatosis of the nose.

CASE HISTORY

Generally, lesions are first noted on the nose and less frequently other sites may become involved. An astute owner may also be aware of a seasonal exacerbation of the clinical signs. The duration of the condition varies between individuals, and it may wax and wane over several weeks or months. Pruritus is variable.

In this case the relevant history was:
- The dog was rehomed by a rescue centre, where it had been held for about 6 months.
- Lesions were present on the nose and the feet at the time the dog was first taken into the rescue centre, and had been investigated. A tentative diagnosis of discoid lupus erythematosus with secondary infection was made based on histopathological examination but a 6-week course of cefalexin had been prescribed to rule out the involvement of mucocutaneous pyoderma, which is indistinguishable from cutaneous lupus on histopathology.
- The condition only partially improved with the cefalexin, so the dog was prescribed 500 mg t.i.d. of oxytetracycline and 500 mg t.i.d. of nicotinamide for several months, again with a poor response.
- The present owner reported that the dog resented pedal examination and was only able to walk for short distances.
- The nasal lesions were prone to haemorrhage if traumatized.
- The dog was not pruritic.
- Appetite was unaffected.

CLINICAL EXAMINATION

Most frequently, lesions will be distributed on the bridge of the nose and the nasal planum. Erythema, ulceration,

303

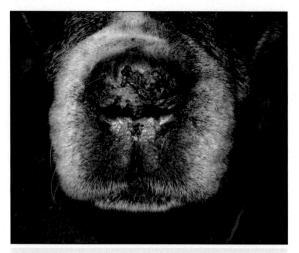

Figure 53.1 Crusting, ulceration and depigmentation on the nasal planum. Note the loss of the cobblestone appearance.

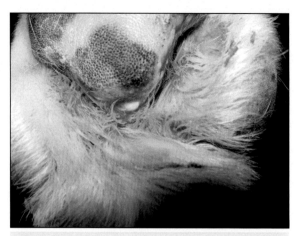

Figure 53.2 Plantar aspect of the foot, showing marked ulceration, crusting and erythema.

crusting, scaling and alopecia are the most common signs on the bridge of the nose. The nasal planum usually loses its cobblestone appearance, becoming smooth with depigmentation, crusting and ulceration. In rare cases, the condition may involve other sites, such as the ears, lip margins, periorbital areas, pinnae, genital areas and the feet.

The examination in this case revealed the following signs:
- Apart from a reactive peripheral lymphadenopathy, involving prescapular and popliteal lymph nodes, the general physical examination was unremarkable.
- Cutaneous lesions were limited to the nasal planum and the feet.
- The nasal planum had lost its cobblestone appearance, leaving a smooth surface with severe crusting, ulceration, hypopigmentation and a deep fissure on the nasal philtrum (Fig. 53.1).
- Painful lesions were present on the plantar aspects of all four feet consisting of well-demarcated ulceration with serpiginous borders at the junction of the central pads and the surrounding skin (Fig. 53.2).
- Crusting and hypopigmentation were evident on the footpads.
- The surrounding skin was markedly erythematous.

DIFFERENTIAL DIAGNOSES

The differential diagnoses included all the ulcerative conditions that affect the mucocutaneous sites:
- Cutaneous lupus erythematosus
- Pemphigus vulgaris
- Vasculitis
- Cutaneous lymphoma (epitheliotropic or non-epitheliotropic)
- Mucocutaneous pyoderma
- Drug eruption
- Erythema multiforme
- Metabolic epidermal necrosis
- Squamous cell carcinoma
- Deep mycoses
- Uveodermatological syndrome.

CASE WORK-UP

Given the previous history and histopathology results, cutaneous lupus erythematosus was still the most likely diagnosis despite the previous poor response to treatment. However, it is possible that a secondary infection was masking some other differential, or that the biopsy samples might have been obtained from inappropriate sites.

It was decided that a thorough work-up was required and the following tests were performed:

- Cytological examination of an impression smear from an ulcerated lesion, which revealed intra- and extracellular coccoid bacteria, but no acantholytic keratinocytes.
- Routine haematology, biochemistry and urinalysis, which were within normal limits.
- An antinuclear antibody test, which was negative.
- Crusts and tissue biopsies were submitted for fungal culture, which was negative.
- *Staphylococcus intermedius* was isolated from a skin swab taken from an ulcerated area (the organism was sensitive to enrofloxacin, amoxicillin/clavulanate, cefalexin, oxytetracycline and cefuroxime, and it was resistant to ampicillin, penicillin and trimethoprim sulphonamide).
- Before undertaking further investigation, antibiotic treatment (cefalexin 20 mg/kg b.i.d. for 4 weeks) was prescribed to resolve the bacterial component. This resulted in little improvement in the cutaneous lesions but no bacteria were found on repeat cytological examination at the end of the course of treatment.
- Seven skin sample (six punch and one elliptical) biopsies were obtained from the pads and the nasal planum under general anaesthesia, for histology.

The elliptical biopsy (2.5 cm in length and 1 cm wide) was taken from the pad at right angles to the ulcerated lesion, which allowed examination of the junction between the ulcerated and non-ulcerated skin. Histology revealed an interface dermatitis, with dense infiltration of mononuclear cells at the dermoepidermal junction and hydropic degeneration and apoptosis of basal keratinocytes (Fig. 53.3). Pigmentary incontinence and focal separation above the basal epidermis were present. This focal clefting was not typical of pemphigus vulgaris, where the basal cells remain attached to the basement membrane, giving the 'tombstone-like appearance to the bottom of the cleft or vesicle'. Uveodermatological syndrome was ruled out on histology because macrophages are the main inflammatory cell type in this condition and hydropic changes of the basal layer are absent. There was no evidence of vasculitis or neoplastic cells in the biopsy material. The histology was consistent with a lupus-type condition, but could not differentiate between the two clinical forms: cutaneous and vesicular lupus erythematosus. However, the latter condition is mostly reported in Shetland sheepdogs, rough collies and collie crosses, and the lesions for this condition are mainly found on the inguinal and axillary areas. Thus, this condition could be ruled out on clinical appearance.

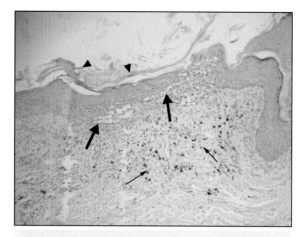

Figure 53.3 Histological section showing hyperkeratosis (arrowheads), hydropic degeneration of the basal layer (bold arrows), pigmentary incontinence (arrows) and inflammatory cells at the dermoepidermal interface.

DIAGNOSIS

The histology was consistent with a lupus-specific disease. A diagnosis of cutaneous lupus erythematosus was made, based on the combination of history, distribution, clinical signs and histological changes.

PROGNOSIS

The prognosis for cutaneous lupus is fair to good; however, most cases wax and wane, and lifelong management of the condition is required. The prognosis also depends on what treatment is required and how well it is tolerated by the individual.

IMMUNOPATHOGENESIS OF CUTANEOUS LUPUS ERYTHEMATOSUS

The cause of cutaneous lupus erythematosus is not fully understood, but because the disease is photoaggravated, it is proposed that ultraviolet light in some way alters the expression of keratinocyte cell surface antigens. These novel antigens lead to an autoimmune response involving the formation of autoantibodies and antibody-dependent cytotoxicity of keratinocytes. In humans, helper T cells are involved in the pathogenesis, whereas in dogs plasma cells predominate in the cellular infiltrate at the dermo-epidermal interface. It is therefore thought that, in dogs, antibody-producing B cells are more important in the pathogenesis.

EPIDEMIOLOGY

There is a higher incidence of this disease in dolicocephalic breeds, such as collies, German sheepdogs, Shetland sheepdogs, Siberian huskies and German short-haired pointers; however, it can occur in any breed. There is a seasonal exacerbation of the clinical signs in the summer. Age predilections have not been reported, but bitches may be more predisposed than dogs.

TREATMENT

There are a number of treatment options for this condition, ranging from benign topical, to aggressive systemic immunosuppressive therapy. The treatment should be individualized in each case, to give maximum effect with the least adverse effects. Cutaneous lupus erythematosus is a relatively benign disease and topical treatment is preferred in most cases to avoid the adverse effects of some systemic therapies.

Topical treatments

A major disadvantage of topical therapy is that the dog can lick it off before it has a chance to penetrate the skin. However, feeding, or otherwise distracting the dog after application, can allow the treatment time to penetrate and licking should not be a reason not to attempt topical therapy. Obviously topical therapies should not carry a risk of systemic adverse effects if ingested.

Glucocorticoids: Topical glucocorticoid ointments or gels are useful for localized early lesions, or for maintaining remission after more aggressive treatments.

Ciclosporin: A 1% ciclosporin solution and 0.1% tacrolimus ointment are also reported as effective topical agents for this condition.

Sun screens: Sun screens with a sun protection factor (SPF) of 30 or more should be applied to the nose if there is likely to be exposure to sun. Exposure to sun should be avoided and affected animals should be kept out of strong sunlight between 10 a.m. and 4 p.m.

Systemic treatments

Vitamin E and essential fatty acids: Some cases may benefit from vitamin E (400–800 IU s.i.d.) and/or essential fatty acid (EFA) supplementation. These treatments have a slow onset of action and should be administered for 2 months before assessing efficacy. For this reason,

additional, more potent therapy may initially be required to achieve lesion resolution, and vitamin E and EFAs may ultimately be sufficient to maintain remission.

Tetracycline and nicotinamide: Combinations of tetracycline and nicotinamide have immunomodulating and immunosuppressive properties that are useful for this condition. The immunomodulating properties of tetracyclines include scavenging of oxygen free radicals, along with decreased production of oxygen free radicals and neutrophil chemotactic factor by neutrophils. Nicotinamide inhibits lymphocyte proliferation, mast cell degranulation and neutrophil functions. Tetracycline (250 mg) and nicotinamide (250 mg) are administered every 8 hours to dogs under 10 kg, and 500 mg of each drug is administered t.i.d. if the dog is over 10 kg in body weight. If beneficial, a response should be evident within 8 weeks.

Glucocorticoids: Prednisolone (2–4 mg/kg s.i.d.) or methylprednisolone (1.6–3.2 mg/kg s.i.d.) are used in refractory cases. The dosage is tapered to the minimum dose on alternate days if long-term maintenance therapy is required. Otherwise, once the condition is in remission, treatment could be switched to topical medication such as 0.1% tacrolimus ointment or a less potent systemic therapy such as tetracycline and nicotinamide.

Azathioprine: Azathioprine (2 mg/kg s.i.d.) can be used in more severe cases during the induction phase. Because of the slow onset of action, it is usually administered as an adjunct to glucocorticoid therapy and may ultimately have a glucocorticoid-sparing effect in the long-term management of the disease. This drug does not have a veterinary licence and should only be used after a discussion with the owner regarding the implications of treatment. Because of its effect on rapidly dividing cells, it can cause serious irreversible bone marrow suppression. The side-effects include anaemia, leucopenia and thrombocytopenia. Other side-effects include vomiting, pancreatitis and hepatic hypersensitivity. Therefore, if this drug is prescribed, routine haematology and biochemistry have to be performed every 2 weeks in the induction stage. The dose can be tapered and reduced to 1 mg/kg on alternate days.

Chlorambucil: Chlorambucil at a dosage of 0.2 mg/kg orally every 24–48 hours can also be used as an adjunct to glucocorticoid therapy in more severely affected cases. It is generally considered a safer alternative to azathioprine, is commonly used in small dogs and is safe for the treatment of cats. However, adverse effects include gradual bone marrow suppression, thrombocytopenia and gastrointestinal disturbance, and appropriate monitoring with regular haematology is indicated (see Chapter 17).

Ciclosporin: Ciclosporin (5 mg/kg s.i.d.) may be an option in dogs with severe disease that are unable to tolerate prednisolone. The use of this drug would be off-label and requires owners' consent.

Treatment in this case

The dog in this case report had failed to respond to oxytetracycline and nicotinamide, even after several months of treatment; therefore, more aggressive immunosuppressive treatments (glucocorticoids, azathioprine and systemic ciclosporin) were considered to achieve remission. After a discussion with the owner, taking into consideration the adverse effects of each medication, the cost of the drugs and the cost of mandatory monitoring of adverse effects with azathioprine, the owner opted for systemic prednisolone, which was started at a dosage of 2 mg/kd s.i.d. After 2 weeks, the lesions on both the nose and the feet had markedly improved (Figs 53.4 and 53.5). At this point, the dog was polyphagic, polydipsic and polyuric. The dosage was then reduced to 2 mg/kg every other day for 2 more weeks. After 4 weeks of treatment, only very small punctate lesions were present on the nasal planum, so the dose was reduced further to 1 mg/kg for 2 more weeks. At this point, 0.1% tacrolimus ointment was prescribed for twice-daily application to the nose and feet, and the prednisolone was reduced again to 0.5 mg/kg on alternate days for a further 2 weeks (Figs 53.6 and 53.7), after which it was tapered off by 0.1 mg/kg a week and eventually maintained on 0.1 mg/kg every other day. During this latter stage, the 0.1% tacrolimus was applied twice daily, just prior to feeding, to minimize licking of the areas. Sun avoidance and sun screen with an SPF of 30 were used concurrently to manage the condition.

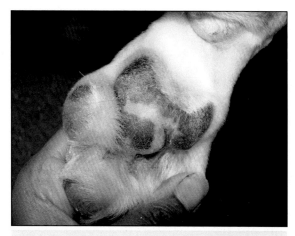

Figure 53.5 The foot after 4 weeks of treatment.

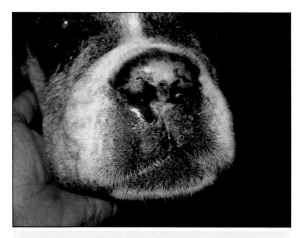

Figure 53.4 Marked improvement of the nose after 4 weeks.

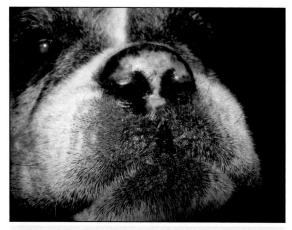

Figure 53.6 The nose 8 weeks after treatment.

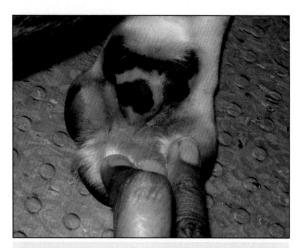

Figure 53.7 The plantar aspect of the foot 8 weeks after treatment.

CLINICAL TIPS

- If there is cytological evidence of bacterial infection in cases with clinical signs resembling cutaneous lupus, it is important to treat the infection before taking samples for histopathology. A lack of response rules out mucocutaneous pyoderma which is indistinguishable from cutaneous lupus erythematosus on histology.
- Sun avoidance and the use of sunblocks is essential in the long-term management of the condition.
- It is always worth prescribing topical treatment for early management of the lesions.
- Always advise owners to wear gloves when applying topical treatments.
- When using unlicensed treatments, the owner's informed consent should be obtained.
- Each case should be individually assessed and on occasion systemic glucocorticoids may be required to achieve remission, either because of previous poor response to other drugs or for welfare reasons because of the slow onset of action of concurrent therapy.

FOLLOW-UP

At the time of writing (6 months on) the dog was maintained on prednisolone (0.1 mg/kg every other day) and topical application of 0.1% tacrolimus once daily. An attempt to reduce the oral prednisolone further resulted in recrudescence of clinical signs on the feet and so the current dosage was maintained.

54 Feline plasma cell pododermatitis

INITIAL PRESENTATION

Swollen and haemorrhaging footpads in a cat.

INTRODUCTION

Feline plasma cell pododermatitis is an uncommon inflammatory disease of the footpads. Its precise aetiology is unknown. The disease results in swollen, discoloured and sometimes haemorrhaging footpads. This case report describes a case of plasma cell pododermatitis in a Maine Coone.

CASE PRESENTING SIGNS

A 2-year-old, neutered male Maine Coone was presented with a 5-month history of footpad swelling and haemorrhage.

CASE HISTORY

On occasion, owners may be unaware of when the lesions first developed, because the cat is only presented when there is evidence of lameness, or haemorrhage, due to footpad ulceration. The disease has a tendency to wax and wane.

The history in this case was as follows:

- There was a 4- to 5-month history of footpad swelling and ulceration, which started in early summer.
- There was no history suggestive of systemic involvement.
- There were three other cats in the household that were unaffected.
- All cats were confined indoors.
- The cat was fed a good quality, complete dried cat food, with meals and water to drink.
- Flea control consisted of monthly applications of fipronil to all cats in the household.

- Routine annual vaccinations and antihelmintic therapy 5 months prior to the onset of skin lesions.
- There had been no visible improvement of the footpad lesions following 3 weeks of broad-spectrum, systemic antibacterial therapy with clavulanic acid potentiated amoxicillin.

CLINICAL EXAMINATION

The characteristic clinical feature of feline plasma cell pododermatitis is soft spongy swelling of multiple footpads. The central tarsal and carpal pads are most frequently affected. The pads often have what is described as a violaceous hue and are cross-hatched with white striae (Fig. 54.1). Initially, the condition is asymptomatic but ulceration may develop in some cases, leading to lameness and sometimes copious haemorrhage. In very long-standing cases where there has been marked footpad ulceration, large masses of granulation tissue may protrude from the ulcerated surface of the footpad. Occasionally, cats may present with concurrent plasma cell stomatitis, manifested by bilateral, proliferative, ulcerated lesions over the palatopharyngeal arches. Swelling over the bridge of the nose and nasal planum due to a plasma cell infiltrate, concurrent immune-mediated glomerulonephritis and renal amyloidosis have also been described.

The clinical signs in this case were:

- No abnormalities were detected on general physical examination.
- Examination of the feet revealed soft swelling of the central footpads on all the feet, with thin white striae over the affected areas (Fig. 54.1).
- The pad on the right forelimb was most severely affected, with a healing ulcerated area (Fig. 54.2).

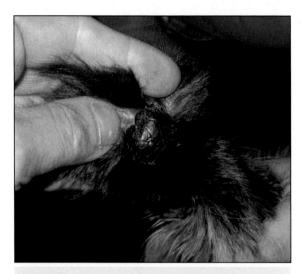

Figure 54.1 Footpad swelling and white striations.

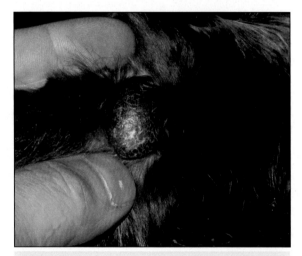

Figure 54.2 Footpad swelling, striations and a crusted ulcerated lesion.

DIFFERENTIAL DIAGNOSES

Although the clinical signs were highly suggestive of feline plasma cell pododermatitis, other possible causes of footpad swelling and/or ulceration include:
- Pemphigus complex
- Lupus erythematosus
- Chemical or physical trauma
- Infectious or sterile pyogranulomas
- Eosinophilic granuloma complex
- Neoplasia, including mastocytoma and lymphosarcoma.

CASE WORK-UP

Cytological examination of fine-needle aspirates from the footpads and surface cytology from any exudative or ulcerated areas would be useful, to look for evidence of plasma cell infiltration (see 'Clinical tips') and to detect secondary bacterial infection. If the history and clinical signs are suggestive of systemic involvement, routine haematology, biochemistry and urinalysis would be indicated. Regenerative anaemia may be evident with long-term footpad haemorrhage, although normocytic, normochromic anaemia is sometimes seen suggesting chronic inflammatory disease or infection. Hyperglobulinaemia may be present and a diagnostically significant polyclonal gammopathy may be evident on serum protein electrophoresis. There are many causes of footpad lesions in cats and even though the clinical presentation is strongly suggestive of the condition, histopathological examination is required to make a definitive diagnosis of plasma cell pododermatitis. In view of the possible association with feline immunodeficiency virus (FIV), serology is also advisable.

The following diagnostic procedures were carried out in this case:
- Cytological examination of a fine-needle aspirate from one affected footpad showed evidence of a mixed inflammatory infiltrate with numerous plasma cells.
- Two 6-mm biopsy punch samples were taken from the footpads for histopathological examination, which showed epidermal acanthosis and a marked perivascular to diffuse infiltration of numerous plasma cells, neutrophils, histiocytes and lymphocytes in the dermis. There were many Mott cells evident.
- FIV serology was negative. In view of the absence of signs of systemic involvement and cost considerations, further blood work and urinalysis were not performed in this case.

DIAGNOSIS

The clinical signs and histopathological examination were consistent with a diagnosis of feline plasma cell pododermatitis.

PROGNOSIS

In general, unless there is concurrent glomerulonephritis or renal amyloidosis, the prognosis for feline plasma cell pododermatitis is favourable. Lesions generally respond to therapy without a tendency to recur.

AETIOPATHOGENESIS

The precise aetiopathogenesis of feline plasma cell pododermatitis is unknown, but the findings of a persistent hypergammaglobulinaemia (a polyclonal gammopathy), tissue infiltration with large numbers of plasma cells and smaller numbers of lymphocytes and neutrophils, and a good response to immunomodulatory therapy all suggest an immune-mediated pathogenesis.

There are reports of a seasonal recurrence of the disease in some cases that might represent an allergic aetiology.

There are conflicting reports regarding the involvement of FIV, but one study found that up to 50% of affected cats were FIV positive on serology.

EPIDEMIOLOGY

In published reports, plasma cell pododermatitis has only been described in cats, although anecdotally a disease with similar histopathological findings has been seen in dogs. There are no age, breed or sex predilections for the disease in cats. In one study, the age of onset ranged from 1 to 12.5 years.

MEDICAL TREATMENT OPTIONS

Asymptomatic lesions may resolve spontaneously without treatment. More severe ulcerated or painful lesions require immunomodulatory therapy with antibacterial treatment if there is evidence of infection.

Prednisolone: Prednisolone (2–4 mg/kg s.i.d., p.o.) is usually effective in resolving the lesions. There should be a clinical response within a few weeks and complete resolution of lesions in 3 months. The prednisolone dosage may then be slowly tapered down and withdrawn altogether over a period of several months.

Triamcinolone and dexamethasone: If prednisolone is ineffective, triamcinolone (0.4–0.6 mg/kg s.i.d., p.o.) or dexamethasone (0.5 mg/kg s.i.d., p.o.) may be used.

Doxycycline: A recent paper described the use of doxycycline in the treatment of feline plasma cell pododermatitis at a dosage of 25 mg/cat s.i.d., p.o. There was complete remission of lesions in 25% of cases after 3–4 weeks of treatment and, after 6–8 weeks, around 80% of cases had either completely resolved or had partially improved. For further information on the use of doxycycline in cats see Chapter 47.

Chrysotherapy: Chrysotherapy has also been reported to be of value in the treatment of feline plasma cell pododermatitis (see Chapter 17).

SURGICAL TREATMENT OPTIONS

Surgical excision is a useful therapy for the treatment of feline plasma cell pododermatitis. Surgical excision of ulcerated or granulomatous lesions, along with systemic antibacterial therapy and subsequent prednisolone, or other immunomodulatory therapy, has been effective in the treatment of ulcerated and granulating lesions. More radical, wide surgical excision of the entire footpad, without the use of additional immunomodulatory therapy, is also an effective treatment and produces a satisfactory cosmetic result without recurrence.

Treatment selected in this case: Ulceration was not severe and initial treatment consisted of doxycycline at a dosage of 10 mg/kg s.i.d.

CLINICAL TIPS

A wedge biopsy specimen, or a deep 6 mm punch biopsy sample, should be obtained from an affected footpad near the pad margin. Small (4 mm) punch biopsy samples may not be suitable, as the sample may not be of adequate depth. If multiple footpads are affected, it is recommended to sample moderately, rather than severely, affected pads, as the latter may not heal well following surgery.

FOLLOW-UP

Re-examination after 6 weeks of treatment revealed a marked improvement, with reduction in the size of the footpads and healing of all ulcerated areas. Treatment was continued for a further 6 weeks until resolution of lesions and then withdrawn.

Long-term follow-up after 3 years revealed that there had been no further recurrence of lesions.

55 Digital squamous cell carcinoma

INITIAL PRESENTATION

Hind limb lameness and a subungual nodule in an English setter.

INTRODUCTION

Nodular lesions of the nail bed may be the result of an inflammatory process, usually with a pyogranulomatous infiltrate, or neoplasia. Squamous cell carcinoma, mast cell tumour and melanoma are three of the more common tumours affecting the nail beds. This case report describes a case of squamous cell carcinoma of the nail bed that was treated by digital amputation.

CASE PRESENTING SIGNS

A 9-year-old, entire female English setter was presented with left hind limb lameness.

CASE HISTORY

- An initial weight-bearing lameness had been noted 1 week previously.
- The patient was now reluctant to bear any weight on the left hind limb and had been licking at the foot.
- There was no history of a previous traumatic wound or foreign body penetration, and no previous history of skin disease or symptoms suggestive of systemic involvement.
- The patient had been annually vaccinated and regularly wormed.
- There were no other animals in the household and no evidence of zoonosis.

CLINICAL EXAMINATION

- General physical examination was unremarkable.
- A 1-cm-diameter, nodular mass with an ulcerated and exudative surface was located subungually on the second digit of the left hind foot (Figs 55.1 and 55.2).
- The digit was swollen and painful, and a purulent discharge exuded from the nail fold and the margins of the mass. The nail was deformed.
- There was left popliteal lymphadenopathy.

DIFFERENTIAL DIAGNOSES

The principal differential diagnoses for a subungual mass are neoplasia or a granulomatous inflammatory lesion. The differential diagnoses included:
- Neoplasia
  - Squamous cell carcinoma
  - Mast cell tumour
  - Malignant melanoma
- Granulomatous inflammation
  - Bacterial or fungal infection
  - Penetrating foreign body.

CASE WORK-UP

Cytological examination of fine-needle aspirates of the mass and also of draining lymph nodes is indicated in nodular diseases. Radiography of the foot can be helpful in identifying foreign bodies and bone lysis that may be evident in neoplastic disease. In suspected neoplasia, survey chest and abdominal radiographs are indicated to look for evidence of metastasis.

The patient was sedated with a combination of medetomidine and butorphanol, and the following diagnostic tests performed:

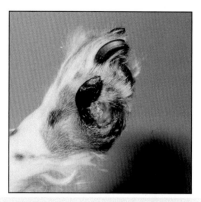

Figure 55.1 Ulcerated nodule with purulent exudation and nail deformity.

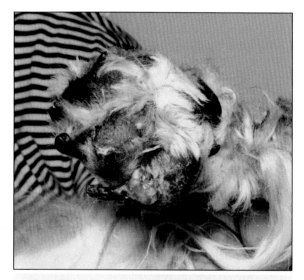

Figure 55.2 Ulcerated nodule with purulent exudation and nail deformity.

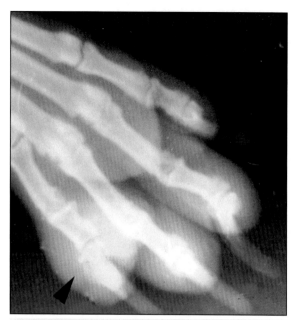

Figure 55.3 Anteroposterior radiograph showing evidence of lysis of P1 (arrowhead).

- Osteolysis of the third phalanx of the second digit was evident on an anteroposterior radiograph of the affected foot (Fig. 55.3).
- There were no abnormalities on thoracic survey radiographs.

A tentative diagnosis of a subungual squamous cell carcinoma was made based on the clinical, radiographic and cytological findings. As squamous cell carcinomas of the canine digit are potentially aggressive and can metastasize early, it has been suggested that radiographic evidence of destruction of the distal phalanx in suspected cases should warrant amputation of the digit. The decision was made to proceed with this procedure even though the diagnosis had not been confirmed histopathologically.

- Under general anaesthesia, the digit was amputated at the level of P3 and submitted for histopathological examination.

DIAGNOSIS

Histopathological examination confirmed that this was a squamous cell carcinoma of high malignancy rating, with cellular atypia and the presence of individual infiltrating cells.

- Cytological examination of a surface impression smear revealed many neutrophils and a mixed population of bacteria with both rods and cocci evident.
- Cytological examination of a fine-needle aspirate from the mass revealed epithelial cells with large nuclei and coarse nuclear chromatin, erythrocytes and occasional inflammatory cells.
- A fine-needle aspirate was taken from the left popliteal lymph node. This was submitted for cytopathological examination and showed a low-level neutrophilia, but no other abnormalities. No epithelial or carcinoma cells were evident.

PROGNOSIS

There is no histological classification that is reliably predictive of the likelihood of local recurrence or distant metastasis, but in general squamous cell carcinoma is locally invasive but slow to metastasize. It is considered that lesions of the claw bed are more aggressive than squamous cell carcinomas in other sites. In around 70% of cases of subungual squamous cell carcinomas, there is radiographic evidence of lysis and periosteal bone formation around P3, and invasion of P3 by neoplastic cells. The incidence of tumour metastasis from subungual squamous cell carcinomas is reported to be between 5% and 29%. It seems to be relatively low following (early) digital amputation.

In this case, there was a wide margin of excision. Nevertheless, the owner was warned of the risk of metastasis and recurrence on other digits.

AETIOPATHOGENESIS OF SQUAMOUS CELL CARCINOMA

Squamous cell carcinomas are common, malignant neoplasms arising from keratinocytes that affect both cats and dogs. Squamous cell carcinoma most commonly affects the trunk, limbs, digits, scrotum, lips, anus and nasal planum. Subungual squamous cell carcinomas arise from the nail-bed epithelium (see Fig. 56.5 in Chapter 56). Lesions may be ulcerative or proliferative and are friable, with a tendency to bleed easily. In general, subungual squamous cell carcinoma affects a single digit, which is swollen, painful, possibly ulcerated, and usually presents as lameness and with nail deformity. Occasionally, multiple digits may be concurrently affected or may be affected sequentially over a period of years. Tumour size is reported to vary from 0.3 to 3 cm; lesions may be well circumscribed or diffusely infiltrative. Histologically, subungual squamous cell carcinomas are unencapsulated, asymmetrical neoplasms with irregular and infiltrative margins. Histological variants of squamous cell carcinomas include well-differentiated and poorly differentiated grades, although the majority of subungual squamous cell carcinomas are of the well-differentiated type.

In man, there are a number of factors that are known to positively influence the development of squamous cell carcinoma, including solar exposure, lack of skin pigmentation, thermal exposure, hydrocarbon exposure (including coal tar and cigarette smoke), chronic radiation exposure, scarring, long-standing benign skin disease, viral factors (in man, many cases of squamous cell carcinomas of the nail bed may be due to human papilloma virus infection) and immunosuppression.

The most commonly identified cause of squamous cell carcinomas in veterinary species is chronic ultraviolet radiation exposure, and many cases of squamous cell carcinoma arise from lesions of actinic keratosis, a solar-induced hyperplastic and dysplastic epidermal lesion occurring in non-pigmented and lightly haired skin. The mechanism by which ultraviolet radiation induces squamous cell carcinomas is considered to be by direct damage to DNA molecules (and resulting DNA mutations) and indirect damage via formation of free radicals. There are known mutations of the tumour suppressor gene p53. The aetiology of subungual squamous cell carcinoma is uncertain, although trauma and chronic infections have been suggested as possible causes.

EPIDEMIOLOGY

Squamous cell carcinoma is diagnosed most commonly in animals that are over 7 years old. It is the most frequently reported nail-bed neoplasia, accounting for 38% of cases in one study, and there is a marked predilection for large breed dogs with black-coloured hair coats – Labradors, Rottweilers, standard poodles, giant schnauzers, Gordon setters and Kerry blue terriers.

TREATMENT OPTIONS

Squamous cell carcinomas may be treated in a number of different ways depending on the anatomical site affected. Surgical excision is the treatment of choice in areas such as the pinna, nasal planum and nail bed. Early digital amputation is the treatment of choice for subungual squamous cell carcinomas. Lesions not amenable to surgery may be treated with photodynamic therapy, laser therapy, hyperthermia, cryosurgery and local therapy with strontium-90.

An alternative way of managing this case if the radiographic and cytological findings were not clear would have been to have excised all or part of the mass and submitted it for histopathological examination, and then performed complete digital amputation following confirmation of the diagnosis.

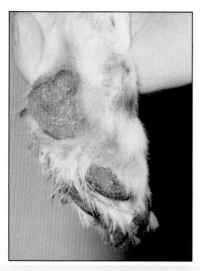

Figure 55.4 Healed amputation site following surgery.

FOLLOW-UP

The wound healed uneventfully following amputation (Fig. 55.4). On follow-up examination 10 months later, there had been no recurrence of the growth and no other digits were affected. The dog remained healthy.

56 Lupoid onychodystrophy

INITIAL PRESENTATION

Claw abnormalities and pain in a Rhodesian ridgeback.

INTRODUCTION

Lupoid onychitis, also known as symmetrical lupoid onychodystrophy, is considered to be an immune-mediated cutaneous reaction pattern. Often, the initial cause leads to secondary paronychia, which further contribute to the ongoing problem. The condition normally affects several claws on the feet, rather than just a single claw or a single foot and is characterized by progressive shedding of nails over a period of weeks to months with associated pain and paronychia. Histologically, it is characterized by a cell-rich interface dermatitis. Claw abnormalities are described using special terms and those used in this chapter are defined in Table 56.1.

CASE PRESENTING SIGNS

A neutered male Rhodesian ridgeback, three and a half years of age, was presented with onycholysis, onychomadesis, onychalgia and paronychia.

CASE HISTORY

Most dogs with lupoid onychitis are presented with a history of lameness, feet licking or pain. The duration of onset varies but commonly there is a history of sloughing of one nail and then over a period of weeks nails are sloughed on the majority, if not all, digits on all four feet. Haemorrhage may be evident from affected digits. Lupoid onychitis does not result in systemic illness and affected dogs are in good general health. The condition is not associated with poor nutrition and most dogs are being fed well-balanced commercial pet foods.

The relevant history in this case was:
- A sudden onset of lameness, about 6 months prior to presentation, which responded to meloxicam analgesia.
- There had been further episodes of lameness and foot licking since the initial episode.
- Onychalgia was observed.
- Frequent feet licking and anal pruritus.
- A previous history of otitis and anal pruritus.
- The familial history was not known.
- The dog was fed on a commercial complete dry diet for large breeds.
- It was prone to gastrointestinal disturbances after dietary changes.

CLINICAL EXAMINATION

Onychomadesis and onychalgia are the most common presenting sign. The claws separate from the claw bed with evidence of exudate. Haemorrhage is not always seen, but when the nail plate comes away the claw may bleed profusely. Previously lost claws regrow in a dystrophic manner, with abnormalities such as brittleness, scaling, dryness and distortion.

Clinical findings in this case included:
- Onycholysis, onychomadesis, onychalgia and erythema of the surrounding claw bed (Fig. 56.1).
- Every claw on all four feet was affected (Fig. 56.2).
- Cutaneous abnormalities and systemic signs were absent.

Table 56.1 Various terms used to describe claw abnormalities in this case report

Term	Visible abnormality of the claw
Onychitis	Inflammation of the claw
Onychodystrophy	Malformation of the claw
Onycholysis	Separation of claw from the claw bed
Onychomadesis	Sloughing of the claw
Paronychia	Inflammation of the claw bed
Onychalgia	Claw pain

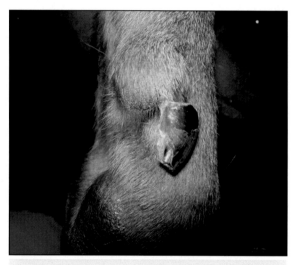

Figure 56.1 Separation of the claw plate from the claw bed.

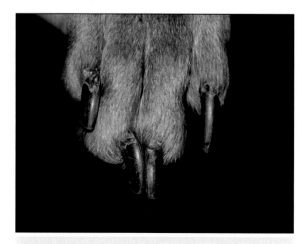

Figure 56.2 All the claws of one foot are affected.

DIFFERENTIAL DIAGNOSES

The history and clinical signs were highly suggestive of lupoid onychitis. Some authors suggest that the combination of nail shedding affecting multiple digits with no evidence of systemic illness is pathognomonic for the disease. However, a number of different conditions were considered, including:

- Trauma
- Infections
  - Bacterial onychitis
  - Fungal onychitis (trichophytosis, malasseziosis, other)
- Immune-mediated diseases
  - Lupoid onychitis
  - Pemphigus complex
  - Bullous pemphigoid
  - Epidermolysis bullosa
  - Vasculitis
  - Adverse drug reaction
- Endocrinopathies
  - Hypothyroidism
  - Hyperadrenocorticism
- Nutritional causes
  - Adverse food reaction
  - Deficiency
- Idiopathic onychomadesis and onychodystrophy.

CASE WORK-UP

Based on the history and the clinical signs, trauma was ruled out because of multiple claw involvement. Several diagnostic tests are needed to rule in or out the many conditions that are responsible for claw disease.

The following tests were performed in this case:

- Cytological examination of impression smears from nail folds revealed numerous cocci and smaller numbers of rods.
- Routine haematological and biochemical parameters were with normal limits, which by and large ruled out metabolic and endocrine diseases.
- Thyroid function tests (total T4, cTSH, free T4 ED, TGAA; see Chapter 22) were performed. The TGAA was raised to 291% (normal reference range <200%). This result did not confirm clinical hypothyroidism, but the presence of autoantibodies was evidence for

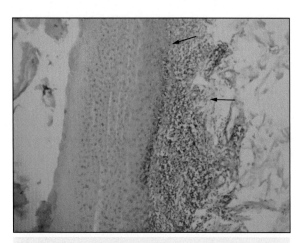

Figure 56.3 Interface dermatitis (arrows) demonstrated on histology.

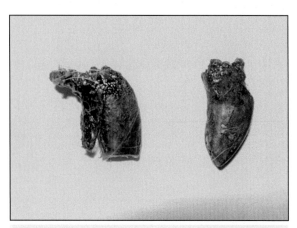

Figure 56.4 Loose claws removed for fungal and bacterial cultures.

lymphocytic thyroiditis and suggested that the dog might, in the future, develop clinical hypothyroidism (the other parameters were within the normal ranges). Six-monthly monitoring of thyroid function was therefore recommended in this case.

- As the dew claws were affected in this case, the third phalanx of one was surgically removed and submitted for histology. Post-surgery analgesia with meloxicam was prescribed. Histology revealed interface dermatitis, with hydropic changes of the basal epithelium and mainly lymphocytes and plasma cells targeting the dermoepidermal junction (Fig. 56.3). These findings supported a diagnosis of immune-mediated lupoid onychitis. Acantholysis and clefting, histological signs of pemphigus, pemphigoid and epidermolysis bullosa, were not evident. There was evidence of mild perivascular dermatitis, but the histological signs associated with vasculitis were absent.

- Some of the shedding claw plates from the same foot as the dew claw biopsy were removed using a haemostat and submitted for bacterial and fungal cultures (Fig. 56.4). The underlying corium was cleaned with chlorhexidine scrub and an electrocautry used to control bleeding. The foot was bandaged and routine postoperative care was provided. *Staphylococcus aureus*, *E. coli* and *Proteus* spp. were isolated from the claw and were considered to be secondary pathogens in the disease process. All three organisms were sensitive to enrofloxacin, clavulanic acid-potentiated amoxicillin, cefovecin, cefalexin and trimethoprim sulphonamides. Fungal culture was negative.

DIAGNOSIS

Lupoid onychitis with secondary bacterial infection.

PROGNOSIS

The prognosis is variable. Some cases respond reasonably well to benign therapy and nail care and have only rare recrudescence of disease. Other cases have repeated episodes of onychomadesis and are much more refractory to treatment. Lifelong treatment is likely to be required in these cases.

ANATOMY AND PHYSIOLOGY REFRESHER

The claw is a specialized horny structure of the skin. It is formed of highly keratinized epidermis and, together with the underlying dermis, is a continuation of the skin covering the digits. The horny layer is formed from the basal layer of the epidermis overlying the dermis (the quick) that covers the distal phalanx.

The nail is supported by the third (distal) phalanx (Fig. 56.5). The distal phalanx is divided into a cone-shaped portion called the ungual process that is surrounded by a thin bony collar, the ungual crest. The claw fold is formed around the ungual crest. The coronary band, where most of the nail growth occurs, is the base of the claw abutting, and partially enclosed by, the ungual crest. Most of the claw's growth is generated at the coronary band, and it is the differential growth rates between the coronary band, the dorsal and the ventral epidermis that produce the curved form of the claw. The

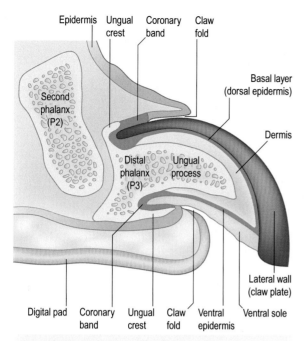

Figure 56.5 Lateral section of a dog's claw.

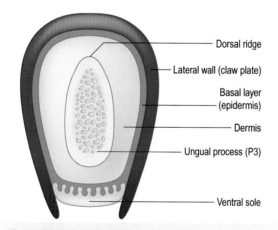

Figure 56.6 Cross-section of a dog's claw.

claw itself is made up of three parts: the coronary band, the lateral and medial walls, and the ventral sole.

The lateral and medial walls are the main body of the nail. They are highly keratinized stratum corneum consisting of hard keratins, rich in cysteine, lipids and water, with little or no stratum granulosum. In cross-section, it is a hooped structure with free edges on its ventral aspect which are joined together by the ventral sole (Fig. 56.6).

The ventral sole is a softer structure that closes the base of the nail. It is stratum corneum but, unlike the walls, it also has distinct granular and clear layers.

The mineral composition of the canine claw includes calcium, magnesium, manganese, iron, potassium, sodium, copper, zinc and phosphorus. The roles of these minerals in maintaining claw condition are not understood, but differences have been noted between the normal and diseased states. However, the higher concentrations of calcium, phosphorus, potassium and sodium found in diseased claws suggest that mineral deficiency is not generally the cause of the disease.

Trauma is the most common cause of damage, when only a single claw is affected. If multiple claws on more than one foot are involved, then numerous aetiologies can be responsible for the clinical disease. They include:

- Autoimmune and immune-mediated conditions (pemphigus complex, bullous pemphigoid, epidermolysis bullosa, systemic and cutaneous lupus erythematosus, drug eruption and vasculitis)
- Infectious diseases (bacterial, fungal)
- Endocrine abnormalities (hypothyroidism, hyperadrenocorticism, diabetes mellitus)
- Protozoa (leishmaniosis)
- Metabolic diseases (metabolic epidermal necrosis, severe nutritional abnormalities).

In many cases, a specific disease may not be identified even after extensive investigations.

Lupoid onychitis, as in this case, is characterized by initial separation of the claw from the claw bed, followed by sloughing and eventually regrowth with variable claw abnormalities. Secondary bacterial infection is common. The disease can take several months to affect all the claws, and when the new claws grow back they are usually dry, brittle and often malformed.

The underlying mechanisms that lead to the immune reaction and nail damage are not clear in the majority of cases and are considered to be idiopathic. However, lupoid onychitis may be a manifestation of an adverse reaction to drug or food administration. Therefore, if there is no history of previous drug administration, a diet trial should be considered to rule out an adverse food reaction, although this was not done in this case.

EPIDEMIOLOGY

There is no age or sex predisposition to the condition, and whilst the condition is not breed specific, it appears to have a greater incidence in larger breeds, e.g. German shepherd dogs, giant schnauzers and Rottweilers. In the author's experience the condition is also over-represented in bearded collies. A genetic predisposition may be inferred, as the condition has been reported in two siblings.

TREATMENT

This can be a challenging disease to treat and most dogs are likely to require long-term, possibly lifelong, therapy.

If presented in the acute stage of the disease, loose (and therefore painful) nails should be removed under heavy sedation or general anaesthesia. Cytology and perhaps culture and sensitivity testing should be performed on any exudate from nail folds and several weeks of antibacterial therapy should be prescribed based on the results of these tests. Appropriate dressings should be applied to the feet if required. Topical therapy in the form of antibacterial soaks in dilute chlorhexidine or similar antiseptic may also be beneficial.

Several anti-inflammatory and immunosuppressive protocols have been reported for the treatment of lupoid onychitis. Less aggressive treatment regimens include high dosage omega-3/omega-6 fatty acid supplementation, vitamin E, biotin and the combination of oxytetracyline and nicotinamide. Biotin supplementation in cattle, pigs, horses and humans has been shown to improve the quality and the growth of hooves and nails respectively.

More severely affected dogs or those that are refractory to treatment may be treated with the immunosuppressive combination of prednisolone and azathioprine. Another protocol described the use of a topical betamethasone mousse combined with systemic treatment using pentoxifylline.

The choice of treatment is based on individual case assessment and discussion with the client. The potential adverse effects of more aggressive therapy with the requirement for haematological and biochemical monitoring and the associated cost, versus the potential benefit of the treatment, should be considered when making a choice for management.

Treatment in this case

In this case, cefalexin was prescribed at a dosage of 20 mg/kg b.i.d. and continued for a total of 6 weeks of treatment. At the same time, the dog was started on vitamine E (400 IU s.i.d.), biotin supplementation and a

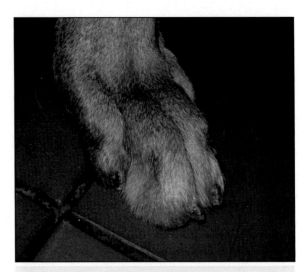

Figure 56.7 The claws after 6 weeks of treatment with cefalexin, Efavet regular, vitamin E and biotin.

commercial essential fatty acid supplement using double the manufacturer's dosage (i.e. 552 mg linoleic acid, 68 mg γ-linolenic acid, 34 mg eicosapentaenoic acid and 22 mg docasahexaenoic acid per 10 kg body weight). Although a combination of oxytetracyline/nocotinamide was considered, it was not prescribed at the first instance. After the initial 6 weeks of antibiotic treatment (Fig. 56.7), a combination of 500 mg of oxytetracycline and 500 mg of nicotinamide t.i.d were prescribed for 3 months.

Advice was given to the owners regarding the necessity of careful nail care. Nails should be regularly clipped and if possible, split nails should be filed to remove sharp edges that could result in further nail fracture.

NURSING ASPECTS

As many owners find nail clipping difficult, nurses should be involved in the nail care of lupoid onychitis cases. Regular clipping and filing of the claws, to reduce the pressure on the claw bed, can be of value in the long-term management of the disease.

CLINICAL TIPS

- Claw disorders can have multiple aetiologies. A definitive diagnosis will improve the chances of successful management of the condition.
- The only useful diagnostic tests possible from a shed claw are fungal and bacterial cultures. The

nail plate by itself will not provide any diagnostic histological information.

- For histology a whole-claw biopsy, taken at P3, is required. Amputation of an affected dew claw minimizes the post-surgical complications.
- A technique for claw biopsy with a biopsy punch without amputation has been described. However, experience has shown that this is not an easy technique.
  - It requires general anaesthesia and experience in the procedure is essential.
  - Cutting through the hard nail with a biopsy punch can prove difficult.
  - The pathology may be present in only part of the claw matrix, so the absence of typical interface changes in the sample does not rule out lupoid onychitis.
  - The procedure may lead to disruption of the tissue.
  - Damage to part of the claw epithelium may lead to permanent distortion of the nail.

FOLLOW-UP

The dog was maintained on the combination of essential fatty acid, vitamin E and biotin supplements long term. The oxytetracycline and nicotinamide combination was withdrawn after 3 months of treatment. The owners were diligent with long-term claw care for the dog; however, the claws continued to grow abnormally and the dog lost another claw after 9 months. A further 8-week course of oxytetracycline and nicotinamide (500 mg of each t.i.d.) was prescribed. Since then there has been no further nail loss.

Total T4 and thyroid-stimulating hormone have been within normal reference ranges when measured on two separate occasions 6 months apart. Thyroglobulin antibodies, however, remain elevated.

A food trial was not undertaken in this case, one reason being the only way the owner was able to administer the supplements was with special treats.

57 Otitis externa and otitis media in a dog

INITIAL PRESENTATION

Purulent otitis externa.

INTRODUCTION

Otitis externa is a common clinical presentation. It is often of multifactorial aetiology and may be part of a generalized skin disease or underlying systemic illness. Although initial symptomatic therapy is appropriate for early, acute cases of otitis externa, a systematic and thorough approach involving detailed history taking, complete physical and dermatological examinations, and appropriate diagnostic work-up is required when investigating and treating chronic otitis externa. This case report describes the investigation and treatment of a case of *Pseudomonas* otitis externa.

CASE PRESENTING SIGNS

A 4-year-old, neutered male springer spaniel was presented with otitis externa.

CASE HISTORY

A detailed history is of paramount importance in understanding the nature of the underlying causes of long-standing otitis externa. It is important to establish the age of onset, seasonality, whether there is evidence of more generalized skin disease or pruritus, and whether there are symptoms of systemic disease. Additional important information is whether the otitis has been unilateral or bilateral, is there aural pruritus or pain, the nature of the aural discharge and whether there are symptoms suggestive of otitis media, such as pain on opening the mouth or neurological signs. Lastly, it is useful to know details of previous treatment and response.

The relevant history in this case was as follows:
- A 3-year history of recurrent tick infestation, otitis externa and intermittent, non-seasonal papulocrustous eruptions over the axillae and groin.
- The dog had received frequent treatment with systemic and topical aural glucocorticoid and antimicrobial therapy, which resulted in an improvement, but the disease always recurred within weeks of treatment withdrawal. Topical antibacterials previously used included framycetin, fucidic acid, polymixin B, gentamycin, marbofloxacin and antifungals, including miconazole and nystatin.
- Over the past year, systemic prednisolone therapy had been more or less continuous in order to control pruritus, but had been withdrawn 4 weeks prior to examination.
- Polydipsia, polyphagia, lethargy and weight gain had been evident over the past year.
- There was no history suggestive of otitis media.
- There were no other animals in the household and no evidence of zoonosis.

CLINICAL EXAMINATION

In addition to examination of the ears, a full physical examination and examination of the entire integument is indicated in a complex case of otitis externa:
- The patient was obese and weighed 37.7 kg.
- There was moderate prescapular and popliteal lymphadenopathy.
- There was mild diffuse erythema of the muzzle and both external ear canals, with a bilateral purulent aural discharge (Fig. 57.1).

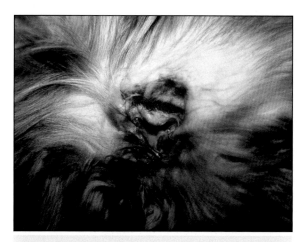

Figure 57.1 *Pseudomonas* otitis externa. Purulent aural discharge and erythema of the external ear canal are seen.

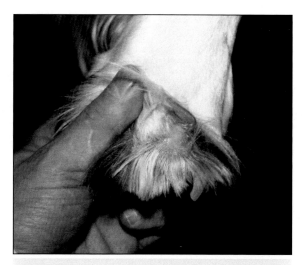

Figure 57.2 The same dog as in Fig. 57.1. Interdigital erythema due to *Malassezia* dermatitis can be observed.

- Otoscopic examination was not performed at this stage because the ears were considered to be too painful.
- A papular eruption and mild scaling were evident over the flexural aspect of the left elbow, with the scaling extending distally over the anterior aspect of the left forelimb.
- Dorsal and plantar interdigital erythema and a greasy discharge were evident over all four feet (Fig. 57.2).

DIFFERENTIAL DIAGNOSES

There was evidence of generalized skin disease as well as otitis externa. The principal differential diagnoses were:
- Bacterial and/or fungal otitis externa/media
- Demodicosis
- Pyoderma
- *Malassezia* dermatitis
- Atopic dermatitis
- Cutaneous adverse food reaction
- Iatrogenic hyperadrenocorticism
- Hypothyroidism.

CASE WORK-UP

Investigation of both the skin disease and otitis was indicated. Full evaluation of chronic otitis externa involves some or all of the following procedures:
- Cytological evaluation of aural discharge from the ear canals and from the tympanic bullae if there is evidence of otitis media.
- Bacterial culture and sensitivity testing.
- Radiographic, ultrasound, CT or MRI evaluation of the ear canals and tympanic bullae.
- Thorough cleaning and hand-held or video-otoscopic examination of the ear canals.
- Full evaluation of underlying diseases, including blood work where necessary, diet trials, and intradermal and/or ELISA testing.

If the ears are painful, general anaesthesia is required to clean and facilitate examination of the ear canals and tympanic membranes. Bulla radiography can be helpful in evaluation of chronic otitis externa and is an aid in deciding whether the ear problem can be managed medically or whether surgery is indicated. The full bulla series consists of ventrodorsal, open-mouth rostrocaudal, lateral, and left and right oblique views. In practice, the first two views usually prove to be the most useful. External ear disease may manifest as calcification of the auricular cartilages and narrowing of the external ear canals. Changes consistent with otitis media include increased density of the air-filled bullae, thickening, lysis or irregularity of the wall of one or both bullae, changes in size and contour, and new bone production. Note that in at least a quarter of cases of otitis media these changes are not present.

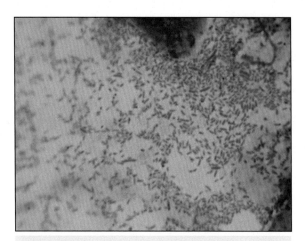

Figure 57.3 *Pseudomonas* otitis externa. Large numbers of rods are seen on cytological examination of discharge. ×1000 original magnification. Diff Quik® stain.

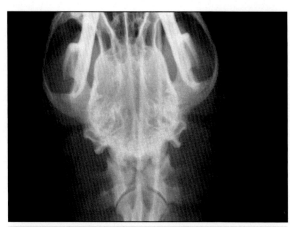

Figure 57.4 Ventrodorsal radiograph of the dog in Fig. 57.1. Stenosis of the proximal horizontal ear canals is apparent.

A diet trial, intradermal testing and blood work were indicated in this case and, as treatment of the otitis was likely to require glucocorticoid therapy, the decision was made to do intradermal testing at this stage.

The results of the work-up were:

- No evidence of ectoparasitism was found on microscopic examination of scale and deep skin scrapes from the pustular areas over the limbs.
- Many *Malassezia* organisms were evident on cytology from the interdigital skin.
- Many rod-shaped bacteria were evident on cytological examination of the aural discharge (Fig. 57.3).
- A swab was taken from both horizontal ear canals for bacterial culture and sensitivity testing, which grew *Pseudomonas aeruginosa* resistant to all the topical antibacterials used, including fluoroquinolones, and sensitive only to ticarcillin *in vitro*.
- Radiographic evaluation of the ear canals and tympanic bullae revealed ear canal stenosis of the proximal horizontal ear canals (Figs 57.4 and 57.5). There was no radiographic evidence of otitis media.
- Flushing and video-otoscopic examination of the ear canals under general anaesthesia revealed markedly erythematous and mildly ulcerated canals with no visible tympanic membranes. The ear canals were moderately stenotic.
- Samples for cytology and culture were collected from both tympanic bullae using a fine-tipped swab. Rods were seen on cytology, and culture and sensitivity testing grew *Pseudomonas aeruginosa* with a similar

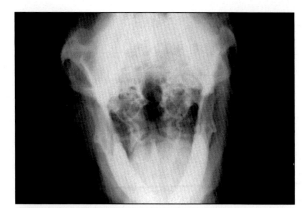

Figure 57.5 Rostrocaudal open-mouth radiograph of the dog in Fig. 57.1. The tympanic bullae appear healthy even though there was otitis media.

sensitivity pattern to the organism cultured from the horizontal canals.
- As prednisolone had been withdrawn 4 weeks previously, an intradermal test was performed that gave positive reactions to *Dermatophagoides farinae*, *Dermatophagoides pteronyssinus* and house dust.
- Routine haematological and biochemical examinations showed neutrophilia, lymphopoenia and elevated serum alkaline phosphatase, results consistent with previous glucocorticoid administration.
- Basal serum thyroxine concentration was 21 nmol/l. This was consistent with normal thyroid function.

DIAGNOSIS

There was evidence of *Pseudomonas* otitis externa and media. There was also evidence of pyoderma and *Malassezia* dermatitis. It was likely that both the skin and ear disease were secondary to an underlying hypersensitivity disorder.

PROGNOSIS

In this case, the ear canals were not irreversibly diseased and it was considered that medical management of the otitis was appropriate. Treatment would require resolution of the bacterial otitis, and identification and management of the underlying allergic disease. The owner was advised that, even with successful resolution of the infection, the patient was likely to require lifelong management of the underlying allergy and was also likely to require lifelong regular ear cleaning. Furthermore, even following apparently successful therapy, *Pseudomonas* otitis may recur in around 20% of cases.

AETIOPATHOGENESIS

The ear canal is a cartilaginous structure lined by skin with hair follicles, sebaceous and modified apocrine (ceruminous) glands (Fig. 57.6). Desquamated cells and glandular secretions form cerumen, which is transported up and out of the ear canal by a 'housekeeping' process of epithelial cell migration. There are a variety of resident commensal bacterial and yeast organisms which colonize the ear canal, including *Malassezia* spp., coagulase-negative staphylococci, streptococci, *Micrococcus*, *Acinetobacter* and others. Under normal circumstances, these organisms are not pathogenic and probably fulfil a useful role in occupying microbial niches, thereby preventing colonization by more pathogenic organisms. Transient organisms such as coagulase-positive staphylococci, *E. coli*, *Proteus* and *Pseudomonas* spp. may also enter the ear canals from the environment, or may be spread from the mouth and anus by licking and grooming.

Both generalized skin disease and systemic illness can lead to otitis externa. Recurrent otitis externa is likely to be a sign of a systemic problem that needs to be identified and corrected, and not a disease entity confined solely to the ear canals.

The underlying causes or factors leading to otitis externa can be divided into three main groups: predisposing factors, primary causes and perpetuating factors (Table 57.1).

Predisposing factors: Predisposing factors are those that place the patient at increased risk of developing ear disease. One of the most important is increased moisture content/humidity within the ear canal, which leads to maceration of the epidermis and breakdown of effective barrier function. These conditions favour colonization and invasion by resident and transient microorganisms.

Primary causes: Primary causes are the factors that cause initial inflammation within the ear canal. The most common primary cause of recurrent otitis externa is atopic dermatitis. Up to 86% of atopic dogs develop otitis externa.

Perpetuating factors: Perpetuating factors arise secondary to the primary process, preventing resolution and resulting in continued disease. Note that yeast and bacterial infections fall into this category. Longer-standing inflammation in the ear causes glandular hyperplasia and increased production of cerumen, increased desquamation and a reduction of epithelial cell migration, resulting in an accumulation of aural discharge. The housekeep-

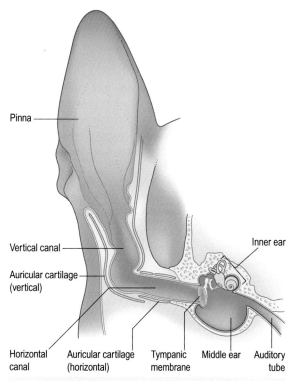

Pinna

Vertical canal

Auricular cartilage (vertical)

Horizontal canal

Auricular cartilage (horizontal)

Tympanic membrane

Middle ear

Inner ear

Auditory tube

Figure 57.6 Diagrammatic representation of the anatomical structures of the ear.

Table 57.1 Predisposing, primary and perpetuating causes of otitis externa

Predisposing	Primary	Perpetuating
Increased environmental temperature	*Otodectes cynotis*	Bacteria
Poor ear conformation	*Sarcoptes scabiei*	Yeasts
Hairy ear canals	*Demodex* spp.	Inappropriate treatment
Congenital ear canal stenosis	Foreign body	Contact dermatitis
Swimming	Atopic dermatitis	Ear canal stenosis
Immunosuppression – hypothyroidism	Adverse food reactions	Calcification
Cushings syndrome	Drug reactions	Cholesteatoma
Obstructive ear disease resulting from neoplasia or	Pemphigus foliaceus	Self-trauma
inflammatory processes (polyps)	Idiopathic seborrhoea	Otitis media
	Sebaceous adenitis	

ing mechanism of epithelial cell migration is unlikely to return to normal after chronic otitis externa, necessitating long-term ear cleaning. Otitis media results from destruction of the tympanic membrane (or occasional ascending infection via the auditory tube) and acts as a reservoir of infection that feeds back out to the external ear, even after apparently successful topical therapy. Repeated empirical topical antibacterial therapy may be a contributory factor in selecting for resistant bacterial infections, in particular *Pseudomonas aeruginosa*.

EPIDEMIOLOGY

Otitis externa is reported to be the third most common dermatological presentation in small animal practice and as such is a common clinical presentation. However, otitis externa is a complex disease, and the wide variety of predisposing and primary factors make the epidemiology difficult to define.

Breeds with ear types that result in increased humidity within the ear canal are predisposed to otitis externa. Floppy-eared breeds and dogs living in warm, humid climates are at increased risk. The Shar Pei is also predisposed due to congenitally stenotic ear canals with a pinna that closes the opening of the ear canal. Breeds such as poodles may also be at increased risk due to hairy ear canals. As atopic dermatitis is the most common primary cause of otitis externa, young dogs and breeds predisposed to atopic dermatitis are likely to be at increased risk. It is recognized that there are certain breeds that are predisposed to develop some forms of otitis externa. For example, *Pseudomonas* otitis is a common presentation in the cocker spaniel, although the reasons for this are not fully understood.

MEDICAL TREATMENT OPTIONS

A full discussion of the treatment of *Pseudomonas* otitis externa is beyond the scope of this chapter. However, cases of otitis externa and otitis media involving *Pseudomonas aeruginosa* present a significant therapeutic challenge. The aims of treatment are to:
- Thoroughly clean and dry the ears
- Treat specific infections
- Reduce inflammation
- Improve ear canal ventilation by resolving stenosis, removing hair and removing obstructive lesions
- Correct predisposing and primary causes of ear disease.

Aggressive topical and systemic antibacterial therapy is indicated, along with flushing of the external ear canals and tympanic bullae (in the case of otitis media) under general anaesthesia.

Ear flushing: Ear flushing, performed under general anaesthesia, is an important part of the treatment of otitis externa. A cuffed endotracheal tube should always be used. The operator should wear gloves, face mask and eye protection to avoid infection from contaminated aerosols, especially if *Pseudomonas* spp. are present. Water and saline are suitable cleaning agents where there is tympanic membrane rupture. The cleaning fluid is delivered via a standard giving set connected to a three-way tap. Also connected to the tap is a 20-ml syringe and a suitable catheter (usually a feeding tube of the appropriate length and diameter; Fig. 57.7). An otoscope is introduced into the canal to the depth of the horizontal canal. The catheter is passed through the cone of the scope and, using the three-way tap to alternately fill the syringe and flush the ear, the ear is continually flushed until all discharge has been removed. If otitis media is present, the catheter should be passed into the tympanic bulla, which may then be thoroughly irrigated to remove any accumulated exudate. Retrograde flushing using this technique is very effective at removing deep material and is the only effective way to clean the middle ear. The use of a video-otoscope dramatically improves visualization of the ear canal during this procedure.

Antimicrobial treatment: Selection of topical and systemic therapy should be based on culture and sensitivity

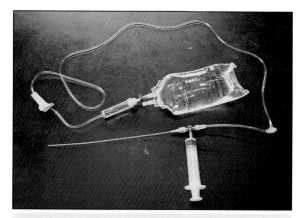

Figure 57.7 Ear flushing. Saline is delivered to the catheter via a syringe and a three-way tap.

testing. Antimicrobial resistance is a major problem and may necessitate the off-licence use of antibiotics. Useful antimicrobials are listed in Table 57.2. Fluoroquinolones are frequently the first choice treatment for *Pseudomonas* otitis. In view of their concentration-dependent killing effects and to minimize the risk of resistance, it has been recommended that enrofloxacin is administered at up to 20 mg/kg s.i.d., p.o. and marbofloxacin at up to 8 mg/kg s.i.d., p.o. Even in the face of a fluoroquinolone-resistant strain of *Pseudomonas* spp., it is worth considering the use of a fluoroquinolone as initial therapy. On occasion, the high *in vivo* concentrations obtained by topical therapy will overcome apparent *in vitro* resistance.

Reduction of inflammation: Glucocorticoids are of great value in the treatment of otitis externa. They reduce swelling and oedema, hyperplasia, glandular secretions and exfoliation, and render the ear canal less favourable for microorganisms. Prednisolone should be administered at a dosage of 1–4 mg/kg/day, depending on the severity of pathological changes, for a period of 1–3 weeks. Once the swelling and inflammation has subsided and the lumen has returned to a normal diameter, therapy should be gradually tapered.

SURGICAL TREATMENT OPTIONS

Surgery should be considered as a last resort when medical treatment has failed or is inappropriate.

Table 57.2 Useful antimicrobials for the treatment of *Pseudomonas* otitis externa

	Systemic	Topical	Notes
Enrofloxacin	5–20 mg/kg s.i.d.	2.5% solution (can dilute 1 : 4 with saline)	Off-licence use at higher dosages
Marbofloxacin	2–8 mg/kg s.i.d.	Proprietary preparation available	Off-licence use at higher dosages
Polymixin B		Proprietary preparation available	Inactivated by debris
Gentamicin	5–10 mg/kg s.c. or i.m., s.i.d.	Proprietary preparation available	Potentially ototoxic and nephrotoxic if used systemically
Silver sulphadiazine		1.5 ml in 13.5 ml distilled water. Applied b.i.d. for 14 days	Unlicensed; inactivated by debris; promotes re-epithelization
Clavulanate-potentiated ticarcillin	15–25 mg/kg t.i.d., i.v.	May be used topically at 10 mg/ml	Unlicensed; unstable after reconstitution
Cefatazidime	25–50 mg/kg i.v., t.i.d.		Not licensed

Lateral ear canal resection: Lateral ear canal resection is indicated in the treatment of otitis externa, and occasionally to gain access to a neoplastic lesion located either on the medial aspect of the vertical ear canal or in the distal horizontal ear canal. Opening the ear canal alters the microenvironment and improves drainage and aeration. To be of use in the treatment of otitis externa, this procedure should be performed early in the course of the disease.

Lateral ear canal resection is contraindicated when the vertical or horizontal ear canals have irreversible disease, and when there is concurrent untreated otitis media that requires surgical intervention. When these are present, the disease has progressed too far for the procedure to be of benefit. In reality, this includes the majority of cases of long-standing otitis externa. The procedure may be of most benefit in the prevention of disease in breeds of dogs with congenitally stenotic ear canals, such as the Shar Pei.

The surgical complications include:
- Wound dehiscence (27%)
- Stenosis of the remaining ear canal
- Failure to alter the progression of otitis externa.

Vertical ear canal resection: This technique is indicated when the epithelium of the vertical ear canal is irreversibly diseased or neoplastic, but the horizontal ear canal is healthy. Vertical ear canal resection is contraindicated when the horizontal ear canal has irreversible disease and when there is concurrent untreated otitis media that requires surgical intervention.

Surgical complications include:
- Wound dehiscence (19%)
- Stenosis of lumen of horizontal ear canal (11%)
- Facial nerve deficits
- Failure to alter the progression of ear disease.

It is important to remember that with both lateral ear canal resection and vertical ear canal resection, the techniques remove chronically diseased tissues, but the underlying skin problems will still need diagnosis and treatment. A poor outcome is associated with failure to address ongoing disease.

There is a high failure rate associated with these techniques due to inappropriate case selection.

Total ear canal ablation and lateral bulla osteotomy: There are a number of indications for total ear canal ablation and lateral bulla osteotomy, including:

- Chronic 'end-stage' otitis externa or media that is non-responsive to medical therapy
- Neoplasms or polyps involving the horizontal canal or tympanic bulla
- Avulsion of the annular cartilage of the ear canals
- Traumatic avulsion of the ear canal
- Para-aural abscessation
- Following failed lateral ear canal resection or vertical ear canal resection.

A total ear canal ablation and lateral bulla osteotomy removes the whole of the ear canal, lateral portion of the tympanic bulla and the mucoperiosteum lining of the middle ear cavity. This radical technique is necessary in most cases of long-standing ear disease affecting the whole ear canal and/or middle ear.

Surgical complications include:
- Wound dehiscence
- Horner's syndrome
- Facial palsy (damage to cranial nerve VII)
- Vestibular syndrome
- Para-aural abscessation.

Apart from potential surgical complications, the main side-effect is loss of hearing. Animals are likely to be hard of hearing rather than deaf, as sound will still be conducted through the bones of the skull. Again, underlying skin disease should still be treated, otherwise disease may persist in the skin fold formed by the pinna.

TREATMENT PLAN

Even though there was *in vitro* fluoroquinolone resistance, initial treatment consisted of:
- Marbofloxacin (8 mg/kg p.o., s.i.d.).
- The owner was going to find three times weekly shampoo therapy difficult and so the *Malassezia* dermatitis was treated with oral ketoconazole (200 mg s.i.d.) for 3 weeks, along with weekly miconazole and chlorhexidine shampoos.
- Prednisolone (20 mg s.i.d.).
- Daily tris-EDTA ear cleaning followed by twice daily, topical applications of injectable marbofloxacin (2%) to both ears.
- In order to exclude the involvement of an adverse food reaction, a proprietary, limited antigen, fish and potato diet was introduced. It would not be possible to assess the response to this diet until withdrawal of glucocorticoid therapy.

Re-examination a week later revealed:

- The pyoderma was resolving. There was no evidence of pruritus.
- There was still a creamy white ceruminous-type discharge evident in both ear canals on otoscopic examination.
- Repeat cytological examination of the discharge revealed small numbers of rods and occasional pyknotic neutrophils.
- Deep ear flushing and flushing of the tympanic bullae under general anaesthesia was repeated. Tympanic membranes could still not be visualized in either ear on examination with the video-otoscope.
- Treatment and the diet were continued as described.

Re-examination after 2 weeks of treatment revealed:

- The pyoderma and *Malassezia* dermatitis had resolved and a small amount of whitish-coloured material was present in both ear canals.
- No rods were seen on ear cytology, but occasional pyknotic neutrophils remained.
- Deep ear flushing and flushing of the tympanic bullae were repeated.
- The diet and all other treatments were continued.

After 3 weeks of therapy:

- A small amount of white-coloured material obscured visualization of the proximal horizontal canal.
- No rods and only occasional pyknotic neutrophils were evident on cytology from the ears.
- Deep ear cleaning and flushing of the tympanic bullae were repeated.

Over the following 3 weeks:

- Prednisolone was tapered and withdrawn.
- Ketoconazole was continued at the same dosage for a further week and then withdrawn, but weekly miconazole and chlorhexidine shampoos were continued.
- Systemic antimicrobial therapy was continued for a further 2 weeks and then withdrawn.
- Topical aural therapy was continued as described.
- The restriction diet was continued.

Re-examination after withdrawal of prednisolone revealed a slight accumulation of white-coloured discharge in both ear canals on otoscopic examination. No inflammatory cells and no microorganisms were evident on cytological examination of this material. There had been recurrence of pedal and ventral pruritus, ruling out the involvement of an adverse food reaction as a sole cause of the pruritus, confirming the diagnosis of underlying atopic dermatitis (see Chapter 6).

Long-term treatment was as follows:

- Daily ear cleaning with a boric acid/acetic acid and hydrocortisone ear cleaner was substituted for the tris-EDTA and marbofloxacin treatments.
- Allergen-specific immunotherapy was started for control of atopic dermatitis.
- Ongoing weekly miconazole and chlorhexidine shampoos.

NURSING ASPECTS

One of the most important aspects when managing otitis externa is to instruct owners on the technique of ear cleaning. In the author's practice, this important task is undertaken by veterinary nurses. Failure of the owner to effectively clean the ear canals is a common reason for accumulation of discharge and recurrence of infection. It is important to try to make the experience as pleasurable as possible for the dog, so gentle handling, avoidance of pain or discomfort and positive reinforcement of good behaviour is important. Many dogs become reluctant to allow ear cleaning because of previous bad experience and this is a major problem when it comes to the long-term management of ear disease.

Ear cleaners should be warmed to body temperature prior to use. The owner should be instructed on how to correctly massage the ear canal after inserting the ear cleaner. The canal should be gently massaged for 30–60 seconds to dislodge and emulsify cerumen within the canal. Cotton buds should not be inserted into the ear canal as this can result in impaction of material into the horizontal canal, but material can be wiped away from the opening of the ear canal using a gauze swan or cotton wool pad.

CLINICAL TIPS

On occasion, marked ear canal stenosis prevents effective examination and cleaning of the ear canals. Glucocorticoid therapy is indicated in these situations and is often effective in resolving the stenosis, and may be used prior to any antimicrobial therapy or further evaluation. Prednisolone should be administered at 1–4 mg/kg s.i.d., p.o., depending on the severity or pathological changes. Failure of the stenosis to resolve indicates a poor prognosis for medical management.

Cytology, culture and flushing of the tympanic bullae are important procedures in the management of otitis media. The clinician should aim to introduce a catheter or swab through the caudoventral quadrant of the opening to the tympanic bulla to avoid damage to the round and oval windows that are situated behind the rostrodorsal quadrant. In reality, in severe cases of otitis media it is not possible to visualize these regions, even with the aid of a video-otoscope, but it is still possible to direct the catheter, or swab, in a caudal and ventral direction.

FOLLOW-UP

Regular re-examinations were scheduled every 4–6 weeks, when otoscopic and cytological examination of both ears was performed. After a further 3 weeks, the frequency of ear cleaning was reduced to alternate-day therapy. Weekly shampoos and monthly immunotherapy injections were continued. There was a further episode of ventral pyoderma 3 months later that responded to 3 weeks of treatment with systemic cefalexin. At that time, otoscopic examination revealed a small amount of cerumen in the right ear which obscured the tympanic membrane. An intact tympanic membrane was visible in the left ear. Ear cytology was unremarkable.

On follow-up a year later, ear cleaning, weekly shampoo treatments and monthly immunotherapy had been continued. There had been no further episodes of *Pseudomonas* otitis or pyoderma. Mild pedal pruritus was evident but was not unacceptable.

APPENDICES

MCQs

1. **At what time of year are rabbits most prone to fly strike?**
   (a) April to October
   (b) August to December
   (c) November to March
   (d) August only
   (e) All year round

2. **Which of the following is not usually involved in leading to fly strike in rabbits?**
   (a) Spinal pain
   (b) Urine scalding
   (c) Obesity
   (d) Dental disease
   (e) Rabbit syphilis

3. **What species of dermatophyte most commonly affects guinea-pigs?**
   (a) *Microsporum gypseum*
   (b) *Trichophyton mentagrophytes*
   (c) *Aspergillus flavus*
   (d) *Trichophyton schoenleinii*
   (e) *Microsporum canis*

4. **What is the colour indicator in dermatophyte test medium kits?**
   (a) Methylene Blue
   (b) Sudan Red
   (c) Periodic acid–Schiff
   (d) Crystal Violet
   (e) Phenol Red

5. **You are presented with an 18-month-old dog with papules, scaling and crusting on the ventrum, pedal pruritus and has had two episodes of otitis externa in the previous 4 months. Which of the following steps would you take to reach a diagnosis of atopic dermatitis in this dog?**
   (a) Perform an intradermal test
   (b) Perform a serum allergy test
   (c) Rule out ectoparasitic conditions, rule in or out any secondary microbial infections and the role of an adverse food reaction with appropriate tests, responses to treatment and to a food trial
   (d) Response to either ciclosporin or prednisolone would support the diagnosis

6. **Which of the following statements is most true of flea allergic dermatitis?**
   (a) It is an immediate type hypersensitivity response
   (b) It is a seasonal condition
   (c) Individuals on monthly flea control do not develop flea allergic dermatitis
   (d) It shows immediate, late and delayed types of hypersensitivity responses

7. **You have a dog with well-managed atopic dermatitis with allergen-specific immunotherapy. When one summer there is an increase in pruritus, do you:**
   (a) Abandon the allergen-specific immunotherapy because it is ineffective
   (b) Reassess the dog with a view to any secondary infections, any parasitic infestations and change in the allergen load, and address the treatment
   (c) Prescribe corticosteroids
   (d) Prescribe ciclosporin

8. **Which of following is true of eosinophilic granuloma complex in cats?**
   (a) It is a multifactorial cutaneous reaction pattern
   (b) It is a single disease
   (c) It is only caused by allergic conditions
   (d) It is only caused by parasitic conditions

9. **Which of these statements is false for feline cowpox virus?**
   (a) It is a zoonotic disease
   (b) The virus is carried by small mammals and the infection occurs during hunting
   (c) It responds to corticosteroid treatment within 4 weeks
   (d) The condition can occur at any time of the year but peak in the autumn

10. **The diagnosis of an adverse food reaction is always based on:**
    (a) Response to a diet trial with a novel protein and carbohydrate only and relapse when re-challenged with the original diet
    (b) Demonstration of IgE specific to dietary proteins on serology
    (c) Demonstration of IgG specific to dietary proteins on serology
    (d) Response to change of diet from one type to another

11. **Which of the following are typical cytological findings on a fine-needle aspirate from a histiocytoma?**
    (a) Round cells with a central round nucleus and cytoplasmic granules
    (b) Round cells with round or oval indented nuclei and pale blue cytoplasm
    (c) Round cells with basophilic staining cytoplasm showing increased anisocytosis and anisokaryosis
    (d) All of the above

12. **Which of these answers best describes cytological findings to describe a pyogranulomatous inflammation?**
    (a) Presence of neutrophils with both intracellular and extracellular coccoid bacteria
    (b) Presence of macrophages, neutrophils, lymphocytes and red blood cells
    (c) Presence of lymphocytes and red blood cells
    (d) Presence of macrophages

13. **Which of the following statements is false?**
    (a) Age, sex, breed, illness and drugs can affect the thyroxin concentration
    (b) The diagnosis of hypothyroidism is confirmed on single assay of total T4 showing a marginally lower than normal reference range

(c) The diagnosis of hypothyroidism is supported by raised thyroid-stimulating hormone (TSH) and lower than normal levels of total T4 and free T4 measured by equilibrium dialysis
(d) Hypothyroidism is generally a non-pruritic condition unless there is a secondary complication

14. **You are presented with a 15-year-old cat with a recent onset of alopecia, shiny skin and mild pruritus on the ventral neck and abdomen. There is also some crusting on the feet. Which of the following diagnostic tests would you consider to be the most appropriate?**
    (a) Give the cat an injection of methyl acetate prednisolone
    (b) Prescribe a short course of corticosteroids and antibiotics and start a food trial
    (c) Perform serum allergy tests
    (d) Do haematology, biochemistry, tape-strips, skin biopsies and consider ultrasound examination

15. **Hepatocutaneous syndrome is a cutaneous manifestation of internal disease. Which of the following conditions is not implicated in the pathogenesis of this syndrome?**
    (a) A glucagon-secreting pancreatic neoplasm
    (b) Hepatic cirrhosis
    (c) Mycotoxins
    (d) Diphenhydramine

16. **You are presented with a 10-year-old cat with a short history of crusting and exfoliation, mainly on the trunk. Skin scrapes are negative and histopathology revealed cell-poor interface dermatitis. Which of the following options would you consider appropriate at that point in this case?**
    (a) Start corticosteroid treatment at immunosuppressive doses
    (b) Do survey thoracic radiographs
    (c) Start treatment with ciclosporin
    (d) Start antibiotic treatment

17. **Which of the following statements is true for cyclical recurrent flank alopecia?**
    (a) The condition only occurs in young dogs under the age of 2

(b) The hair always grows back by the end of the winter in all cases

(c) The hair loss can occur either in the spring or autumn

(d) The affected dogs are lethargic and obese

18. **Which of the following clinical signs are associated with a superficial pyoderma?**
    (a) Papules and pustules
    (b) Lichenification
    (c) Scaling
    (d) All of the above

19. **Which of the following stains are used to identify acid-fast organisms such as mycobacteria both on cytological and histological preparations?**
    (a) Periodic acid–Schiff
    (b) Ziehl–Neelsen stain
    (c) Gram stain
    (d) Methenamine silver stain

20. **Which of the following statements is false with regard to discoid (cutaneous) lupus erythematosus?**
    (a) Dolicocephalic breeds are predisposed to the condition
    (b) It is not affected by sunlight
    (c) Topical and/or systemic treatment should be individually tailored to suit the patient
    (d) The condition has a tendency to wax and wane

21. **The optimum sample for culture and sensitivity testing in cases of deep pyoderma is:**
    (a) A swab taken from the skin surface
    (b) A swab taken from the skin surface after surgical preparation of the site
    (c) A biopsy sample of skin subcutis after surgical preparation
    (d) A swab of pus squeezed from deep within the lesion after surgical preparation

22. **Which of the following breeds are predisposed to develop syndrome 1 zinc-responsive dermatitis:**
    (a) Labrador retriever
    (b) Alaskan malamute
    (c) Border terrier
    (d) Chow-chow

23. **Which of the following statements is true regarding canine demodicosis?**
    (a) Juvenile-onset demodicosis is usually a marker for an underlying immunosuppressive disorder
    (b) Trial amitraz therapy is indicated in suspected cases of demodicosis when mites cannot be found on skin scraping
    (c) An underlying immunosuppressive disease may be identified in approximately 50% of cases of adult-onset demodicosis
    (d) Adult-onset demodicosis is due solely to a specific T-cell deficit, allowing an increase in the numbers of *Demodex* mites

24. **Which of the following are most likely to result in circular spreading patches of alopecia?**
    (a) A hair growth cycle abnormality
    (b) Hypothyroidism
    (c) Self-trauma
    (d) Folliculitis

25. **Anagen hair bulbs are:**
    (a) Club shaped and non-pigmented
    (b) Club shaped and pigmented
    (c) Spear shaped and pigmented
    (d) Spear shaped and non-pigmented

26. **Which of the following statements is not true. Cheyletiellosis is a difficult disease to treat because:**
    (a) All in-contact cats, dogs and rabbits need to be treated in a household
    (b) Adult mites can survive for up to 10 days within the environment
    (c) Adult mites live in tunnels in the epidermis and are protected from topical acaricides
    (d) The 35-day life cycle requires at least 6 weeks of treatment

27. **Amongst the imidazoles, itraconazole has a lesser potential for adverse effects compared to ketoconazole because:**
    (a) It is more active against fungal enzymes compared to mammalian enzymes
    (b) It is more active against mammalian enzymes compared to fungal enzymes
    (c) It is less hepatotoxic than ketoconazole
    (d) It binds more readily to fungal rather than mammalian cell walls

28. Which of the following statements regarding pemphigus foliaceus is incorrect?
(a) Pemphigus foliaceus is a sterile pustular skin disease
(b) Pemphigus foliaceus may be exacerbated by exposure to ultraviolet light
(c) Desmoglein-1 is a minor antigen in pemphigus foliaceus
(d) An accurate diagnosis of pemphigus foliaceus may be made on finding neutrophils and acantholytic keratinocytes on pustule cytology

29. Follicular casts are:
(a) Accumulations of keratosebaceous material surrounding hair shafts that represent hair follicle pathology
(b) Accumulations of crust surrounding hair shafts that are seen in folliculitis
(c) Circular rims of scale on the skin representing the end stage of pustule evolution
(d) Plugs of material blocking hair follicle ostia

30. Which of the following is not a recognized side-effect of retinoid therapy?
(a) Teratogenicity
(b) Decreased tear production
(c) Elevated serum creatine kinase
(d) Hyperlipidaemia

31. Which of the following statements is inaccurate?
(a) Visible scale may be due to a failure of enzymatic degradation of intercorneocyte adhesion
(b) Crust is formed when layers of stratum corneum are separated from the underlying epidermis as a result of pustule formation
(c) Crust represents a breach of epithelial integrity
(d) Scale may accumulate because of an increased rate of epithelial turnover

32. Pruritus in cats is most commonly manifested by which of the following symptoms?
(a) Symmetrical alopecia, eosinophilic granuloma complex, miliary dermatitis, head and neck pruritus
(b) Symmetrical alopecia, miliary dermatitis, head and neck dermatitis, paronychia
(c) Miliary dermatitis, head and neck pruritus, eosinophilic granuloma complex, head shaking
(d) Symmetrical alopecia, head and neck pruritus, otitis externa, miliary dermatitis

33. Leucotrichia be seen in which of the following diseases?
(a) Colour dilution alopecia and alopecia areata
(b) Alopecia areata and cyclical flank alopecia
(c) Alopecia areata and vitiligo
(d) Vitiligo and colour dilution alopecia

34. Which of the following statements regarding macromelanosomes is incorrect?
(a) Macromelanosomes are the result of abnormal melanosome storage and transfer from melanocyte to keratinocyte
(b) They are found in the hair shafts of all dilute coat colour breeds
(c) They are only found in the hair shafts of dogs suffering from colour dilution alopecia
(d) They can result in hair shaft fracture and alopecia

35. Which of the following statements is correct?
(a) Castration would be the treatment of choice for alopecia X in an intact male dog
(b) Alopecia X is a growth hormone deficiency
(c) Alopecia X affects mainly short-coated breeds of dog
(d) A trichogram from a dog with alopecia X would show mainly club-shaped hair bulbs

36. Which combination would be considered the treatment of choice for the management of a pruritic dog with demodicosis?
(a) Prednisolone and ivermectin
(b) Amitraz and cefalexin
(c) Amitraz and prednisolone
(d) Amitraz and chlorpheniramine

37. Which of the following is correct?
(a) Vasculitis results from infection of endothelial cells with endothelioptropic pathogens
(b) Vasculitis is a type III hypersensitivity reaction to exogenous antigens
(c) Vasculitis can result in a variety of cutaneous lesions, including oedema, erythema, purpura, scaling and ulceration
(d) All of the above

38. **Pentoxifylline is useful in the treatment of dermatomyositis because:**
    (a) It improves blood flow through damaged blood vessels and has a mild immunomodulatory effect
    (b) It is a potent immunosuppressive agent
    (c) It has a protective effect against ultraviolet light
    (d) It has an antiviral effect

39. **Which of the following is correct regarding erythema multiforme?**
    (a) It is caused by the formation of antibodies to intercorneocyte adhesion molecules and results in vesicle and bulla formation
    (b) It is a neoplastic disease resulting in lymphocytic invasion of the epidermis
    (c) It is a lymphocyte-mediated immune response against keratinocytes most commonly associated with viral infection
    (d) It is a lymphocyte-mediated immune response against keratinocytes most commonly associated with a drug reaction

40. **Diagnostic features of plasma cell pododermatitis include:**
    (a) Swollen footpads, mixed inflammatory cell infiltrate on cytology and histopathology, all cats are FIV positive and show polyclonal hypergammaglobulinaemia
    (b) Swollen footpads, mixed inflammatory cell infiltrate on cytology and histopathology, up to 50% cats are FIV positive and show polyclonal hypergammaglobulinaemia
    (c) Swollen footpads, mixed inflammatory cell infiltrate on cytology and histopathology, up to 50% cats are FIV positive and show monoclonal hypergammaglobulinaemia
    (d) Swollen footpads; solely plasma cell infiltrate on cytology and histopathology, 100% cats are FIV positive and show polyclonal hypergammaglobulinaemia

41. **With regard to treatment of acral lick dermatitis, which of the following are false?**
    (a) The first line of treatment in acral lick dermatitis is systemic antibacterial therapy
    (b) The first line of treatment in acral lick dermatitis is systemic glucocorticoid therapy
    (c) Glucocorticoids are frequently contraindicated in acral lick dermatitis because of the presence of deep pyoderma
    (d) Glucocorticoids may be helpful to break the lick–itch cycle in acral lick dermatitis

42. **Which of the following statements is incorrect regarding squamous cell carcinoma (SCC)?**
    (a) SCC is locally invasive but slow to metastasize
    (b) SCC of the digit carries a more favourable prognosis than SCC of the trunk
    (c) Digital SCC most commonly affects black dogs
    (d) The treatment of choice for SCC of the digit is early digital amputation

43. **When treating *Pseudomonas* otitis externa:**
    (a) Fluoroquinolones should be administered systemically at up to four times data sheet dose because they are concentration-dependent antibacterials
    (b) Fluoroquinolones should only be used at up to double data sheet dose because above this dosage they can induce neurotoxicity
    (c) Topical fluoroquinolones should not be used if there is evidence of in vitro resistance
    (d) Selecting the correct antibacterial is the single most important therapeutic consideration

44. **Which of the following is true?**
    (a) Buffy coat smears are a sensitive and specific method of detecting mast cell tumour (MCT) metastasis
    (b) Pulmonary metastasis of MCT can be ruled out in the absence of 'cannon-ball' metastases on thoracic radiography
    (c) Cytological evaluation of fine-needle aspirates is usually diagnostic for cases of MCT
    (d) Injections of deionized water have been shown to be a reliable method of prevent local recurrence of MCT

45. **Mechanisms for hyperpigmentation in endocrinopathy might include:**
    (a) Ultraviolet tanning of sun-exposed alopecic skin
    (b) Post-inflammatory hyperpigmentation due to secondary bacterial or yeast infection
    (c) Stimulation of melanocytes by increased concentrations of ACTH
    (d) All of the above

MCQs – Answers

1. **(a)** April to October

2. **(e)** Rabbit syphilis

3. **(b)** *Trichophyton mentagrophytes*

4. **(e)** Phenol Red

5. **(c)** Rule out ectoparasitic conditions, rule in or out any secondary microbial infections and the role of an adverse food reaction with appropriate tests, responses to treatment and to a food trial

6. **(d)** It shows immediate, late and delayed types of hypersensitivity responses

7. **(b)** Reassess the dog with a view to any secondary infections, any parasitic infestations and change in the allergen load, and address the treatment

8. **(a)** It is a multifactorial cutaneous reaction pattern

9. **(c)** It responds to corticosteroid treatment within 4 weeks

10. **(a)** Response to a diet trial with a novel protein and carbohydrate only and relapse when re-challenged with the original diet

11. **(b)** Round cells with round or oval indented nuclei and pale blue cytoplasm

12. **(b)** Presence of macrophages, neutrophils, lymphocytes and red blood cells

13. **(b)** The diagnosis of hypothyroidism is confirmed on single assay of total T4 showing a marginally lower than the normal reference range

14. **(d)** Do haematology, biochemistry, tape-strips, skin biopsies and consider ultrasound examination

15. **(d)** Diphenhydramine

16. **(b)** Do survey thoracic radiographs

17. **(c)** The hair loss can occur either in the spring or autumn

18. **(d)** All of the above

19. **(b)** Ziehl–Neelsen stain

20. **(b)** It is not affected by sunlight

21. **(c)** A biopsy sample of skin subcutis after surgical preparation

22. **(b)** Alaskan malamute

23. **(c)** An underlying immunosuppressive disease may be identified in approximately 50% of cases of adult-onset demodicosis

24. **(d)** Folliculitis

25. **(b)** Club shaped and pigmented

26. **(c)** Adult mites live in tunnels in the epidermis and are protected from topical acaricides

27. **(a)** It is more active against fungal enzymes compared to mammalian enzymes

28. **(d)** An accurate diagnosis of pemphigus foliaceus may be made on finding neutrophils and acantholytic keratinocytes on pustule cytology

29. **(a)** Accumulations of keratosebaceous material surrounding hair shafts that represent hair follicle pathology

30. **(c)** Elevated serum creatine kinase

31. **(b)** Crust is formed when layers of stratum corneum are separated from the underlying epidermis as a result of pustule formation

32. **(a)** Symmetrical alopecia, eosinophilic granuloma complex, miliary dermatitis, head and neck pruritus

33. **(c)** Alopecia areata and vitiligo

34. **(c)** They are only found in the hair shafts of dogs suffering from colour dilution alopecia

35. **(a)** Castration would be the treatment of choice for alopecia X in an intact male dog

36. **(b)** Amitraz and cefalexin

37. **(d)** All of the above

38. **(a)** It improves blood flow through damaged blood vessels and has a mild immunomodulatory effect

39. **(c)** It is a lymphocyte-mediated immune response against keratinocytes most commonly associated with viral infection

40. **(b)** Swollen footpads, mixed inflammatory cell infiltrate on cytology and histopathology, up to 50% cats are FIV positive and show polyclonal hypergammaglobulinaemia

41. **(b)** The first line of treatment in acral lick dermatitis is systemic glucocorticoid therapy

42. **(b)** SCC of the digit carries a more favourable prognosis than SCC of the trunk

43. **(a)** Fluoroquinolones should be administered systemically at up to four times data sheet dose because they are concentration-dependent antibacterials

44. **(c)** Cytological evaluation of fine-needle aspirates is usually diagnostic for cases of MCT

45. **(d)** All of the above

APPENDIX
Antibacterials used in veterinary dermatology

Many agents used in veterinary dermatology are not licensed for use in animal species. According to UK legislation, if a licensed product is available it must be used first, but under the Cascade system it is acceptable to use a licensed human product should there be no veterinary alternative. Owners must sign appropriate forms to this effect.

Antibacterials are classified as time dependent or concentration dependent in action. Time-dependent antibiotics require the plasma concentration to be above the minimum inhibitory concentration (MIC) for as long as possible, whereas for concentration-dependent antibiotics the time above the MIC is not so critical, but the dose should be adjusted to maximize the peak plasma concentration.

Aminoglycosides and fluoroquinolones are concentration-dependent antibiotics, whereas penicillins and cephalosporins are time dependent.

Only 4% of cardiac output reaches the dermis and subcutis, and the epidermis is entirely dependent on diffusion of the antibiotic from the underlying dermis. The cutaneous concentration of cefalexin is only 20% of plasma concentration. Therefore, high doses of systemic antibacterial agents are required in order to reach therapeutic concentrations in the dermis and epidermis.

Superficial pyoderma generally requires a minimum of 21 days of systemic antibacterial therapy and at least 7 days' use past the clinical cure. Deep pyoderma requires a minimum of 42 days' treatment, with at least 14 days past the clinical cure.

Ideally, a narrow-spectrum antibacterial should be used in preference to one with a broad spectrum of activity.

Table A1.1 Systemic antibacterials for treatment of pyoderma

	Dosage	Spectrum	Advantages	Disadvantages	Adverse effects
First-line antibacterials	Indications: Treatment of canine and feline bacterial skin disease at first presentation.				
Macrolides					
Tylosin	10–20 mg/kg b.i.d., p.o.	Narrow (Gram positives)	Inexpensive	Lincosamide cross-resistance	GI disturbance
Erythromycin	15 mg/kg t.i.d., p.o. With food	Narrow (Gram positives)	Inexpensive	Three times daily administration. Cross-resistance with lincosamides	Vomiting
Lincosamides					
Clindamycin	5–11 mg/kg b.i.d. Use at higher dosage in immunocompromised patients	Narrow (Gram positives and anaerobes)	Excellent first-line antibacterial for pyoderma	Cross-resistance with macrolides	
Lincomycin	20 mg/kg b.i.d. Empty stomach	Narrow (Gram positives)		Cross-resistance with macrolides	Diarrhoea. Potentially hepatotoxic
Potentiated sulphonamides					
Trimethoprim/ sulphadiazine	15–30 mg/kg b.i.d.	Broad	Inexpensive	Decreased efficacy in deep pyoderma. Not recommended for extended treatment. 10–25% of strains of *S. intermedius* are resistant to potentiated sulphonamides	Keratoconjunctivitis sicca, Type 3 hypersensitivities: hepatotoxicity, hypothyroidism, crystaluria/ haematuria
Second-line antibacterials	Indications: Second-line antibacterials should ideally be reserved for the treatment of bacterial skin conditions that have responded poorly, or are expected to respond poorly, to first-line antibacterials. These drugs are also suitable for long-term or pulse therapy if required.				
Cephalosporins					
Cefalexin	15–30 mg/kg b.i.d.	Broad spectrum	Safe for long-term therapy. Very effective	Over, and inappropriate, use may result in emergence of staphylococcal resistance	Occasional GI disturbance. Hypersensitivity (cross-reaction with penicillins)
Cefovecin	8 mg/kg s.c.	Broad spectrum	Long-acting injection. Very convenient	Over, and inappropriate, use may result in emergence of staphylococcal resistance	Possible hypersensitivity reactions (cross-reaction with penicillins)

Continued

Table A1.1 Systemic antibacterials for treatment of pyoderma—cont'd

	Dosage	Spectrum	Advantages	Disadvantages	Adverse effects
Penicillins					
Amoxycillin and clavulanic acid	12.5–22 mg/kg b.i.d.	Broad spectrum	Safe for long-term therapy		Occasional GI disturbance. Hypersensitivity disorders (cross-reaction with cephalosporins)
Third-line antibacterials	Indications: Otitis externa due to *Pseudomonas aeruginosa* susceptible to fluoroquinolones. Pyoderma due to Gram-negative infections. Pyoderma due to *Staphylococcus intermedius* where other antibiotics are contraindicated or ineffective. Arguably should be reserved for infections involving both Gram-negative rods and cocci				
Fluoroquinolones					
Enrofloxacin	5–20 mg/kg s.i.d., p.o. Use at higher dosages when treating *Pseudomonas* spp.	Broad spectrum	Once daily dosing. Effective against many Gram negatives, including *Pseudomonas* spp.	Expensive. Overusage has resulted in emergence of resistant staphylococci and *Pseudomonas* spp.	Contraindicated in young growing dogs. Retinal blindness in cats at high dosages. CNS disturbance at high dosages
Marbofloxacin	2–8 mg/kg s.i.d. Use at higher dosages when treating *Pseudomonas* spp.	Broad spectrum	Once daily dosing. Effective against many Gram negatives, including *Pseudomonas* spp.	Expensive. Over and inappropriate usage will result in bacterial resistance	Occasional GI disturbance

Note that dosages given in some cases are up to four times the data sheet recommendations.

2 APPENDIX
Basic list of equipment required

The basic equipment required for dealing with dermatological conditions is as follows:

- Binocular microscope with a good quality, ×100 oil immersion objective
- Immersion oil
- Lens cleaning tissue
- Otoscope with different speculum sizes (3.5 V halogen light source is ideal)
- Microscope slides – frosted ends are useful for writing details on slides
- Coverslips
- Haemostat forceps with jaws protected by drip tubing for trichography
- Diff Quik® or Rapi-Diff® stains
- Tape for cytology (Cellux®, Diamond White® or Scotch pressure tape® work best)
- Clippers
- Curved scissors
- Scalpel blades, No. 10
- Flea comb
- Staining jars
- 4-, 6- and 8-mm biopsy punches
- Local anaesthetic without adrenaline (Lidocaine®)
- Swabs for bacterial culture, including mini-tip swabs for obtaining samples from the middle ear
- New toothbrushes for fungal culture
- Wood's lamp (240 V, with two UV strip bulbs and magnifier).

APPENDIX
List of diseases by presenting signs

Table A3.1

Presenting sign	Disease (Chapter)
Pruritus	Canine scabies (4) Flea allergy dermatitis (5) Cheyletiellosis (8) Atopic dermatitis/pyoderma (6) *Malassezia* dermatitis (7) Trichophytosis (9) Dermatophytosis in a guinea-pig (10) Cutaneous adverse food reaction (11) Cutaneous lymphoma in a hamster (30) Feline head and neck pruritus (37) Hormonal hyperpigmentation (43) Acral lick dermatitis (45) Sterile pyogranulomatous dermatitis (46) Eosinophilic furunculosis (52)
Erythema	Canine scabies (4) Flea allergy dermatitis (5) Atopic dermatitis/pyoderma (6) *Malassezia* dermatitis (7) Trichophytosis (9) Cutaneous adverse food reaction (11) Paraneoplastic exfoliative dermatosis (14) Metabolic epidermal necrosis (18) Canine demodicosis (26) Feline paraneoplastic alopecia (31) Vasculitis (34) Dermatomyositis (35) Cat pox (51) Cutaneous lupus erythematosus (53) Sterile pyogranulomatous dermatitis (46)
Papules	Canine scabies (4) Flea allergy dermatitis (5) Atopic dermatitis/pyoderma (6) Cheyletiellosis (8) Cutaneous adverse food reaction (11)

Continued

Table A3.1—cont'd

Presenting sign	Disease (Chapter)
Crusting	Canine scabies (4)
	Malassezia dermatitis (7)
	Trichophytosis (9)
	Dermatophytosis in a guinea-pig (10)
	Cutaneous adverse food reaction (11)
	Paraneoplastic exfoliative dermatosis (14)
	Cutaneous epitheliotropic lymphoma (15)
	Zinc-responsive dermatosis (19)
	Canine demodicosis (26)
	Feline paraneoplastic alopecia (31)
	Vasculitis (34)
	Dermatomyositis (35)
	Cat pox (51)
	Erythema multiforme (33)
	Uveodermatological syndrome (41)
	Cutaneous lupus erythematosus (53)
Scaling	Canine scabies (4)
	Flea allergy dermatitis (5)
	Cheyletiellosis (8)
	Trichophytosis (9)
	Dermatophytosis in a guinea-pig (10)
	Cutaneous adverse food reaction (11)
	Sebaceous adenitis (13)
	Paraneoplastic exfoliative dermatosis (14)
	Cutaneous epitheliotropic lymphoma (15)
	Hypothyroidism (22)
	Canine recurrent flank alopecia (25)
	Dermatophytosis – *M. canis* in a cat (28)
	Feline paraneoplastic alopecia (31)
	Vasculitis (34)
	Uveodermatological syndrome (41)
	Hormonal hyperpigmentation (43)
	Cutaneous lupus erythematosus (53)
Erosions/ulcers	Pemphigus foliaceus (17)
	Zinc-responsive dermatosis (19)
	Erythema multiforme (33)
	Vasculitis (34)
	Dermatomyositis (35)
	Feline eosinophilic plaque (36)
	Feline head and neck pruritus (37)
	Mast cell tumour (48)
	Eosinophilic furunculosis (52)
	Plasma cell pododermatitis (54)
	Squamous cell carcinoma (55)
Fissuring	Metabolic epidermal necrosis (18)

Table A3.1—cont'd

Presenting sign	Disease (Chapter)
Hyperpigmentation	Flea allergy dermatitis (5) Trichophytosis (9) Hypothyroidism (22) Alopecia X (24) Canine recurrent flank alopecia (25) Canine demodicosis (26) Feline paraneoplastic alopecia (31) Lentigo simplex (42) Hormonal hyperpigmentation (43)
Hypopigmentation	Cutaneous epitheliotropic lymphoma (15) Vitiligo (40) Uveodermatological syndrome (41) Cutaneous lupus erythematosus (53)
Alopecia	Atopic dermatitis/pyoderma (6) *Malassezia* dermatitis (7) Trichophytosis (9) Dermatophytosis in a guinea-pig (10) Cutaneous epitheliotropic lymphoma (15) Feline symmetrical alopecia (21) Hypothyroidism (22) Colour dilution alopecia (23) Alopecia X (24) Canine recurrent flank alopecia (25) Canine demodicosis (26) Staphylococcal pyoderma (27) Dermatophytosis – *M. canis* in a cat (28) Alopecia areata (29) Cutaneous lymphoma in a hamster (30) Feline paraneoplastic alopecia (31) Vasculitis (34) Dermatomyositis (35) Uveodermatological syndrome (41) Hormonal hyperpigmentation (43) Acral lick dermatitis (45) Sterile pyogranulomatous dermatitis (46) Feline mycobacterial disease (47)
Nodules and swellings	Acral lick dermatitis (45) Sterile pyogranulomatous dermatitis (46) Feline mycobacterial disease (47) Mast cell tumour (48) Cutaneous histiocytoma (49) Plasma cell pododermatitis (54) Squamous cell carcinoma (55)
Epidermal collarettes	Atopic dermatitis/pyoderma (6) Erythema multiforme (33)
Lichenification	*Malassezia* dermatitis (7)
Otitis externa	Cutaneous adverse food reaction (11) Otitis externa (57)

Continued

Table A3.1—cont'd

Presenting sign	Disease (Chapter)
Nail involvement/paronychia	Pemphigus foliaceus (17) Squamous cell carcinoma (55) Lupoid onychodystrophy (56)
Footpad lesions	Zinc-responsive dermatosis (19) Erythema multiforme (33) Vitiligo (40) Cutaneous lupus erythematosus (53) Plasma cell pododermatitis (54) Squamous cell carcinoma (55)
Head and neck involvement	Trichophytosis (9) Pemphigus foliaceus (17) Dermatomyositis (35) Feline head and neck pruritus (37) Cat pox (51) Eosinophilic furunculosis (52)
Nasal planum involvement	Vitiligo (40) Uveodermatological syndrome (41) Cutaneous lupus erythematosus (53)
Lip involvement	Lentigo simplex (42)
Leucotrichia	Alopecia areata (29) Vitiligo (40)
Shiny skin	Feline paraneoplastic alopecia (31)
Oral lesions	Erythema multiforme (33)
Necrosis	Vasculitis (34) Cat pox (51)
Draining sinus tracts	Sterile pyogranulomatous dermatitis (46) Feline mycobacterial disease (47)

4 APPENDIX
Shampoo therapy

Shampoo therapy is frequently of value in the management of skin disease, either as a sole therapy or used as an adjunct to systemic treatment.

There are a wide variety of shampoos available and shampoo selection depends on the therapeutic goal.

The most common uses for shampoo therapy are:
1. Cleansing
2. Soothing and antipruritic effects
3. Scaling disorders
4. Fungal skin disease, including *Malassezia* dermatitis and dermatophytosis
5. Adjunctive treatment for pyoderma.

A shampoo may be required to address more than one of these indications at a time.

SHAMPOO TERMINOLOGY

Moisturizers increase the water content of the stratum corneum, and by doing so soften the skin and hair coat. There are two types of moisturizers: humectants and emollients. Humectants are hygroscopic; they draw water into the skin by absorbing many times their own molecular weight of water. Emollients are oils or other occlusive substances which trap water next to the skin. They work best if applied immediately after bathing.

Antiseborrhoeics reduce scaling and have keratoplastic and/or keratolytic activity. Keratoplastic products reduce scaling by slowing down epithelial turnover time, whereas keratolytics break down adhesions between corneocytes, increasing desquamation.

Microvesicle. Many shampoos contain microvesicle technology. These are microscopic, layered spheres that have greatly benefited shampoo treatments by giving a sustained release of the active ingredient over time. The microvesicle binds to skin and hair and is not rinsed away.

Table A4.1 shows a list of the more common ingredients and actions of shampoos currently available in the UK. The list is not comprehensive and there are additional, effective products that are not listed.

Table A4.1 Common ingredients and actions of shampoos currently available in the UK

Active ingredient	Product	Actions	Clinical indication	Side-effects/contraindications
Benzoyl peroxide	Paxcutol®	Bactericidal Keratolytic Keratoplastic Potent degreaser	Greasy scaling skin disorders Pyoderma with crusting Pustular demodicosis	Irritant in a small number of dogs Very drying Bleaches hair coat and carpets
Ethyl lactate	Etiderm®	Antibacterial Keratoplastic	Superficial pyoderma where there is dry scaling	
Chlorhexidine	Malaseb® Nolvasan®	Antibacterial Antifungal	Superficial pyoderma with dry skin *Malassezia* dermatitis (at >3% concentration)	
Miconazole	Malaseb®	Antifungal	*Malassezia* dermatitis	
Acetic acid/boric acid	Malacetic®	Antibacterial Antifungal	*Malassezia* dermatitis Pyoderma	
Salicylic acid	Sebolytic®	Keratolytic Keratoplastic Bacteriostatic	Scaling disorders	
Selenium sulphide	Seleen®	Keratolytic Keratoplastic Degreasing Antibacterial Antiparasitic Antifungal	Greasy skin disorders Scaling Pyoderma *Malassezia* dermatitis	Unpleasant odour to some owners May turn white hair coats a red–brown colour
Ketoconazole	Ketoconazole shampoo®; Millpledge	Antifungal	*Malassezia* dermatitis	
Piroctone olamine	Sebolytic® Sebomild® Allermyl®	Antibacterial Antifungal	Pyoderma	
Colloidal oatmeal	Episoothe® Coatex Aloe and Oatmeal®	Humectant Antipruritic	Dry pruritic skin disorders, particularly atopic dermatitis	
Lactic acid, sodium lactate, urea and chitosanide	Various	Humectants	Dry pruritic skin disorders, particularly atopic dermatitis	
Coconut oil, safflower oil, cottonseed oil, vitamin E, lanolin	Various	Emollients	Dry pruritic skin disorders, particularly atopic dermatitis	
Hexetidine	Hexocil®	Skin cleansing		

5 APPENDIX
Zoonoses

Despite the close proximity that pets live with their owners, zoonotic skin disease is a relatively uncommon occurrence (see Figs A5.1, A5.2 and A5.3), but knowledge of the zoonotic skin diseases affecting both pets and owners is essential because of public health considerations, but also of great help from a diagnostic viewpoint. The dermatology history should always include questions about whether in-contact people have been affected (see Chapter 1).

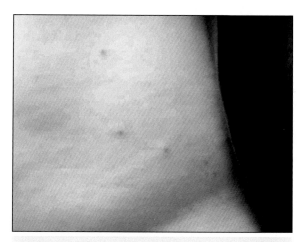

Figure A5.1 Pruritic papules over the trunk of an owner whose dog was affected by scabies.

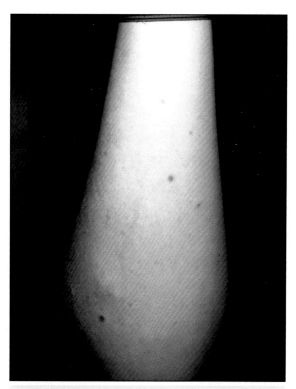

Figure A5.2 Pruritic papules over the forearm of an owner whose dog was affected by cheyletiellosis.

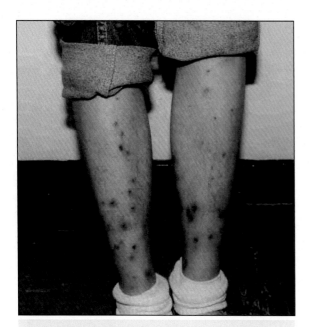

Figure A5.3 Pruritic papules over the lower legs of an owner resulting from cat flea bites.

Factors affecting the likelihood of zoonosis occurring include the number of animals in the household, the infectious burden of the animal, their proximity to owners and the health status of the owners. Young, elderly and immunosuppressed owners are more likely to be affected by zoonotic disease. In general, keeping pets clean, healthy and free of parasites, and good household and personal hygiene, particularly good handwashing practice, will greatly reduce the likelihood of zoonotic skin disease.

Table A5.1 Diseases responsible for skin lesions in both pets and humans

Disease	Aetiology	Animal spp. affected	Signs in humans	Action
Canine scabies	*Sarcoptes scabiei* var. *canis*	Dogs, cats (rare), ferrets	30–50% of in-contact people develop pruritus/papules over trunk and limbs (Fig. A5.1)	Usually resolves once animal disease treated. Seek medical attention if persistently affected
Notoedric mange	*Notoedres cati*	Cats (rare)	Pruritic papular disease. Rare zoonosis	As above
Otodectic mange	*Otodectes cynotis*	Dogs, cats, ferrets	Pruritus. Otitis	As above
Cheyletiellosis	*Cheyletiella* spp.	Dogs, cats, rabbits and other mammals	30–50% of in-contact people develop pruritus/papules over trunk and limbs (Fig. A5.2)	As above
Flea infestation	*Ctenocephalides* spp.	Dogs, cats rabbits and other mammals	Pruritic papules and macules on lower limbs (Fig. A5.3)	Bites resolve once infestation treated
Tropical rat mite	*Liponyssus bacoti*	Rats	Pruritic papular dermatosis	Usually resolves once animal disease treated. Seek medical attention if persistently affected
Dermatophytosis	Usually *Microsporum canis* infection	Cats, dogs, rabbits, ferrets and other small mammals	Various lesions, including variably pruritic, erythematous and scaling macules, and patches over exposed areas of skin	Advise seek medical attention
Malassezia dermatitis	*Malassezia* spp.	Dogs, cats	Low risk, rare zoonosis. Consideration in hospitals/nursing homes where in-contact people are immunosuppressed or have indwelling catheter	Seek urgent medical attention if suspected
Mycobacterial infection	*Mycobacterium bovis, M. tuberculosis, M. avium*	Dogs (very rare), cats	Tuberculosis	Seek medical attention
Cowpox	*Orthopoxvirus*	Cats, rodents	Painful cutaneous nodules to systemic disease	Owners should wear gloves when handling infected cats. Seek medical attention

Further reading

Chapter 2: Laboratory tests

Foster A, Foil C (2003): Investigation and laboratory techniques. In: BSAVA Manual of Small Animal Dermatology. Blackwell Publishing, London.

Harvey RG, Harari J, Delauche AJ (2001): Cytological characteristics of normal and abnormal ears. In: Ear Diseases of the Dog and Cat. Manson Publishing, London, pp. 50–57.

Hill PB (2002): Small Animal Dermatology, A practical guide to diagnosis. Butterworth-Heinemann, London.

Scott DW, Miller WH, Griffin CE (2001): Diagnostic methods. In: Muller and Kirk's Small Animal Dermatology, 6th Edition. WB Saunders, Philadelphia, pp. 71–206.

Chapter 3: Introduction to pruritus – pathogenesis and evolution of lesions

Hill P, Lo A, Edin CA, et al. (2006): Survey of the prevalence, diagnosis and treatment of dermatological conditions in small animals in general practice. Vet Rec 158, 533–539.

Chapter 4: Sarcoptic mange

Arlian LG, Morgan MS, Rapp CM, et al. (1996): The development of protective immunity in canine scabies. Vet Parasitol 62, 133–142.

Arlian LG, Morgan MS (2000): Serum antibody to *Sarcoptes scabiei* and house dust mite prior to and during infestation with *S. scabiei*. Vet Parasitol 90, 315–326.

Bornstein S, Thebo P, Zakrisson G (1996): Evaluation of an enzyme-linked immunosorbent assay (ELISA) for the serological diagnosis of canine sarcoptic mange. Vet Dermatol 7, 21–28.

Curtis CF (2001): Evaluation of a commercially available enzyme-linked immunosorbent assay for the diagnosis of canine sarcoptic mange. Vet Rec 24 (148), 238–239.

Curtis CF (2004): Current trends in the treatment of *Sarcoptes*, *Cheyletiella* and *Otodectes* mite infestations in dogs and cats. Vet Dermatol 15, 108–114.

Fourie LJ, Heine J, Horak IG (2006): The efficacy of an imidacloprid/moxidectin combination against naturally acquired *Sarcoptes scabiei* infestations on dogs. Aus Vet J 84, 17–21.

Lower KS, Medleau LM, Hnilica K (2001): Evaluation of an enzyme-linked immunosorbent assay (ELISA) for the serological diagnosis of sarcoptic mange in dogs. Vet Dermatol 12, 315–320.

Pin D, Bensignor E, Carlotti DN, et al. (2006): Localised sarcoptic mange in dogs: a retrospective study of 10 dogs. J Small Anim Pract 47, 611–614.

Chapter 5: Flea allergic dermatitis

Dickin SK, McTier TL, Murphy MG, et al. (2003): Efficacy of selamectin in the treatment and control of clinical signs of flea allergy dermatitis in dogs and cats experimentally infested with fleas. J Am Vet Med Assoc 223, 639–644.

Dryden MW, Denenberg TM, Bunch S (2000): Control of fleas on naturally infested dogs and cats and in private residences with topical spot applications of fipronil or imidacloprid. Vet Parasitol 93, 69–75.

Frank GR, Hunter SW, Stiegler GI, et al. (1998): Salivary allergens of *Ctenocephalides felis*: collection, purification and evaluation by intradermal skin testing in dogs. In: Kwochkwa KW, Willemse T, von Tscharner C, Eds. Advances in Veterinary Dermatology, Volume 3. Butterworth-Heinemann, Oxford, pp. 201–212.

Laffort-Dassot C, Carlotti DN, Pin D, et al. (2004): Diagnosis of flea allergy dermatitis: comparison of intradermal testing with flea allergens and a FcepsilonRI alpha-based IgE assay in response to flea control. Vet Dermatol 15, 321–330.

Medleau L, Hnilica KA, Lower K, et al. (2002): Effect of topical application of fipronil in cats with flea allergic dermatitis Am Vet Med Assoc 221, 254–257.

Medleau L, Clekis T, McArthur TR, et al. (2003): Evaluation of fipronil spot-on in the treatment of flea allergic dermatitis in dogs. J Small Anim Pract 44, 71–75.

Ritzhaupt LK, Rowan TG, Jones RL (2000): Evaluation of efficacy of selamectin and fipronil against *Ctenocephalides felis* in cats. J Am Vet Med Assoc 217, 1666–1668.

Rust MK (2005): Advances in the control of *Ctenocephalides felis* (cat flea) on cats and dogs. Trends Parasitol 21, 232–236.

Scott DW, Miller WH, Griffin CE (2001): Muller and Kirk's Small Animal Dermatology, 6th Edition. WB Saunders, Philadelphia, pp. 543–666.

Wilkerson MJ, Bagladi-Swanson M, Wheeler DW, et al. (2004): The immunopathogenesis of flea allergy dermatitis in dogs, an experimental study. Vet Immunol Immunopathol 99, 179–192.

Wuersch K, Brachelente C, Doherr M, et al. (2006): Immune dysregulation in flea allergy dermatitis – a model for the immunopathogenesis of allergic dermatitis. Vet Immunol Immunopathol 110, 311–323.

Chapter 6: Atopic dermatitis

Day MJ (1999): Clinical Immunology of the Dog and Cat. Manson Publishing, London.

Ferguson EA, Littlewood JD, Carlotti DN, et al. (2006): Management of canine atopic dermatitis using the plant extract PYM00217: a randomized, double-blind, placebo-controlled clinical study. Vet Dermatol 17, 236–243.

Guaguere E, Steffan J, Olivery T (2004): Cyclosporin A: a new drug in the field of canine dermatology. Vet Dermatol 15, 61–74.

Marsella R, Nicklin C, Saglio S, et al (2004): Investigation on the clinical efficacy and safety of 0.1% tacrolimus ointment (Protopic®) in canine atopic dermatitis: a randomised, double-blinded, placebo-controlled, cross-over study. Vet Dermatol 15, 294–303.

Marsella R, Nicklin C, Lopez J (2006): Studies on the role of routes of allergen exposure in high IgE-producing beagle dogs sensitized to house dust mites. Vet Dermatol 17, 306–312.

Nuttall TJ, Hill PB, Bensignor E, et al. (2006): House dust and forage mite allergens and their role in human and canine atopic dermatitis. Vet Dermatol 17, 223–235.

Olivry T (Ed.) (2001): The American College of Veterinary Dermatology Task Force on canine atopic dermatitis. Veterinary Immunology and Immunopathology, Volume 81. Elsevier, Amsterdam.

Prelaud P, Guaguere E, Alhaidari Z, et al. (1998): Re-evaluation of diagnostic criteria of canine atopic dermatitis. Rev Med Vet 149, 1057–1064.

Reedy LM, Miller WH, Willemse T (1997): Allergic Skin Diseases of Dogs and Cats, 2nd Edition. WB Saunders, Philadelphia.

Scott DW, Miller WH, Griffin CE (2001): Muller and Kirk's Small Animal Dermatology, 6th Edition. WB Saunders, Philadelphia.

Chapter 7: *Malassezia* dermatitis

Bond R, Ferguson EA, Curtis CF, et al. (1996): Factors associated with elevated cutaneous *Malassezia* in population of dogs with pruritic skin disease. J Small Anim Pract 37, 103–107.

Bond R, Elwood CM, Littler RM, et al. (1998): Humoral and cell-mediated responses to *Malassezia pachydermatis* in healthy dogs and dogs with *Malassezia* dermatitis. Vet Rec 143, 381–384.

Bond R, Curtis CF, Hendricks A, et al. (2002): Intradermal test reactivity to *Malassezia pachydermatis* in atopic dogs. Vet Rec 150, 448–449.

Chen TA, Halliwell REW, Pemberton AD, et al. (2002): Identification of major allergens of *Malassezia pachydermatis* in dogs with atopic dermatitis and *Malassezia* overgrowth. Vet Dermatol 13, 141–150.

Guillot J, Bond R (1999): *Malassezia pachydermatis*: a review. Med Mycol 37, 295–306.

Morris DO, Olivier NB, Rosser EJ (1998): Type-1 hypersensitivity reactions to *Malassezia* extracts in atopic dogs. Am J Vet Res 59, 836–841.

Nuttall, TJ, Halliwell REW (2001): Serum antibodies to *Malassezia* yeasts in canine atopic dermatitis. Vet Dermatol 12, 327–332.

Chapter 8: Cheyletiellosis

Chadwick AJ (1997): Use of a 0.25% fipronil pump spray formulation to treat canine cheyletiellosis. J Small Anim Pract 38 (6), 261–262.

Mueller RS, Bettenay SV (2002): Efficacy of selamectin in the treatment of canine cheyletiellosis. Vet Rec 151 (25), 773.

Saevik BK, Bredal W, Ulstein TL (2004): Cheyletiella infestation in the dog: observations on diagnostic methods and clinical signs. J Small Anim Pract 45, 495–500.

Scarampella F, Pollmeier M, Visser M, Boeckh A, Jeannin P (2005): Efficacy of fipronil in the treatment of feline cheyletiellosis. Vet Parasitol 129 (3), 333–339.

Scott DW, Miller WH, Griffin CE (2001): Parasitic skin diseases. In: Muller and Kirk's Small Animal Dermatology, 6th Edition. WB Saunders, Philadelphia, pp. 455–457.

Chapter 9: Dermatophytosis in a Jack Russell terrier

Bond R (2002): Canine dermatophytosis associated with *Trichophyton* species and *Microsporum persicolor*. In Practice 24 (7), 388–395.

Hill PB, Moriello KA, Shaw SE (1995): A review of systemic antifungal agents. Vet Dermatol 6 (2), 59–66.

Moriello KA (2004): Treatment of dermatophytosis in dogs and cats: review of published studies (Special Issue: Therapeutics). Vet Dermatol 15 (2), 99–107.

Paterson S (1999): Miconazole/chlorhexidine shampoo as an adjunct to systemic therapy in controlling dermatophytosis in cats. J Small Anim Pract 40 (4), 163–166.

Perrins N, Bond R (2004): Differential diagnosis and treatment of facial skin diseases in dogs. In Practice 26 (10), 522–529.

Scott DW, Miller WH, Griffin CE (2001): Fungal skin diseases. In: Muller and Kirk's Small Animal Dermatology, 6th Edition. WB Saunders, Philadelphia, pp. 336–422.

Chapter 10: Dermatophytosis in a guinea-pig

Carpenter JW (2005): Exotic Animal Formulary, 3rd Edition. Elsevier Saunders, Missouri.

Ellis C, Mori M (2001): Skin diseases of rodents and small exotic mammals. Vet Clin North Am Exotic Anim Pract 4 (2), 493–542.

O'Rourke DP (2004). Disease problems of guinea pigs. In: Quesenberry KE, Carpenter JW, Eds. Ferrets, Rabbits and Rodents. Clinical Medicine and Surgery. Elsevier Saunders, Missouri.

Scott DW, Miller WH, Griffin CE (2001): Muller and Kirk's Small Animal Dermatology, 6th Edition. WB Saunders, Philadelphia.

Chapter 11 Adverse food reaction

Cave NJ (2006): Hydrolyzed protein diets for dogs and cats. Vet Clin North Am Small Anim Pract 36, 1251–1268.

Hillier A, Griffin C (2001): The ACVD task force on canine atopic dermatitis (X): is there a relationship between canine atopic dermatitis and cutaneous adverse food reactions? Vet Immunol Immunopathol 20, 227–231.

Jackson HA, Jackson MW, Coblentz L, et al. (2003): Evaluation of the clinical and allergen specific serum IgE response to oral challenge with cornstarch, corn, soy and a soy hydro-lysate in dogs with spontaneous food allergy. Vet Dermatol 14, 181–187.

Loeffler A, Soares-Magalhaes R, Bond R, et al. (2006): A retrospective analysis of case series using home-prepared and chicken hydrolysate diets in the diagnosis of adverse food reactions in 181 pruritic dogs. Vet Dermatol 17, 273–279.

Martin A, Sierra MP, Gonzalez JL, et al. (2004): Identification of allergens responsible for canine cutaneous adverse food reactions to lamb, beef and cow's milk. Vet Dermatol 15, 349–356.

Chapter 12: Introduction to crusting and scaling

Scott DW, Miller WH, Griffin CE (1995): Diagnostic methods. In: Muller and Kirk's Small Animal Dermatology, 5th Edition. WB Saunders, Philadelphia, pp. 55–173.

Chapter 13: Sebaceous adenitis

DeManuelle T, Rothstein E (2002): Food allergy and nutritionally related skin disease. In: Thoday KL, Foil CS, Bond R, Eds. Advances in Veterinary Dermatology, Volume 4. Blackwell Science, Oxford, pp. 224–230.

Lee Gross T, Ihrke PJ, Walder EJ, Affolter VK (2005): Diseases with abnormal cornification. In: Skin Diseases of the Dog and Cat. Clinical and Histopathological Diagnosis. Blackwell Science, Oxford, pp. 186–188.

Linek M, Boss C, Haemmerling R, Hewicker-Trautwein M, Mecklenburg L (2005): Effects of cyclosporine A on clinical and histologic abnormalities in dogs with sebaceous adenitis. J Am Vet Med Assoc 226 (1), 59–64.

Noli C, Toma S (2006): Three cases of immune-mediated adnexal skin disease treated with cyclosporin. Vet Dermatol 17 (1), 85–92.

Power HT, Ihrke PJ (1990): Synthetic retinoids in veterinary dermatology. Vet Clin North Am Small Anim Pract 20 (6), 1525–1539.

Rybnicek J, Affolter VK, Moore PF (1998): Sebaceous adenitis: an immunohistological examination. In: Kwochka KW, Willemse T, von Tscharner C, Eds. Advances in Veterinary Dermatology, Volume 3. Butterworth-Heinemann, Oxford, pp. 539–540.

Sousa CA (2006): Sebaceous adenitis. Vet Clin North Am Small Anim Pract 36 (1), 243–249, ix.

Stewart LJ, White SD, Carpenter JL (1991): Isotretinoin in the treatment of sebaceous adenitis in two vizslas. J Am Anim Hosp Assoc 27 (1), 65–71.

White SD, Rosychuk RA, Scott KV, Hargis AM, Jonas L, Trettien A (1995): Sebaceous adenitis in dogs and results of treatment with isotretinoin and etretinate: 30 cases (1990–1994). J Am Vet Med Assoc 207 (2), 197–200.

Chapter 14: Exfoliative dermatitis with thymoma

Affolter VK, Moore PF, Sandmaier BM (1998): Immunohisto-chemical characterisation of canine acute graft-versus-host disease and erythema multiforme. In: Kwochka KW, Willemse T, von Tscharner C, Eds. Advances of Veterinary Dermatology, Volume 3. Butterworth-Heinemann, Oxford, pp. 103–115.

Day MJ (1997): Review of thymic pathology in 30 cats and 36 dogs. J Small Anim Pract 38, 393–403.

Forster-van-Hijfte MA, Curtis CF, White RN (1997): Resolution of exfoliative dermatitis and Malassezia pachydermatis overgrowth in a cat after surgical thymoma resection. J Small Anim Pract 38, 451–454.

Godfrey DR (1999): Dermatosis and associated systemic signs in a cat with thymoma and recently treated with an imidacloprid preparation. J Small Anim Pract 40, 333–337.

Gross TL, Ihrke PJ, Walder EJ, et al. Skin Diseases of the Cat and Dog: Clinical and Histopathologic Diagnosis, 2nd Edition. Blackwell Science, Oxford, pp. 68–70.

Mauldin EA, Morris DO, Goldschmidt MH (2002): Retrospec-tive study: the presence of Malassezia in feline skin biopsies. A clinicopathological study. Vet Dermatol 13, 7–13.

Rottenberg S, von Tscharner C, Roosje PJ (2004): Thymoma associated exfoliative dermatitis in cats. Vet Pathol 41, 429–433.

Yager JA, Wilcock BP (1994): Colour Atlas and Text of Surgical Pathology of the Dog and Cat. Mosby Year Book, London, pp. 100–101.

Chapter 15: Epitheliotrophic lymphoma

Beale KM, Bolon B (1993): Canine cutaneous lymphosarcoma: epitheliotropic and non epitheliotropic, a retrospective study. In: Ihrke PJ, et al., Eds. Advances in Veterinary Dermatology, Volume 2. Pergamon Press, Oxford, pp. 273–284.

de Lorimer LP (2006): Updates on the management of canine epitheliotropic cutaneous T-cell lymphoma. Vet Clin North Am Small Anim Pract 36, 213–228.

Gross TL, Ihrke PJ, Walder EJ, et al. (2006): Lymphocytic Tumours in Skin Diseases of the Dog and Cat: Clinical and Histo-pathologic Diagnosis, 2nd Edition. Blackwell Science, Oxford, pp. 866–893.

Moore PE, Olivry T, Naydan D (1994): Canine cutaneous epitheliotropic lymphoma (mycosis fungoides) is a pro-liferative disorder of CD8+ T cells. Am J Pathol 144, 421–429.

Risbon RE, de Lorimer LP, Skorupski K, et al. (2006): Response to canine cutaneous epitheliotropic lymphoma to lomus-tine (CCNU): a retrospective study of 46 cases (1999–2004). J Vet Intern Med 20, 1389–1397.

White SD, Rosychuk RA, Scott KV, et al. (1993): Use of isotreti-noin and etretinate for the treatment of benign cutaneous neoplasia and cutaneous lymphoma in dogs. J Am Vet Med Assoc 202, 387–391.

Williams LE, Rassnick KM, Power HT, et al. (2006): CCNU in the treatment of canine epitheliotropic lymphoma. J Vet Intern Med 20, 136–143.

Chapter 16: Cheyletelliosis in a rabbit

Harcourt-Brown F (Ed.) (2002): Skin diseases. In: Textbook of Rabbit Medicine. Butterworth-Heinemann, Oxford, pp. 224–248.

Harcourt-Brown F (Ed.) (2002): Infectious diseases of domestic rabbits. In: Textbook of Rabbit Medicine. Butterworth-Heinemann, Oxford, pp. 361–385.

Hess LH (2004): Dermatologic diseases. In: Quesenberry KE, Carpenter JW, Eds. Ferrets, Rabbits and Rodents: Clinical Medicine and Surgery, 2nd Edition. WB Saunders, Philadelphia, pp. 194–202.

Jenkins JR (2001): Skin disorders of the rabbit. Vet Clin North Am Exotic Anim Pract 4 (2), 543–563.

Scarff DH (1991): Skin disorders of small mammals. J Small Anim Pract 32, 408–412.

Scarff DH (2003): Rabbits and rodents. In: Foster AP, Foil CS, Eds. BSAVA Manual of Small Animal Dermatology. BSAVA, Gloucester, pp. 242–251.

Scott DW, Miller WH, Griffin CE (2001): Dermatoses of pet rodents, rabbit and ferrets. In: Muller and Kirk's Small Animal Dermatology, 6th Edition., WB Saunders, Philadelphia, pp. 1415–1458.

Smith S (2005): Small mammal therapeutics. Proceedings of the British Veterinary Dermatology Study Group, Autumn Meeting, pp. 43–50.

Wilkinson GT, Harvey RG (Eds) (1994): Parasitic disease. In: Colour Atlas of Small Animal Dermatology – A guide to diagnosis. Mosby-Wolfe, London, pp. 53–87.

Chapter 17: Pemphigus in a cat

Gross TL, Ihrke PJ, Walder EJ, Affolter VK (2006): Pemphigus foliaceus. In: Skin Diseases of the Dog and Cat – Clinical and Histopathologic Diagnosis. Blackwell Science, Oxford, pp. 13–18.

Olivry T (2006): A review of autoimmune skin diseases in domestic animals: I – Superficial pemphigus. Vet Dermatol 17 (5), 291–305.

Preziosi DE, Goldschmidt MH, Greek JS, Jeffers JG, Shanley KS, Drobatz K, et al. (2003): Feline pemphigus foliaceus: a retrospective analysis of 57 cases. Vet Dermatol 14 (6), 313–321.

Rosenkrantz WS (2004): Pemphigus: current therapy (Special Issue: Therapeutics). Vet Dermatol 15 (2), 90–98.

Scott DW, Miller WH, Griffin CE (2001): Immune-mediated disorders. In: Muller and Kirk's Small Animal Dermatology, 6th Edition. WB Saunders, Philadelphia, pp. 667–779.

Smith SA, Tobias AH, Fine DM, Jacob KA, Ployngam T (2004): Corticosteroid-associated congestive heart failure in 12 cats. J Appl Res Vet Med 2 (3), 159–170.

Chapter 18: Metabolic epidermal necrosis

Allenspach K, Arnold P, Glaus T, et al. (2000): Glucagon-producing neuroendocrine tumour associated with hypoaminoacidaemia and skin lesions. J Small Anim Pract 41, 402–406.

Bond R, McNeil PE, Evans H, et al. (1995): Metabolic epidermal necrosis in two dogs with different underlying diseases. Vet Rec 136, 466–471.

Byrne KP (1999): Metabolic epidermal necrosis-hepatocutaneous syndrome. Vet Clin North Am Small Anim Pract 29, 1337–1355.

Doyle JA, Schoeter AL, Rogers RS (1979): Hyperglucagonaemia and necrolytic migratory erythema in cirrhosis – possible pseudoglucagonoma syndrome. Br J Dermatol 100, 581–587.

Gross TL, O'Brien TD, Davies AP, et al. (1990): Glucagon producing tumours in two dogs with superficial necrolytic dermatitis. J Am Vet Med Assoc 197, 1619–1622.

Hill PB, Auxilia ST, Munro E, et al. (2000): Resolution of skin lesions and long-term survival in a dog with superficial necrolytic dermatitis and liver cirrhosis. J Small Anim Pract 41, 519–523.

March PA, Hillier A, Weisbrode SE, et al. (2004): Superficial necrolytic dermatitis in 11 dogs with a history of phenobarbital administration (1995–2002). J Vet Intern Med 18, 65–74.

Miller WH, Scott DW, Buerger RG, et al. (1990): Necrolytic migratory erythema in dogs: a hepatocutaneous syndrome. J Am Anim Hosp Assoc 26, 573–581.

Miller WH, Anderson WJ, McCann JP (1991): Necrolytic migratory erythema in a dog with glucagon secreting tumour. Vet Dermatol 2, 179–181.

Outerbridge CA, Marks SL, Rogers OR (2002): Plasma amino acid concentrations in 36 dogs with histologically confirmed superficial necrolytic dermatitis. Vet Dermatol 13, 177–186.

Torres SM, Caywood DD, O'Brien TD, et al. (1997): Resolution of superficial necrolytic dermatitis following excision of a glucagon-secreting pancreatic neoplasm in a dog. J Am Anim Hosp Assoc 33, 313–319.

Turek MM (2003): Cutaneous paraneoplastic syndromes in dogs and cats: a review of the literature. Vet Dermatol 14, 279–296.

Chapter 19: Zinc-responsive dermatosis

Broek AHM vd, Stafford WL (1988): Diagnostic value of zinc concentrations in serum, leucocytes and hair of dogs with zinc-responsive dermatosis. Res Vet Sci 44 (1), 41–44.

Burton G, Mason KV (1998): The possible role of prednisolone in 'zinc responsive dermatosis' in the Siberian husky. Aust Vet Pract 28, 20.

Gross TL, Ihrke PJ, Walder EJ, Affolter VK (2006): Zinc responsive dermatosis. In: Skin Diseases of the Dog and Cat – Clinical and Histopathologic Diagnosis. Blackwell Science, Oxford, pp. 188–191.

Kunkle GA (1980): Zinc responsive dermatoses in dogs. In: Kirk RW, Ed. Current Veterinary Therapy VII. WB Saunders, Philadelphia, pp. 472–476.

Scott DW, Miller WH, Griffin CE (2001): Nutrional skin diseases. In: Muller and Kirk's Small Animal Dermatology, 6th Edition. WB Saunders, Philadelphia, pp. 1119–1122.

Chapter 20: Introduction to alopecia

Lloyd DH, Patel AP (2003): Structure and function of the skin. In: Foster AP, Foil C, Eds. BSAVA Manual of Small Animal Dermatology, 2nd Edition. BSAVA, Gloucester, pp. 1–10.

Chapter 21: Feline symetrical alopecia

Alhaidari Z (2000): Diagnostic approach to alopecia. In: Guaguere E, Prelaud P, Eds. A Practical Guide to Feline Dermatoses. Blackwell Science, Oxford, pp. 19.1–19.7.

Barrs VR, Martin P, Beatty JA (2006): Antemortem diagnosis and treatment of toxoplasmosis in two cats on cyclosporin therapy. Aust Vet J 84 (1/2), 30–35.

Bettenay S (1998): Response to hyposensitization in 29 atopic cats. In: Kwochka KW, Willemse T, von Tscharner C, Eds. Advances in Veterinary Dermatology, Volume 3. Proceedings of the Third World Congress of Veterinary Dermatology, Edinburgh, Scotland, 11–14 September 1996. Butterworth-Heinemann, Oxford, p 517.

Last RD, Suzuki Y, Manning T, Lindsay D, Galipeau L, Whitbread TJ (2004): A case of fatal systemic toxoplasmosis in a cat being treated with cyclosporin A for feline atopy. Vet Dermatol 15 (3), 194–198.

Miller WH, Scott DW (1990): Efficacy of chlorpheniramine maleate for management of pruritus in cats. J Am Vet Med Assoc 197 (1), 67–70.

O'Dair HA, Markwell PJ, Maskell IE (1996): An open prospective investigation into aetiology in a group of cats with suspected allergic skin disease. Vet Dermatol 7 (4), 193–202.

Ployngam T, Tobias AH, Smith SA, Torres SME, Ross SJ (2006): Hemodynamic effects of methylprednisolone acetate administration in cats. Am J Vet Res 67 (4), 583–587.

Prost C (1998): Diagnosis of feline allergic diseases: a study of 90 cats. In: Kwochka KW, Willemse T, von Tscharner C, Eds. Advances in Veterinary Dermatology, Volume 3. Proceedings of the Third World Congress of Veterinary Dermatology, Edinburgh, Scotland, 11–14 September 1996. Butterworth-Heinemann, Oxford, p 516.

Scott DW, Miller WH (1995): The combination of antihistamine (chlorpheniramine) and an omega-3/omega-6 fatty acid-containing product for the management of pruritic cats: results of an open clinical trial. N Z Vet J 43 (1), 29–31.

Scott DW, Miller WH, Griffin CE (2001): Skin immune system and allergic skin diseases. In: Muller and Kirk's Small Animal Dermatology. WB Saunders, Philadelphia, pp. 543–666.

Smith SA, Tobias AH, Fine DM, Jacob KA, Ployngam T (2004): Corticosteroid-associated congestive heart failure in 12 cats. J Appl Res Vet Med 2 (3), 159–170.

Vercelli A, Raviri G, Cornegliani G (2006): The use of oral cyclosporin to treat feline dermatoses: a rerospective analysis of 23 cases. Vet Dermatol 17 (3), 201–206.

Chapter 22: Hypothyroidism

Dixon RM, Mooney CT (1999): Evaluation of serum free thyroxine and thyrotropin concentrations in the diagnosis of canine hypothyroidism. J Small Anim Pract 40, 72–78.

Dixon RM, Reid SWJ, Mooney CT (1999): Epidemiological, clinical, haematological and biochemical characteristics of canine hypothyroidism. Vet Rec 145, 481–487.

Frank L (1996): Comparison of thyrotropin releasing hormone (TRH) to thyrotropin (TSH) stimulation for evaluating thyroid function in dogs. J Am Anim Hosp Assoc 32, 481–487.

Panicera DL (1990): Canine hypothyroidism. Part II. Thyroid function, tests and treatment. Compend Contin Ed Pract Vet 12, 843–857.

Panicera DL (1998): Canine hypothyroidism In: Torrance AG, Mooney CT, Eds. Manual of Small Animal Endocrinology, 2nd Edition. BSAVA, Cheltenham, pp. 103–113.

Panicera DL (1998): Monitoring thyroid replacement. In: Torrance AG, Mooney CT, Eds. Manual of Small Animal Endocrinology, 2nd Edition. BSAVA, Cheltenham, pp. 225–228.

Peterson ME, Melian C, Nichols R (1997): Measurement of serum total thyroxine, triiodothyronine, free thyroxine, and thyrotropin concentrations for diagnosis of hypothyroidism in dogs. J Am Vet Med Assoc 211, 1396–1402.

Scott-Moncrieff JCR, Nelson RW, Bruner JM, et al. (1998): Comparison of serum concentrations of thyroid stimulating hormone in healthy dogs, hypothyroid dogs, and euthyroid dogs with concurrent illness. J Am Vet Med Assoc 212, 387–391.

Chapter 23: Colour dilution alopecia

Beco L, Fontaine J, Gross TL, Charlier G (1996): Colour dilution alopecia in seven dachshunds. A clinical study and the hereditary, microscopical and ultrastructural aspect of the disease. Vet Dermatol 7 (2), 91–97.

Bomhard Wv, Mauldin EA, Schmutz SM, Leeb T, Casal ML (2006): Black hair follicular dysplasia in Large Munsterlander dogs: clinical, histological and ultrastructural features. Vet Dermatol 17 (3), 182–188.

Carlotti DN (1990): Canine hereditary black hair follicular dysplasia and colour mutant alopecia: clinical and histopathological aspects. In: Advances in Veterinary Dermatology, Volume 1. Bailliere Tindall, London, pp. 43–46.

Laffort-Dassot C, Beco L, Carlotti DN (2002): Follicular dysplasia in five Weimaraners. Vet Dermatol 13 (5), 253–260.

Lee Gross T, Ihrke PJ, Walder EJ, Affolter VK (2006): Colour dilution alopecia and black hair follicular dysplasia. In: Skin Diseases of the Dog and Cat: Clinical and Histopathologic Diagnosis. Blackwell Science, Oxford, pp. 518–522.

Roperto F, Cerundolo R, Restucci B, Vincensi MR, Caprariis Dd, Vico Gd, et al. (1995): Colour dilution alopecia (CDA) in ten Yorkshire Terriers. Vet Dermatol 6 (4), 171–178.

Scott DW, Miller WH, Griffin CE (2001): Color dilution alopecia. In: Muller and Kirk's Small Animal Dermatology. WB Saunders, Philadelphia, pp. 966–970.

Chapter 24: Alopecia X in a Pomeranian

Cerundolo R, Lloyd DH, Persechino A, Evans H, Cauvin A (2004): Treatment of canine Alopecia X with trilostane. Vet Dermatol 15 (5), 285–293.

Frank LA, Hnilica KA, Oliver JW (2004): Adrenal steroid hormone concentrations in dogs with hair cycle arrest (Alopecia X) before and during treatment with melatonin and mitotane. Vet Dermatol 15 (5), 278–284.

Lee Gross T, Ihrke PJ, Walder EJ, Affolter VK (2006): Alopecia X. In: Skin Diseases of the Dog and Cat: Clinical and

Histopathologic Diagnosis. Blackwell Science, Oxford, pp. 494–497.

Leone F, Cerundolo R, Vercelli A, Lloyd DH (2005): The use of trilostane for the treatment of Alopecia X in Alaskan malamutes. J Am Anim Hosp Assoc 41 (5), 336–342.

Schmeitzel LP, Lothrop CD, Jr (1990): Hormonal abnormalities in Pomeranians with normal coat and in Pomeranians with growth hormone-responsive dermatosis. J Am Vet Med Assoc 197 (10), 1333–1341.

Scott DW, Miller WH, Griffin CE (2001): Endocrine and metabolic diseases. In: Muller and Kirk's Small Animal Dermatology. WB Saunders, Philadelphia, pp. 780–885.

Chapter 25: Canine recurrent flank alopecia

Curtis CF, Evans H, Lloyd DH (1996): Investigation of the reproductive and growth hormone status of dogs affected by idiopathic recurrent flank alopecia. J Small Anim Pract 37, 417–422.

Daminet S, Paradis M (2000): Evaluation of thyroid function in dogs suffering from recurrent flank alopecia. Can Vet J 41, 699–703.

Miller WA, Dunstan RW (1993): Seasonal flank alopecia in boxers and Airedale terriers: 24 cases (1985–1992). J Am Vet Med Assoc 203, 1567–1572.

Chapter 26: Demodicosis

Duclos DD, Jeffers JG, Shanley KJ (1994): Prognosis for treatment of adult-onset demodicosis in dogs: 34 cases (1979–90). J Am Vet Med Assoc 204 (4), 616–619.

Gortel K (2006): Update on canine demodicosis (Updates in dermatology). Vet Clin North Am Small Anim Pract 36 (1), 229–241.

Lemarie SL, Hosgood G, Foil CS (1996): A retrospective study of juvenile- and adult-onset generalized demodicosis in dogs (1986–91). Vet Dermatol 7 (1), 3–10.

Mozos E, Perez J, Day MJ, Lucena R, Ginel PJ (1999): Leishmaniosis and generalized demodicosis in three dogs: a clinicopathological and immunohistochemical study. J Comp Pathol 120 (3), 257–268.

Mueller RS (2004): Treatment protocols for demodicosis: an evidence-based review. Vet Dermatol 15 (2), 75–89.

Scott DW, Miller WH, Griffin CE (2001): Parasitic skin diseases. In: Muller and Kirk's Small Animal Dermatology, 6th Edition. WB Saunders, Philadelphia, pp. 423–516.

Chapter 27: Staphylococcal pyoderma

Allaker RP, Lloyd DH, Simpson A (1992): Occurrence of Staphylococcus intermedius on hair and skin of normal dogs. Res Vet Sci 52, 174–176.

Bes M, Guerin-Faublee V, Freney J, et al. (2002): Isolation of Staphylococcus schleiferi subspecies coagulans from two cases of canine pyoderma. Vet Rec 150, 487–488.

Carlotti DN, Guaguere E, Pin D, et al. (1999): Therapy in difficult cases of canine pyoderma with marbofloxacin: a report of 39 dogs. J Small Anim Pract 40, 265–270.

Carlotti DN, Jasmin P, Gardey L, et al. (2005): Evaluation of cephalexin intermittent therapy (weekend therapy) in the control of recurrent idiopathic pyoderma in dogs: a randomised, double-blinded, placebo-controlled study. In: Hillier A, Foster AP, Kwochka KW, Eds. Advances in Veterinary Dermatology, Volume 5. Blackwell Science, Oxford, pp. 137–146.

Chesney CJ (1993): Water: its form, function and importance in the skin of domestic animals. J Small Anim Pract 34, 65–71.

Chesney CJ (1996): Mapping the canine skin: a study of coat relative humidity in Newfoundland dogs. Vet Dermatol 7, 35–41.

Chesney CJ (1997): The microclimate of the canine coat: the effects of heating on coat and skin temperature and relative humidity. Vet Dermatol 8, 183–190.

Curtis CF, Lamport AI, Lloyd DH (2006): Masked, controlled study to investigate the efficacy of a Staphylococcus intermedius autogenous bacterin for the control of canine idiopathic recurrent pyoderma. Vet Dermatol 17, 163–168.

Harvey RG, Lloyd DH (1994): The distribution of Staphylococcus intermedius and coagulase-negative staphylococci in the hair, skin surface, within the hair follicles and on the mucous membranes of dogs. Vet Dermatol 5, 75–81.

Harvey RG, Lloyd DH (1995): The distribution of bacteria (other than staphylococci and Propionibacterium acnes) on hair, at the skin surface and within hair follicles of dogs. Vet Dermatol 6, 79–84.

Hillier A, Alcorn JR, Cole LK, et al. (2006): Pyoderma caused by Pseudomonas aeruginosa infection in dogs. Vet Dermatol 17, 432–439.

Littlewood JD, Lakhami KH, Paterson S, et al. (1999): Clindamycin hydrochloride and clavulanate–amoxycillin in the treatment of canine superficial pyoderma. Vet Rec 44, 662–625.

Lloyd DH, Allaker RP, Pattison A (1991): Carriage of Staphylococcus intermedius on the ventral abdomen of clinically normal dogs and those with pyoderma. Vet Dermatol 2, 161–164.

Lloyd DH, Carlotti DN, Koch HJ, et al. (1997): Treatment of canine pyoderma with co-amoxyclav: a comparison of two dose rates. Vet Rec 25, 439–441.

Mason IS, Mason KV, Lloyd DH (1996): A review of the biology of canine skin with respect to the commensals Staphylococcus intermedius, Demodex canis and Malassezia pachydermatis. Vet Dermatol 7, 119–132.

McEwan NA (2000): Adherence by Staphylococcus intermedius to canine keratinocytes in atopic dermatitis. Res Vet Sci 68, 279–283.

Pin D, Carlotti DN, Jasmin P, et al. (2006): Prospective study of bacterial overgrowth syndrome in eight dogs. Vet Rec 158, 437–441.

Ruedisueli FL, Eastwood NJ, Gunn NK, et al. (1998): The measurement of skin pH in normal dogs of different breeds. In: Kwochka KW, Willemse T, von Tscharner C, Eds. Advances in Veterinary Dermatology, Volume 3. Butterworth Heinemann, Oxford, pp. 521–522.

Saijonmaa-Koulumies L, Parsons E, Lloyd DH (1998): Elimination of Staphylococcus intermedius in healthy dogs by topical treatment with fusidic acid. J Small Anim Pract 39, 341–347.

Scott DW, Miller WH, Griffin CE (2001): Muller and Kirk's Small Animal Dermatology, 6th Edition. WB Saunders, Philadelphia, pp. 274–335.

Chapter 28: Dermatophytosis

DeBoer DJ, Moriello KA, Volk L, et al. (2003): Effects of Lufenuron treatment in cats on the establishment and course of *Microsporum canis* infection following exposure to infected cats. J Am Vet Med Assoc 222, 1216–1220.

Mancianti F, Nardoni S, Corazza M, et al. (2003): Environmental detection of *Microsporum canis* arthrospores in the households of infected cats and dogs. J Feline Med Surg 5, 323–328.

Moriello KA (2003): Feline dermatophytosis: topical and systemic treatment recommendations. Vet Med 98, 877–884.

Moriello KA (2003): Important factors in the pathogenesis of feline dermatophytosis. Vet Med 98, 845–856.

Moriello KA (2003): Monitoring treatment and preventing reinfection in cats with dermatophytosis. Vet Med 98, 886–890.

Moriello KA (2003): Practical diagnostic testing for dermatophytosis in cats. Vet Med 98, 859–876.

Moriello KA (2003): Symposium on feline dermatophytosis. Vet Med 98, 844.

Moriello KA, Deboer DJ (1991): Fungal flora of the coat of pet cats. Am J Vet Res 52, 602–606.

Patel A, Lloyd DH, Lamport AI (2005): Survey of dermatophytes on clinically normal cats in the southeast of England. J Small Anim Pract 46, 436–439.

Paterson S (1999). Miconazole/Chlorhexidine shampoo as an adjunct to systemic therapy in controlling dermatophytosis in cats. J Small Anim Pract 40, 163–166.

Sparks AH, Gruffydd-Jones TJ, Shaw SE, et al. (1993): Epidemiological and diagnostic features of canine and feline dermatophytosis in the United Kingdom from 1956 to 1991. Vet Rec 133, 57–61.

Sparks AH, Werrett G, Stokes CR, et al. (1994): Microsporum canis: inapparent carriage by cats and the viability of arthrospores. J Small Anim Pract 35, 397–401.

Zaror L, Fischmann O, Borges M, et al. (1986): The role of cats and dogs in the epidemiological cycle of *Microsporum canis*. Mykosen 29, 185–188.

Chapter 29: Alopecia areata

Gross T-L, Ihrke PJ, Walder EJ, Affolter VK (2005): Mural diseases of the hair follicle. In: Skin Diseases of the Dog and Cat: Clinical and Histopathological Diagnosis, 2nd Edition. Blackwell Science, Oxford, pp. 460–479.

Jonghe SRd, Ducatelle RV, Mattheeuws DR (1999): Trachyonychia associated with alopecia areata in a Rhodesian Ridgeback. Vet Dermatol 10, 123–126.

Olivry T, Moore PF, Naydan DK, Puget BJ, et al. (1996): Antifollicular cell-mediated and humoral immunity in canine alopecia areata. Vet Dermatol 7, 67–79.

Tobin DJ, Fenton DA, Kendall MD (1990): Ultrastructural observations on the hair bulb melanocytes and melanosomes in acute alopecia areata. J Invest Dermatol 94, 803–807.

Tobin DJ, Olivry T, Bystryn J-C (1998): Anti-trichohyalin antibodies in canine alopecia areata. In: Kwochka KW, Willemse T, von Tscharner C, Eds. Advances in Veterinary Dermatology, Volume 3. Butterworth-Heinemann, Oxford, pp. 355–362.

Tobin DJ, Gardner SH, Luther PB, Dunston SM, et al. (2003): A natural canine homologue of alopecia areata in humans. Br J Dermatol 149, 938–950.

Chapter 30: Lymphoma in a hamster

Capello V (2002): Pet hamster medicine and surgery. Part III: Infectious, parasitic and metabolic diseases. Exotic DVM 3 (6), 27–32.

Carpenter JW (2005): Exotic Animal Formulary, 3rd Edition. Elsevier Saunders, Missouri.

Donnelly TM (2004): Disease problems of small rodents. In: Quesenberry KE, Carpenter JW, Eds. Ferrets, Rabbits and Rodents. Clinical Medicine and Surgery, 2nd Edition. Elsevier Saunders, Missouri.

Ellis C, Mori M (2001): Skin diseases of rodents and small exotic mammals. Vet Clin North Am Exotic Anim Pract 4 (2), 493–542.

Goodman G (2002): Hamsters. In: Redrobe S, Meredith A, Eds. BSAVA Manual of Exotic Pets, 4th Edition. BSAVA, Gloucester.

Kent MS (2004): The use of chemotherapy in exotic animals. Vet Clin North Am Exotic Anim Pract 7, 807–820.

Scott DW, Miller WH, Griffin CE (2001): Muller and Kirk's Small Animal Dermatology, 6th Edition. WB Saunders, Philadelphia.

Chapter 31: Feline paraneoplastic alopecia

Brooks DG, Campbell KL, Dennis JS, et al. (1994): Paraneoplastic alopecia in three cats. J Am Anim Hosp Assoc 30, 557–563.

Godfrey DR (1998): Dermatosis and associated systemic signs in a cat with thymoma and recently treated with an imidacloprid preparation. J Small Anim Pract 40, 333–337.

Pascal-Tenorio A, Olivry T, Gross TL, et al. (1997): Paraneoplastic alopecia associated with internal malignancies in the cat. Vet Dermatol 8, 47–52.

Patel A, Whitbread TJ, McNeil PE (1996). A case of metabolic epidermal necrosis in a cat. Vet Dermatol 7, 221–226.

Tasker S, Griffon DJ, Nuttall TJ, et al. (1999): Resolution of paraneoplastic alopecia following surgical removal of a pancreatic carcinoma in a cat. J Small Anim Pract 40, 16–19.

Chapter 33: Erythema multiforme

Byrne KP, Giger U (2002): Use of human immunoglobulin for treatment of severe erythema multiforme in a cat. J Am Vet Med Assoc 220 (2), 197–201.

Delmage DA, Payne-Johnson CE (1991): Erythema multiforme in a Dobermann on trimethoprim–sulphamethoxazole therapy. J Small Anim Pract 32 (12), 635–639.

Favrot C, Olivry T, Dunston SM, Degorce-Rubiales F, Guy JS (2000): Parvovirus infection of keratinocytes as a cause of canine erythema multiforme. Vet Pathol 37 (6), 647–649.

Hanley CS, Simmons HA, Wallace RS, Clyde VL (2005): Erythema multiforme in a spotted hyena (*Crocuta crocuta*). J Zoo Wildlife Med 36 (3), 515–519.

Hees Jv, Mason KV, Gross TL, Burren VS (1985): Levamisole-induced drug eruptions in the dog. J Am Anim Hosp Assoc 21 (2), 255–260.

Hinn AC, Olivry T, Luther PB, Cannon AG, Yager JA (1998): Erythema multiforme, Stevens–Johnson syndrome, and toxic epidermal necrolysis in the dog: clinical classification, drug exposure, and histopathological correlations. J Vet Allergy Clin Immunol 6 (1), 13–20.

Itoh T, Nibe K, Kojimoto A, Mikawa M, Mikawa K, Uchida K, et al. (2006): Erythema multiforme possibly triggered by food substances in a dog. J Vet Med Sci 68 (8), 869–871.

Noli C, Koeman JP, Willemse T (1995): A retrospective evaluation of adverse reactions to trimethoprim–sulphonamide combinations in dogs and cats. Vet Quart 17 (4), 123–128.

Noli C, von Tscharner C, Suter MM (1998): Apoptosis in selected skin diseases. Vet Dermatol 9 (4), 221–229.

Nuttall TJ, Malham T (2004): Successful intravenous human immunoglobulin treatment of drug-induced Stevens–Johnson syndrome in a dog. J Small Anim Pract 45 (7), 357–361.

Scott DW, Miller WH, Jr (1999): Erythema multiforme in dogs and cats: literature review and case material from the Cornell University College of Veterinary Medicine (1988–96). Vet Dermatol 10 (4), 297–309.

Taga N, Morishima T, Asai T, Ishida T, Naganawa T, Matsamoto K, et al. (2006): Erythema multiforme in a dog with an intrathoracic malignant lymphoma [in Japanese]. J Vet Med Japan 59 (7), 577–579.

Chapter 34: Vasculitis

Cowan LA, Hertzke DM, Fenwick BW, Andreasen CB (1997): Clinical and clinicopathologic abnormalities in Greyhounds with cutaneous and renal glomerular vasculopathy: 18 cases (1992–1994). J Am Vet Med Assoc 210 (6), 789–793.

Felsburg PJ, HogenEsch H, Somberg RL, Snyder PW, Glickman LT (1992): Immunologic abnormalities in canine juvenile polyarteritis syndrome: a naturally occurring animal model of Kawasaki disease. Clin Immunol Immunopathol 65 (2), 110–118.

Fondati A, Fondevila MD, Minghelli A, Romano E, Varazzani B (1998): Familial cutaneous vasculopathy and demodicosis in a German Shepherd dog. J Small Anim Pract 39 (3), 137–139.

Lee Gross T, Ihrke PJ, Walder EJ, Affolter VK (2006): Vascular diseases of the dermis. In: Skin Diseases of the Dog and Cat: Clinical and Histopathological Diagnosis, 2nd Edition. Blackwell Science, Oxford, pp. 238–260.

Malik R, Foster SF, Martin P, Canfield PJ, Mason KV, Bosward KL, et al. (2002): Acute febrile neutrophilic vasculitis of the skin of young Shar-Pei dogs. Aust Vet J 80 (4), 200–206.

Morris DO, Beale KM (1999): Cutaneous vasculitis and vasculopathy. Vet Clin North Am Small Anim Pract 29 (6), 1325–1335.

Nichols PR, Morris DO, Beale KM (2001): A retrospective study of canine and feline cutaneous vasculitis. Vet Dermatol 12 (5), 255–264.

Parker WM, Foster RA (1996): Cutaneous vasculitis in five Jack Russell Terriers. Vet Dermatol 7 (2), 109–115.

Pedersen K, Scott DW (1991): Idiopathic pyogranulomatous inflammation and leukocytoclastic vasculitis of the nasal planum, nostrils and nasal mucosa in Scottish Terriers in Denmark. Vet Dermatol 2 (2), 85–89.

Randell MG, Hurvitz AI (1983): Immune-mediated vasculitis in five dogs. J Am Vet Med Assoc 183 (2), 207–211.

Rest JR, Forrester D, Hopkins JN (1996): Familial vasculopathy of German Shepherd Dogs. Vet Rec 138, p. 4 ref.

Scott DW, Miller WH, Griffin CE (2001): Immune-mediated disorders. In: Muller and Kirk's Small Animal Dermatology, 6th Edition. WB Saunders, Philadelphia, pp. 667–779.

Snyder PW, Kazacos EA, Scott-Moncrieff JC, HogenEsch H, Carlton WW, Glickman LT, et al. (1995): Pathologic features of naturally occurring juvenile polyarteritis in Beagle dogs. Vet Pathol 32 (4), 337–345.

Wilcock BP, Yager JA (1986): Focal cutaneous vasculitis and alopecia at sites of rabies vaccination in dogs. J Am Vet Med Assoc 188 (10), 1174–1177.

Chapter 35: Familial canine dermatomyositis

Ferguson EA, Cerundolo R, Lloyd DH, et al. (2000): Dermatomyositis in five Shetland sheepdogs in the United Kingdom. Vet Rec 146, 214–217.

Hargis AM, Mundell AC (1992): Familial canine dermatomyositis. Compend Continuing Educ Practic Vet 14, 855–864.

Hargis AM, Prieur DJ, Haupt KH, et al. (1986): Postmortem findings in four litters of dogs with familial canine dermatomyositis. Am J Pathol 123, 480–496.

Haupt KH, Prieur DJ, Moore MP, et al. (1985): Familial canine dermatomyositis: clinical, electrodiagnostic, and genetic studies. Am J Vet Res 46, 1861–1869.

Lee Gross T, Ihrke PJ, Walder EJ, Affolter VK (2006): Ischaemic dermatopathy/canine dermatomyositis. In: Skin Diseases of the Dog and Cat: Clinical and Histopathological Diagnosis, 2nd Edition. Blackwell Science, Oxford, pp. 49–52.

Chapter 36: Feline eosinophilic plaque

Bardagi M, Fondanti A, Fondevila D, et al. (2003): Ultrastructural study of cutaneous lesions in feline eosinophilic granuloma complex. Vet Dermatol 14, 297–303.

Bloom PB (2006): Canine and feline eosinophilic skin diseases. Vet Clin North Am Small Anim Pract 36, 141–160.

Fondanti A, Fondevila D, Ferrer L (2001): Histopathological study of feline eosinophilic dermatoses. Vet Dermatol 12: 333–338.

Fondanti A, Fondevila D, Ferrer L (2003): Piecemeal degranulation (PMD) morphology in feline circulating eosinophils. Res Vet Sci 75, 127–132.

Kimura T, Kano R, Maeda S, et al. (2003): Expression of RANTES mRNA in skin lesions of feline eosinophilic plaque. Vet Dermatol 14, 269–273.

Lilliehook I, Tyedten H (2003): Investigation of hypereosinophilia and potential treatments. Vet Clin North Am Small Anim Pract 33, 1359–1378.

Power HT, Ihrke PJ (1995): Selected feline eosinophilic skin diseases. Vet Clin North Am Small Anim Pract 25, 833–850.

Prost C. (1998): Diagnosis of feline allergic diseases: a study of 90 cats. In: Kwochka KW, Willemse T, von Tscharner C, Eds. Advances in Veterinary Dermatology, Volume 3. Butterworth-Heinemann, Boston, pp 516–517.

Vercelli A, Rayiri G, Cornegliani L (2006): The use of oral ciclo-sporin to treat feline dermatoses: a retrospective analysis of 23 cases. Vet Dermatol 17, 201–206.

Chapter 37: Head and neck pruritus

Medleau L, Blue JL (1988): Frequency and antimicrobial suscep-tibility of staphylococcal sp. isolated from feline skin lesions. J Am Vet Med Assoc 193, 1080–1081.

Patel A (2006): In: August JR, Ed. Bacterial Pyoderma in Con-sultations of Feline Internal Medicine. WB Saunders, St Louis, pp. 251–259.

Patel A, Lloyd DH, Lamport AI (1999): Antimicrobial resistance of feline staphylococci in south-eastern England. Vet Der-matol 10, 257–261.

Patel A, Lloyd DH, Lamport AI (2002): Prevalence of feline staphylococci with special reference to *Staphylococcus felis* among domestic and feral cats in the south-east of England. In: Thoday KL, et al., Eds. Advances in Veterinary Dermatology, Volume 4, pp. 85–91.

Patel A., Lloyd DH, Howell SA, et al. (2002): Investigation into the potential pathogenicity of *Staphylococcus felis* in a cat. Vet Rec 150, 668–669.

Scott DW, Miller WH, Griffin CE (2001): Muller and Kirk's Small Animal Dermatology, 6th Edition. WB Saunders, Philadelphia, pp. 1148–1153.

Stegemann MR, Passmore CA, Sherington J, et al. (2006): Anti-microbial activity and spectrum of cefovecin, a new extended-spectrum cephalosporin against pathogens col-lected from dogs in Europe and North America. Antimi-crob Agents Chemother 50, 2286–2292.

Stegemann MR, Sherrington J, Coati N, et al. (2006): Pharma-cokinetics of cefovecin in cats. J Vet Pharmacol Ther 29, 513–524.

Chapter 38: Fly strike in a rabbit (myiasis)

Anderson GS (2000): Minimum and maximum development rates of some forensically important Calliphoridae (Diptera). J Forensic Sci 45, 824–832.

Cosquer G (2006): Veterinary care of rabbits with myiasis. In Practice 28, 342–349.

Harcourt-Brown F (Ed.) (2002): Textbook of Rabbit Medicine. Butterworth-Heinemann, Oxford.

Harcourt-Brown F (Ed.) (2002): Infectious diseases of domestic rabbits. In: Textbook of Rabbit Medicine. Butterworth-Heinemann, Oxford, pp. 361–385.

Harcourt-Brown F (Ed.) (2002): Skin diseases. In: Textbook of Rabbit Medicine. Butterworth-Heinemann, Oxford, pp. 224–248.

Hess LH (2004): Dermatologic diseases. In: Quesenberry KE, Carpenter JW, Eds. Ferrets, Rabbits and Rodents: Clinical Medicine and Surgery, 2nd Edition. WB Saunders, Phila-delphia, pp. 194–202.

Jenkins JR (2001): Skin disorders of the rabbit. Vet Clin North Am Exotic Anim Pract 4 (2), 543–563.

Kamal AS (1958): Comparative study of thirteen species of sarcosaprophagous Calliphoridae and Sarcophagidae (Diptera). I. Bionomics. Ann Entomol Soc Am 51, 261–270.

Meredith A, Flecknall P (Eds) (2006): Manual of Rabbit Medicine and Surgery, 2nd Edition. BSAVA, Gloucester.

Scarff DH (1991): Skin disorders of small mammals. J Small Anim Pract 32, 408–412.

Scarff DH (2003): Rabbits and rodents. In: Foster AP, Foil CS, Eds. BSAVA Manual of Small Animal Dermatology. BSAVA, Gloucester, pp. 242–251.

Scott DW, Miller WH, Griffin CE (2001): Dermatoses of pet rodents, rabbit and ferrets. In: Muller and Kirk's Small Animal Dermatology, 6th Edition. WB Saunders, Philadel-phia, pp. 1415–1458.

Smith S (2005): Small mammal therapeutics. Proceedings of the British Veterinary Dermatology Study Group, Autumn Meeting, pp. 43–50.

Wilkinson GT, Harvey RG (Eds) (1994): Parasitic disease. In: Colour Atlas of Small Animal Dermatology – A Guide to Diagnosis. Mosby-Wolfe, London, pp. 53–87.

Chapter 39: Introduction to skin and hair pigmentation

Alhaidari Z, Olivry T, Ortonne J-P (1999): Melanocytogenesis and melanogenesis: genetic regulation and comparative clinical diseases. Vet Dermatol 10, 3–16.

Jimbow K, Quevedo WC, Prota G, et al. (1999): In: Freedberg IM, Eisen AZ, Wolff K, et al., Eds. Fitzpatrick's Dermatology in General Medicine. McGraw-Hill, New York, pp. 192–220.

Chapter 40: Vitiligo in two dogs

Alhaidari Z, Olivry T, Ortonne JP (1999): Melanocytogenesis and melanogenesis: genetic regulation and comparative clinical diseases. Vet Dermatol 10 (1), 3–16.

Lee Gross T, Ihrke PJ, Walder EJ, Affolter VK (2006): Vitiligo. In: Skin Diseases of the Dog and Cat: Clinical and Histopatho-logical Diagnosis, 2nd Edition. Blackwell Science, Oxford, pp. 231–234.

Mosher DB, Fitzpatrick TB., Ortonne J-P, Hori Y (1999): Hypomelanoses and hypermelanoses. In: Freedberg IM, et al., Eds. Fitzpatrick's Dermatology in General Medicine. McGraw-Hill, New York, pp. 945–1017.

Scott DW, Miller WH, Griffin CE (2001): Pigmentary abnor-malities. In: Muller and Kirk's Small Animal Dermatology, 6th Edition. WB Saunders, Philadelphia, pp. 1005–1024.

Chapter 41: Uveodermatological syndrome

Carter W, Crispin SM, Gould DJ, et al. (2005): An immunohis-tochemical study of uveodermatologic syndrome in two Japanese Akita dogs. Vet Ophthalmol 8, 17–24.

Griffin CE, Kwochka, KW, MacDonald JM (1993): Current Vet-erinary Dermatology: The science and art of therapy. Mosby, St Louis, pp. 217–222.

Gross TL, Ihrke PJ, Walder EJ, et al. (2005): Skin Diseases of the Dog and Cat: Clinical and Histopathologic Diagnosis, 2nd Edition. Blackwell Science, Oxford, pp. 266–268.

Scott DW, Miller WH,, Griffin CE (2001): Muller and Kirk's Small Animal Dermatology, 6th Edition. WB Saunders, Philadelphia, pp. 756–759.

Chapter 42: Lentigo simplex

Gross TL, Ihrke PJ, Walder EJ, et al. (2005): Skin Diseases of the Dog and Cat: Clinical and Histopathologic Diagnosis, 2nd Edition. Blackwell Science, Oxford, p 814.

Scott DW, Miller WH, Griffin CE (2001): Muller and Kirk's Small Animal Dermatology, 6th Edition. WB Saunders, Philadelphia, pp. 1006–1007.

Chapter 43: Hyperpigmentation due to hypothyroidism

Daminet S, Ferguson DC (2003): Influence of drugs on thyroid function in dogs. J Vet Intern Med 17 (4), 463–472.

Dixon R (2001): Recent developments in the diagnosis of canine hypothyroidism. In Practice 23 (6), 328–335.

Dixon RM, Reid SWJ, Mooney CT (1999): Epidemiological, clinical, haematological and biochemical characteristics of canine hypothyroidism. Vet Rec 145 (17), 481–487.

Dixon RM, Reid SWJ, Mooney CT (2002): Treatment and therapeutic monitoring of canine hypothyroidism. J Small Anim Pract 43 (8), 334–340.

Lee Gross T, Ihrke PJ, Walder EJ, Affolter VK (2006): Hypothyroidism. In: Skin Diseases of the Dog and Cat: Clinical and Histopathological Diagnosis, 2nd Edition. Blackwell Science, Oxford, pp. 481–484.

Scott DW (1982): Histopathologic findings in endocrine skin disorders of the dog. J Am Anim Hosp Assoc 18 (1), 173–183.

Scott DW, Miller WH, Griffin CE (2001): Endocrine and metabolic disease. In: Muller and Kirk's Small Animal Dermatology, 6th Edition. WB Saunders, Philadelphia, pp. 780–885.

Tobin DJ (2000): The biology of pigmentation. In: Forsythe PJ, Ed. British Veterinary Dermatology Study Group Autumn Meeting, Harrogate.

Chapter 45: Acral lick dermatitis

Dodman NH, Shuster L, White SD, Court MH, Parker D, Dixon R (1988): Use of narcotic antagonists to modify stereotypic self-licking, self-chewing, and scratching behavior in dogs. J Am Vet Med Assoc 193 (7), 815–819.

Goldberger E, Rapoport JL (1991): Canine acral lick dermatitis: response to the antiobsessional drug clomipramine. J Am Anim Hosp Assoc 27 (2), 179–182.

Hewson CJ, Luescher UA, Parent JM, Conlon PD, Ball RO (1998): Efficacy of clomipramine in the treatment of canine compulsive disorder. J Am Vet Med Assoc 213 (12), 1760–1766.

Koutinas AF (1990): Topical treatment for canine lick acral dermatitis: clinical evaluation of nine cases [in Greek]. Deltion tes Ellenikes Kteniatrikes Etaireias=Bull Hellenic Vet Med Soc 41 (3), 148–155.

MacDonald JM, Bradley D (2000): Acral lick dermatitis. In: Bonagura JD, Ed. Kirk's Current Veterinary Therapy XIII: Small Animal Practice. WB Saunders, Philadelphia, pp. 551–556.

Pavicic Z, Potocnjak D, Krsnik B, Zubcic D, Petak I, Hadina S, et al. (2001): Effective use of acupuncture in treating acral lick dermatitis in a dog [in German]. Tierarztliche Umschau 56 (4), 200–205.

Scott DW, Miller WH, Griffin CE (2001): Psychogenic skin diseases. In: Muller and Kirk's Small Animal Dermatology. WB Saunders, Philadelphia, pp. 1055–1072.

White SD (1990): Naltrexone for treatment of acral lick dermatitis in dogs. J Am Vet Med Assoc 196 (7), 1073–1076.

Chapter 46: Sterile pyogranulomatous nodular dermatitis

German A, Foster AP, Holden D, et al. (2003): Sterile nodular panniculitis and pansteatitis in three Weimaraners. J Small Anim Pract 44, 449–455.

Gross T, Ihrke PJ, Walder EJ, et al. (2005): The Skin Diseases of the Dog and Cat: Clinical and Histopathological Diagnosis. Blackwell Science, Oxford, pp. 320–341.

Hughes D, Goldschmidt MH, Washabau RJ, et al. (1996): Serum α_1-antitrypsin concentrations in dogs with panniculitis. J Am Vet Med Assoc 9, 1582–1584.

Mellanby RJ, Stell A, Baines E, et al. (2003): Panniculitis associated with pancreatitis in a cocker spaniel. J Small Anim Pract 44, 24–28.

Scott DW, Anderson W (1985): Panniculitis in dogs and cats. J Am Anim Hosp Assoc 21, 551–559.

Scott DW, Miller WH, Griffin CE (2001): Muller and Kirk's Small Animal Dermatology. WB Saunders, Philadelphia, pp. 1156–1162.

Torres SMF (1999): Sterile nodular dermatitis in dogs. Vet Clin North Am Small Anim Pract 6, 1311–1323.

Yager JA, Wilcock BP (1994): Colour Atlas and Text of Surgical Pathology of the Dog and Cat. Mosby Year Book, London, pp. 199–215.

Chapter 47: Feline mycobacterial disease

Beale KM (1995): Nodules and draining tracts. Vet Clin North Am Small Anim Pract 25, 887–900.

Cavanagh R, Begon M, Bennett M, et al. (2002): *Mycobacterium microti* infection (vole tuberculosis) in wild rodent populations. J Clin Microbiol 40, 3281–3285.

Davies JL, Sibley JA, Myers S, et al. (2006): Histological and genotypical characterisation of feline cutaneous mycobacteriosis: a retrospective study of formalin-fixed paraffin-embedded tissues. Vet Dermatol 17, 155–162.

Fairley RA, Fairley NM (1999): *Rhodococcus equi* infections in cats. Vet Dermatol 10, 43–46.

Gunn-Moore D, Shaw S (1997): Mycobacterial disease in the cat. In Pract 19, 493–501.

Gunn-Moore DA, Jenkins PA (1996): Feline tuberculosis: a literature review and discussion of 19 cases caused by an unusual mycobacterial variant. Vet Rec 138, 53–58.

Lemarie SL (1999): Mycobacterial dermatitis. Vet Clin North Am Small Anim Pract 29, 1291–1301.

Malik R (2005): Mycobacterial disease in cats and dogs. In: Hillier A, Foster AP, Kwochka K, Eds. Advances in Veterinary Dermatology, Volume 5. Blackwell, Oxford, pp. 219–237.

Malik R, Martin P, Mitchell DH, et al. (1998): Subcutaneous granuloma caused by *Mycobacterium avium* complex infection in a cat. Aus Vet J 76, 604–607.

Malik R, Wigney DI, Dawson D, et al. (2000): Infection of the subcutis and skin of cats with rapidly growing mycobacteria: a review of microbiological and clinical findings. J Feline Med Surg 2, 35–48.

Papich MG (1995): Antimicrobial drugs. In: Ettinger SJ, et al., Eds. Textbook of Veterinary Internal Medicine, 4th Edition. WB Saunders, Philadelphia, pp. 272–283.

Patel A (2002): Pyogranulomatous skin disease and cellulitis in a cat caused by *Rhodococcus equi*. J Small Anim Pract 43, 129–132.

Reinke SI, Ihrke PJ, Reinke JD, et al. (1986): Actinomycotic mycetoma in a cat. J Am Vet Med Assoc 189, 446–448.

Yager JA, Wilcock BP (1994): Colour Atlas and Text of Surgical Pathology of the Dog and Cat. Mosby Year Book, London, pp. 136–138.

Chapter 48: Multiple mast cell tumours

Bray J (2001): Dealing with canine mast cell tumours. Veterinary Times 3rd December, 16–18.

Jaffe MH, Hosgood G, Kerwin SC, Hedlund CS, Taylor HW (2000): Deionised water as an adjunct to surgery for the treatment of canine cutaneous mast cell tumours. J Small Anim Pract 41 (1), 7–11.

Kravis L, Vail D, Kisseberth W, et al. (1996): Frequency of argyrophilic nucleolar organiser regions in fine needle aspirates and biopsy specimens from mast cell tumors in dogs. J Am Vet Med Assoc 209, 1418–1420.

LaDue T, Price GS, Dodge R, Page RL, Thrall DE (1998): Radiation therapy for incompletely resected canine mast cell tumors. Vet Radiol Ultrasound 39 (1), 57–62.

McManus P (1999): Frequency and severity of mastocytemia in dogs with and without mast cell tumors: 120 cases (1995–1997). J Am Vet Med Assoc 215, 355–357.

Michels GM, Knapp DW, DeNicola DB, Glickman N, Bonney P (2002): Prognosis following surgical excision of canine cutaneous mast cell tumors with histopatholgically tumor-free versus nontumor-free margins: a retrospective study of 33 cases. J Am Anim Hosp Assoc 38, 458–466.

Miller DM (1995): The occurrence of mast cell tumors in young Shar Peis. J Vet Diagnost Invest 7, 360.

Murphy S (2001): Canine mast cell tumours. In: Forsythe PJ, Ed. British Veterinary Dermatology Study Group, Autumn Meeting, Chester.

Murphy S, Sparkes AH, Blunden AS, Brearley MJ, Smith KC (2004): Relationships between the histologic grade of cutaneous mast cell tumours in dogs, their survival and the efficacy of surgical resection. Vet Rec 154, 743–746.

Murphy S, Sparkes, AH, Blunden AS, Brearley MJ, Smith KC (2006): Effect of stage and numbers of tumours on prognosis of dogs with cutaneous mast cell tumours. Vet Rec 158, 287–291.

Neyens IJS, Kirpenstejin J, Grinwis GCM, Teske E (2004): Pilot study of intraregional deionised water adjunct therapy for mast cell tumours in dogs. Vet Rec 154, 90–91.

Ogilvie K, Moore AS (1995): Mast cell tumours. In: Managing the Veterinary Cancer Patient: A Practice Manual. Veterinary Learning Systems, Trenton, pp. 503–510.

O'Keefe DA (1990): Canine mast cell tumors. Vet Clin North Am Small Anim Pract 20 (4), 1105–1115.

Owen LN (1980): TNM Classification of Tumors in Domestic Animals. World Health Organization, Geneva.

Patnaik AK, Ehler WJ, MacEwen EG (1984): Canine cutaneous mast cell tumor: morphologic grading and survival time in 83 dogs. Vet Pathol 21 (5), 469–474.

Poirier VJ, Adams WM, Forrest LJ, Green EM, Dubielzig RR, Vail DM (2006): Radiation therapy for incompletely excised grade II canine mast cell tumors. J Am Anim Hosp Assoc 42 (6), 430–434.

Seguin B, Leibman NF, Bregazzi VS, Ogilvie GK, Powers BE, Dernell WS, et al. (2001): Clinical outcome of dogs with grade-II mast cell tumors treated with surgery alone: 55 cases (1996–1999). J Am Vet Med Assoc 218 (7), 1120–1123.

Turrel JM, Kitchell BE, Miller LM, Theon A (1988): Prognostic factors for radiation treatment of mast cell tumor in 85 dogs. J Am Vet Med Assoc 193 (8), 936–940.

Chapter 49: Histiocytoma

Affolter VK (2002): Histiocytes in skin disease In: Thoday KL, Foil CS, Bond R, Eds. Advances in Veterinary Dermatology, Volume 4. Blackwell Science, Oxford, pp. 111–130.

Gross TL, Ihrke PJ, Walder EJ, et al. (2005): Skin Diseases of the Dog and Cat: Clinical and Histopathologic Diagnosis. Blackwell Science, Oxford, pp. 837–850.

Scott DW, Miller WH, Griffin CE (2001): Muller and Kirk's Small Animal Dermatology, 6th Edition. WB Saunders, Philadelphia, pp. 1236–1413.

Chapter 50: Dermatoses of specific sites

Scott DW, Miller WH, Griffin CE (2001): Diseases of eyelids, claws, anal sacs and ears. In: Muller and Kirk's Small Animal Dermatology, 6th Edition. WB Saunders, Philadelphia, pp. 1185–1235.

Chapter 51: Feline cowpox virus infection

Baxby D, Bennett M, Getty B (1994): Human cowpox; a review based on 54 cases, 1969–93. Br J Dermatol 131, 598–607.

Bennett M, Gaskell CJ, Baxby D, et al. (1990): Feline cowpox virus infection. J Small Anim Pract 31, 167–173.

Bennett M, Gaskell CJ, Gaskell RM, et al. (1996): Poxvirus infection in the domestic cat; some clinical and epidemiological observations. Vet Rec 118, 387–390.

Brown A, Bennett M, Gaskell CJ (1989): Fatal poxvirus infection in association with FIV infection. Vet Rec 124, 19–20.

Chantrey J, Meyer H, Baxby D, et al. (1999): Cowpox: reservoir hosts and geographic range. Epidemiol Infect 122, 455–460.

Godfrey DR, Blundell CJ, Essbauer S, et al. (2004): Unusual presentations of cowpox infection in cats. J Small Anim Pract 45, 202–205.

Hawrenek, T, Tritscher M, Muss WH, et al. (2003): Feline ortho-poxvirus infection transmitted from cat to human. J Am Acad Dermatol 49, 513–518.

Hazel SM, Bennett M, Chantrey J, et al. (2000): A longitudinal study of endemic disease in its wildlife reservoir: cowpox and wild rodents. Epidemiol Infect 124, 551–562.

Kaplan C, Healing TD, Evans N, et al. (1980): Evidence of infection by viruses in small British field rodents. J Hygiene 84, 285–294.

Pfeffer M, Pfleghaar S, von Bomhard D, Kaader OR, Meyer H (2002): Retrospective investigation of feline cowpox in Germany. Vet Rec 150, 50–51.

Chapter 52: Eosinophilic folliculitis and furunculosis

Curtis CF, Bond R, Blunden AS, et al. (1995): Canine eosinophilic folliculitis and furunculosis in three cases. J Small Anim Pract 36, 119–123.

Gross TL (1993): Canine eosinophilic furunculosis of the face. In: Ihrke PJ, Mason IS, White SD, Eds. Advances of Veterinary Dermatology, 2nd Edition. Pergamon Press, Oxford, pp. 239–246.

Gross TL, Ihrke PJ, Walder EJ, et al. (2006): Skin Diseases of the Dog and Cat: Clinical and Histopathologic Diagnosis, 2nd Edition. Blackwell, Oxford, pp. 406–459.

Scott DW, Miller WH, Griffin CE (2001): Muller and Kirk's Small Animal Dermatology, 6th Edition. WB Saunders, Philadelphia, pp. 641–642.

Chapter 53: Cutaneous lupus erythematosus

Font A, Bardagi M, Mascort J, et al. (2006): Treatment with oral ciclosporin A of a case of vesicular cutaneous lupus erythematosus in a rough collie. Vet Dermatol 17, 440–442.

Gerhauser I, Strothmann-Luerssen A, Baumgarter W (2006): A case of interface perianal dermatitis in a dog: is this an unusual manifestation of lupus erythematosus? Vet Pathol 43, 761–764.

Griffies JD, Mendelsohn CL, Rosenkrantz WS, et al. (2004): Topical 0.1% tacrolimus for the treatment of discoid lupus erythematosus and pemphigus erythematosus in dogs. J Am Anim Hosp Assoc 40, 29–41.

Gross TL, Ihrke PJ, Walder EJ, et al. (2005): Skin Diseases of the Dog and Cat: Clinical and Histopathologic Diagnosis. Blackwell Science, Oxford, pp. 49–74.

Jackson HA (2004): Eleven cases of vesicular cutaneous lupus erythematosus in Shetland sheepdogs and rough collies: clinical management and prognosis. Vet Dermatol 15, 37–41.

Jackson HA, Olivry T (2001): Ulcerative dermatosis of Shetland Sheepdog and rough collie dog may represent a novel vesicular variant of cutaneous lupus erythematosus. Vet Dermatol 12, 19–27.

Schrauwen E, Junius G, Swinen C, et al. (2004): Dyschezia in dogs with discrete erosive anal disease and histological lesions suggestive of mucocutaneous lupus erythematosus. Vet Rec 154, 752–754.

Scott DW, Miller WH, Griffin CE (2001): Muller and Kirk's Small Animal Dermatology, 6th Edition. WB Saunders, Philadelphia, pp. 667–779.

Weimelt SP, Goldschmidt MH, Greek JS, et al. (2004): A retrospective study comparing the histopathological features and response to treatment in two canine nasal dermatoses, DLE and MCP. Vet Dermatol 15, 341–348.

White SD, Rosychuk, RA, Reinke SI, et al. (1992): Use of tetracycline and niacinamide for treatment of autoimmune skin disease in 31 dogs. J Am Vet Med Assoc 200, 497–500.

Chapter 54: Feline plasma cell pododermatitis

Bettenay SV, Mueller RS, Dow K, Friend S (2003): Prospective study of the treatment of feline plasmacytic pododermatitis with doxycycline. Vet Rec 152 (18), 564–566.

Gruffydd-Jones TJ, Orr CM, Lucke VM (1980): Food pad swelling and ulceration in cats: a report of five cases. J Small Anim Pract 21 (7), 381–389.

Guaguere E, Hubert B, Delabre C (1992): Feline pododermatoses. Vet Dermatol 3 (1), 1–12.

Lee Gross T, Ihrke PJ, Walder EJ, Affolter VK (2006): Plasma cell pododermatitis. In: Skin Diseases of the Dog and Cat: Clinical and Histopathological Diagnosis. Blackwell, Oxford, pp. 363–364.

Scott DW, Miller WH, Griffin CE (2001): Feline plasma cell pododermatitis. In: Muller and Kirk's Small Animal Dermatology. WB Saunders, Philadelphia, pp. 1129–1130.

Simon M, Horvath C, Pauley D, King N, Hunt R, Ringler D (1993): Plasma cell pododermatitis in feline immunodeficiency virus-infected cats. Vet Pathol 30, 477.

Chapter 55: Digital squamous cell carcinoma

Lee Gross T, Ihrke PJ, Walder EJ, Affolter VK (2006): Nailbed squamous cell carcinoma. In: Skin Diseases of the Dog and Cat, 2nd Edition. Blackwell, Oxford, pp. 700–702.

Madewell BR, Pool RR, Theilen GH, Brewer WG (1982): Multiple subungual squamous cell carcinomas in five dogs. J Am Vet Med Assoc 180 (7), 731–734.

Marino DJ, Matthiesen DT, Stefanacci JD, Moroff SD (1995): Evaluation of dogs with digit masses: 117 cases (1981–1991). J Am Vet Med Assoc 207 (6), 726–728.

O'Brien MG, Berg J, Engler SJ (1992): Treatment by digital amputation of subungual squamous cell carcinoma in dogs. J Am Vet Med Assoc 201 (5), 759–761.

Paradis M, Scott DW, Breton L (1989): Squamous cell carcinoma of the nail bed in three related Giant Schnauzers. Vet Rec 125 (12), 322–324.

Schwartz RA, Stoll HL (1999): Squamous cell carcinoma. In: Freedberg IM, et al., Eds. Fitzpatrick's Dermatology in General Medicine, 5th Edition. McGraw-Hill, New York, pp. 840–856.

Scott DW, Miller WH (1992): Disorders of the claw and clawbed in dogs. Compend Continuing Educ Pract Vet 14 (11), 1448–1454, 1456–1458.

Chapter 56: Lupoid onychodystrophy

Bergvall K (1998): Treatment of symmetrical onychomadesis and onychodystrophy in five dogs with omega-3 and omega-6 fatty acids. Vet Dermatol 9, 263–268.

Buffa EA, van Den Berg SS, Verstraete FJ, et al. (1992): Effect of dietary biotin supplement on equine hoof horn growth rate and hardness. Equine Vet J 24, 472–474.

Colombo VE, Gerber F, Bronhofer M, et al. (1990): Treatment of brittle fingernails and onychoschizia with biotin: scanning electron microscopy. J Am Acad Dermatol 23, 1127–1132.

Harvey RG, Markwell PJ (1996): The mineral composition of nails in normal dogs and comparison with shed nails in canine idiopathic onychomadesis. Vet Dermatol 7, 29–34.

Higuchi H, Maeda T, Nakamura A, et al. (2004): Effects of biotin supplementation on serum biotin levels and physical properties of samples of solar horn of Holstein cows. Can Vet J 68, 93–97.

Hochman LG, Scher RK, Meyerson MS (1993): Brittle nails: response to daily biotin supplementation. Cutis 51, 303–305.

Johnston AM, Penny RH (1989): Rate of claw horn growth and wear in biotin-supplemented and non-supplemented pigs. Vet Rec 125, 130–132.

Mueller RS, Sterner-Kock A, Stannard AA (1993): Microanatomy of the canine claw. Vet Dermatol 4, 5–11.

Muller RS (1999): Diagnosis and management of canine claw diseases. Vet Clin North Am Small Anim Pract 29, 1357–1371.

Muller RS, Olivry T (1999): Onychobiopsy without onychectomy: description of a new biopsy technique for canine claws. Vet Dermatol 10, 55–58.

Scott DW, Miller WH, Griffin CE (2001): Muller and Kirk's Small Animal Dermatology, 6th Edition. WB Saunders, Philadelphia, pp. 1185–1235.

Verde MT, Basurco A (2000): Symmetrical lupoid onychodystrophy in a crossbred pointer dog: long-term observations. Vet Rec 146, 376–378.

Chapter 57: Otitis externa and otitis media in a dog

Cole LK, Kwochka KW, Kowalski JJ, Hillier A (1998): Microbial flora and antimicrobial susceptibility patterns of isolated pathogens from the horizontal ear canal and middle ear in dogs with otitis media. J Am Vet Med Assoc 212 (4), 534–538.

Dickie AM, Doust R, Cromarty L, Johnson VS, Sullivan M, Boyd JS (2003): Comparison of ultrasonography, radiography and a single computed tomography slice for the identification of fluid within the canine tympanic bulla. Res Vet Sci 75 (3), 209–216.

Foster AP, DeBoer DJ (1998): The role of *Pseudomonas* in canine ear disease. Compend Continuing Educ Pract Vet 20 (8), 909–919.

Gotthelf L (2000): Small Animal Ear Diseases. WB Saunders, Philadelpia.

Griffiths LG, Sullivan M, O'Neill T, Reid SWJ (2003): Ultrasonography versus radiography for detection of fluid in the canine tympanic bulla. Vet Radiol Ultrasound 44 (2), 210–213.

Harvey RG, Harari J, Delauche AJ (2001): A Colour Handbook of Ear Diseases of the Dog and Cat. Manson, London.

Nuttall TJ (1998): Use of ticarcillin in the management of canine otitis externa complicated by *Pseudomonas aeruginosa*. J Small Anim Pract 39 (4), 165–168.

Palmeiro BS, Morris DO, Wiemelt SP, Shofer FS (2004): Evaluation of outcome of otitis media after lavage of the tympanic bulla and long-term antimicrobial drug treatment in dogs: 44 cases (1998–2002). J Am Vet Med Assoc 225 (4), 548–553.

Remedios AM, Fowler JD, Pharr JW (1991): A comparison of radiographic versus surgical diagnosis of otitis media. J Am Anim Hosp Assoc 27 (2), 183–188.

Siemering GH (1980): Resection of the vertical ear canal for treatment of chronic otitis externa. J Am Anim Hosp Assoc 16 (5), 753–758.

Nuttall T, Cole LK (2004): Ear cleaning: the UK and US perspective (Special Issue: Therapeutics). Vet Dermatol 15 (2), 127–136.

Appendix 5

Chitty J, Hendricks A (2007): Zoonotic skin disease in small animals. In Practice 29 (2), 92–97.

Index

Notes

Page numbers in **bold** refer to figures and tables.

Readers are advised to refer to specific breeds for real-life studies related to each condition within this book.

Printed in the United States
By Bookmasters